Clinical Management of Bowel Endometriosis

Simone Ferrero · Marcello Ceccaroni

Editors

Clinical Management of Bowel Endometriosis

From Diagnosis to Treatment

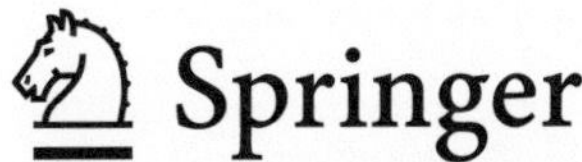

Editors
Simone Ferrero
Division of Obstetrics and Gynaecology,
Department of Neurosciences,
Rehabilitation, Ophthalmology,
Genetics, Maternal
and Child Health (DiNOGMI)
University of Genova
Genova
Italy

Marcello Ceccaroni
Department of Obstetrics and
Gynaecology, Gynecologic Oncology
and Minimally-Invasive Pelvic Surgery
International School of Surgical
Anatomy, IRCCS Sacro Cuore Don
Calabria Hospital
Negrar di Valpolicella
Verona
Italy

ISBN 978-3-030-50448-9   ISBN 978-3-030-50446-5   (eBook)
https://doi.org/10.1007/978-3-030-50446-5

This Springer imprint is published by the registered company Springer Nature Switzerland AG
The registered company address is: Gewerbestrasse 11, 6330 Cham, Switzerland

Contents

Part III Treatment

List of Videos

Video 5.1 Bulky rectosigmoid nodule (AVI 14,159 kb)
Video 5.2 Rectosigmoid nodule with absence of sliding (AVI 12,075 kb)
Video 5.3 Normal sliding of the uterus in absence of POD occlusion
           (AVI 5648 kb)
Video 9.1 (MP4 9967 kb)
Video 10.1 (MOV 1658605 kb)

Electronic supplementary material is available in the online version of the related chapter
on SpringerLink: http://link.springer.com/

Part I

Bowel Endometriosis

Pathogenesis of Bowel Endometriosis

Jessica Ottolina, Ludovica Bartiromo, Matteo Schimberni, Paola Viganò, and Massimo Candiani

1.1 Definition and Epidemiology

Deep infiltrating endometriosis (DIE) is a specific entity defined by the presence of an endometriotic lesion extending more than 5 mm underneath the peritoneum, including the infiltrative forms that involve vital structures, such as the bowel, ureters, bladder, and rectovaginal lesions. The choice of 5 mm of extension was made in light of epidemiologic observation [1]. Current data are insufficient to estimate the true incidence of endometriosis causing bowel obstruction, since literature consists almost exclusively of case reports. Differences in the estimated incidence may be due to different definitions of bowel endometriosis, or may be a reflection of missed diagnosis. Furthermore, a number of women with bowel endometriosis are diagnosed with other disorders such as irritable bowel syndrome and may never actually be diagnosed with or treated for bowel endometriosis [2]. Despite this, endometriosis causing intestinal obstruction is extremely rare with reported incidence between 0.1% and 0.7% [3].

1.2 Anatomical Distribution and Classification

Intestinal endometriosis is the most common extra-pelvic site [4]. Among women with endometriosis, the reported prevalence of rectovaginal or bowel involvement ranges widely from 5% to 25%, followed by localizations of the rectum, ileum, appendix, and cecum [5, 6]. Moreover, few case reports of lesions found in the upper abdomen including the stomach and transverse colon are reported [7, 8]. Multifocality is one of the main characteristics of DIE, especially when the intestinal tract is involved. When DIE affects the recto-sigmoid, multifocal bowel lesions are observed in about 40% of patients [9]. As reported by Kavallaris et al., with regard to rectal endometriosis, multifocal involvement (defined as presence of deep lesions within 2 cm area from the main lesions) was observed in 62% of the cases while multicentric involvement (defined as a satellite deep nodule found 2 cm from the main lesions) was found in 38% of the cases [10]. Markham et al. published a classification system dividing extra-pelvic lesions into four classes: Class I: endometriosis of the gastrointestinal

J. Ottolina · L. Bartiromo · M. Schimberni
M. Candiani
Gynecology and Obstetrics Unit,
San Raffaele Scientific Institute, Milan, Italy
e-mail: ottolina.jessica@hsr.it;
bartiromo.ludovica@hsr.it;
schimberni.matteo@hsr.it; candiani.massimo@hsr.it

P. Viganò (✉)
Reproductive Sciences Lab, Gynecology and
Obstetrics Unit, San Raffaele Scientific Institute,
Milan, Italy
e-mail: vigano.paola@hsr.it

© Springer Nature Switzerland AG 2020
S. Ferrero, M. Ceccaroni (eds.), *Clinical Management of Bowel Endometriosis*,
https://doi.org/10.1007/978-3-030-50446-5_1

tract; Class U: endometriosis of the urinary tract; Class L: endometriosis of the lungs and thorax; and Class O: endometriosis involving all other sites. A further staging includes the classification of the lesions based on the exact location and dimension of the defect [11]. Although isolated bowel involvement can be observed, the majority of patients with bowel endometriosis show evidence of disease elsewhere [12]. Remorgida and colleagues suggested a system for staging gastrointestinal tract endometriosis correlating with patients' symptoms and based on bowel specimen. They divided the disease into four stages: stage 0, the endometriotic tissue is only affecting the peritoneum and the subserosal connective tissue (not reaching the subserous plexus); stage 1, endometriotic foci are located in the subserous fat tissue or adjacent to the neurovascular branches (subserous plexus), rarely involving the external muscle layer; stage 2, the muscular wall and the Auerbach plexus are involved; stage 3, the infiltration reaches the submucosal nervous plexus or the mucosa [13]. Most of the endometriotic lesions of the gastrointestinal tract are confined to the serosal layer and surrounding connective tissue (stage 0). According to this, diagnosis of deep gastrointestinal endometriosis can be made only when invasion of the muscularis layer is established, while deeper lesions are uncommon with only few reports of endometriosis penetrating the bowel lumen [14–16]. Lymph node involvement can be observed ranging between 26% and 42% of the cases and it seems to correlate with the size of the bowel lesion and the percentage of the intestinal wall affected by the deep nodule; its presence may contribute to postoperative recurrences [17]. The incidence of lymph node involvement may be underestimated since the definitive diagnosis is obtainable only on bowel specimens after segmental bowel resection for deep endometriosis [17–19].

1.3 Theories Surrounding Pathogenesis

Multiple theories exist regarding the pathogenesis of endometriosis, the main being the retrograde menstruation and metaplasia theories, but nowadays it is well known that the pathogenesis of the disease is complex and likely multifactorial.

1.3.1 Retrograde Menstruation

The retrograde menstruation was the first and the most commonly cited theory [20]. The "implantation" theory proposes that endometrial tissue from the uterus is shed during menstruation and transported through the fallopian tubes (retrograde menstruation), thereby gaining access to and implanting on pelvic structures, including the bowel. Numerous studies have demonstrated that reflux of endometrial cells into the peritoneal cavity is a very common physiologic condition occurring during normal menstruation in most women with patent tubes [21, 22]. Therefore, anatomic alterations of the pelvis that increase tubal reflux of menstrual endometrium should increase a woman's chance of developing endometriosis. This is supported by the evidence that incidence of endometriosis is increased in girls with genital tract obstructions that prevent the expulsion of menses into the vagina increasing the likelihood of tubal reflux [23]. However, since up to 90% of women have retrograde menstruation, most women do not develop endometriosis suggesting that additional factors are involved [24]. According to Sampson's theory, endometriotic lesions affect the recto-sigmoid starting from the serosa, invade toward the lumen of the bowel and finally infiltrate the rectal wall [20]. The pathogenetic pathway leads to superficial implantation of endometrial cells triggering a strong inflammatory stimulus. When the process involves the sigmoid or, more rarely, the cecum, a distinct, large, and hard nodule forms. This lesion most often consists of duplicated and invaginated intestinal wall with very limited endometriotic tissue. Supporting this theory, evidence showed that the bowel endometriosis is not an isolated disease and that the subserosal layer is most commonly involved, with only few reports reporting deeper involvement [16]. Another observation supporting the theory of retrograde menstruation refers to the anatomical distribution of pelvic DIE, presenting in a double asymmetry: lesions

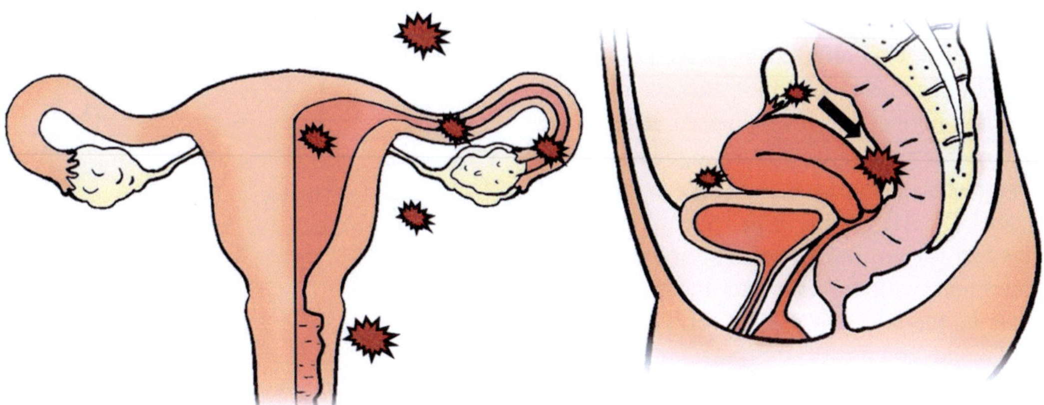

Fig. 1.1 The retrograde menstruation theory (Sampson theory)

are more frequently observed in the posterior compartment and most often located in the left side because of the gravity and the presence of the sigmoid colon on the left side close to the left adnexa [9]. This also explains why pelvic DIE lesions are more frequently observed in the low than in the high abdomen, and why intestinal lesions are preferentially located on the rectum and recto-sigmoid junction [9]. This is the so-called anatomical shelter theory. The retrograde menstruation theory is illustrated in Fig. 1.1.

1.3.2 Coelomic Metaplasia

The second theory supposed to explain the pathogenesis of endometriosis is that of "metaplasia", reported by Meyer in 1919 [25], subsequently developed as either coelomic (peritoneal) metaplasia by Gruenwald in 1942 [26] or Müllerian remnants metaplasia proposed by Donnez in 1995 [27]. The first hypothesis is based on embryologic studies demonstrating that all pelvic organs, including the endometrium, derived from cells lining the coelomic cavity. According to Donnez [27], deep lesions of the posterior cul-de-sac correspond to adenomyotic nodules originating from metaplasia of Müllerian remnants located in the rectovaginal septum, thus constituting a different entity from peritoneal endometriosis [28]. This hypothesis is based on the typical histological aspect of the different localizations and types.

In fact, endometriotic rectovaginal nodules show a histological aspect similar to adenomyotic nodules: differently from peritoneal endometriosis, in which epithelial glands are surrounded systematically by endometrial-type stroma, they consist in proliferating smooth muscle cells with active glandular epithelium and scanty stroma [29]. Indeed, several authors agree that there are three different types of endometriosis based on their histological presentation, with different pathogenetic mechanisms: peritoneal, ovarian, and DIE [28]. It has to be noticed that the vast majority of fibrotic rectovaginal plaques are found in the retrocervical area [30]. The rectovaginal septum is located caudally with respect to the posterior vaginal fornix and, since the base of the posterior cul-de-sac extends to at least the level of the middle third of the posterior vaginal fornix, it may not be the real site of deep nodular endometriosis [31]. If the mullerian remnants metaplasia theory is true, the anatomy of the pouch of Douglas should be similar in women with and without the so-called "adenomyotic nodules" because these lesions, if they really originate in the rectovaginal septum, should be located extraperitoneally. On the other hand, if deep foci are a manifestation of intraperitoneal disease, the pouch of Douglas should be partially or completely obliterated in affected women. Vercellini et al. studied whether the depth and volume of the pouch of Douglas differed in patients affected by endometriosis, with or without DIE, compared to normal controls (or patients affected by other pelvic diseases). The mean depth of the rectovaginal pouch in normal women, as measured from the upper border of the uterosacral ligaments to its base, has been demonstrated to be slightly over 5 cm [32]. All women with rectovaginal nodules had various degrees of anterior rectal displacement with adhesion to the peritoneum covering the posterior vaginal fornix: the mean depth and volume of the pouch of Douglas were significantly reduced in the deep endometriosis group, with about a one-third reduction in depth of the pouch of Douglas. No significant difference has been reported in women without deep lesions compared to controls (those with diseases other than endometriosis and those with a normal pelvis). The partial obliteration by the anterior rectal wall seems to be the cause of this apparent depth reduction and may give the false impression that nodules are subperitoneal. In other words, the authors concluded that endometriotic plaques and nodules found in the posterior vaginal fornix, cranially with respect to the rectovaginal septum may instead be a massive disease of the deepest portion of the pouch of Douglas that has been buried and excluded from the remaining pelvis by adhesions [32]. Moreover, various forms of peritoneal and ovarian disease are usually present in patients with rectovaginal endometriosis, suggesting that the pathogenesis may not be different. In this regard, Anaf et al. demonstrated (using immunochemical techniques with a monoclonal antibody against alfa-smooth muscle actin (α-SMA)) that a smooth muscle component is present in all types of endometriotic lesions but it is absent in disease-free peritoneum [33]. They hypothesize that the smooth muscle component may result from the metaplastic capacity of the mesothelium to differentiate into smooth muscle cells in response to the implanted endometrium. This metaplastic response might differ from one location to the other, thus explaining histological differences among the various forms of endometriosis [34].

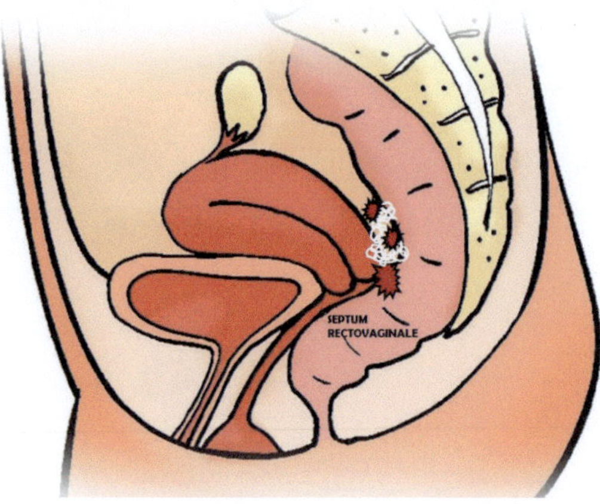

Fig. 1.2 The coelomic metaplasia (Müllerian remnants)

The coelomic metaplasia theory is illustrated in Fig. 1.2.

1.3.3 Stem Cells

The endometrial regeneration after menstrual shedding and the endometrial re-epithelialization after delivery or surgical curettage support the existence of a stem cell pool [35]. Since the endometrial basalis layer remains after the monthly menstrual shedding of the functional layer, the stem cells are thought to reside in the basalis layer of the endometrium [36]. Recently, endometrial-derived clonogenic cells (the stem cell population in the human endometrium) have been identified and proposed to be involved in the development of ectopic endometrial lesions [37]. According to Brosens et al., the neonatal uterine bleeding contains a high amount of endometrial progenitor cells [38]. Leyendecker et al. proposed that women affected by endometriosis abnormally shed the endometrial basalis tissue initiating endometriotic deposits after retrograde menstruation [39]. The possibility of an increased shedding of the stem cell from the basalis layer in patients affect by endometriosis as compared to healthy women, together with the similarity observed between ectopic lesions and the basalis layer, may support the theory of retrograde menstruation as providing an access for the endometrial stem cells to extrauterine structures [39]. Otherwise, these stem cells may be transported by the lymphatic or vascular pathways to ectopic sites [40]. Moreover, the fact that some of the endometrial stem cells possibly derive from the bone marrow further supports the hematogenous dissemination theory of these cells [41]. However, since stem cells are normally expected to differentiate into mature cells in concordance with the environmental niche, the supposedly multipotential endometrial stem cells in the peritoneal cavity should differentiate in peritoneal-type cells. It is possible that the deposition of endometrial tissue fragments containing both endometrial stem cells and their niche cells in the peritoneal cavity promote regeneration of endometrium-like tissue, thanks to the signals received by the stem cells from the surrounding endometrial niche cells. On the other hand, the relocation of an aberrant or committed stem cell from the endometrium to an ectopic site may also generate endometrium-like lesions. Endometrial tissue produces several chemokines and angiogenic factors causing neovascularisation in the ectopic site that ensure the establishment of these lesions [42]. Although possible, the reasons for such specific differentiation of stem cells into endometrium-like tissue remain unexplained.

1.3.4 Genetic Factors

Genetic factors probably play a role on individual's susceptibility to endometriosis [43–45]. The possibility of a familiarity for endometriosis has been recognized for several decades and concordance in twins has also been observed [43]. A study analyzing exome sequencing of DIE lesions reported somatic mutations in 79% of lesions and more specifically, mutations for the known cancer driver genes ARID1A, PIK3CA, KRAS, and PPP2R1A in 26% of lesions. The presence of cancer driver mutations in nonmalignant cells may partially explain the aggressive nature of deeply invasive lesions compared with superficial peritoneal lesions.

Moreover, these mutations were only found in the epithelial cells suggesting a unique selective pressure [46].

1.4 Histopathologic Findings

1.4.1 The Profibrotic Nature of Endometriosis

In the last years, advances in knowledge regarding the histological definition of endometriosis occurred. These changes have been consistent enough to require a reconceptualization of endometriosis, which is no more considered just as the mere presence of endometrial epithelial and stromal cells in ectopic sites, involving the profibrotic nature of the disease inside its "new" definition [47]. Although the presence of endometrial cells in ectopic sites is probably the starting point in the pathogenesis of endometriosis, it has been widely demonstrated in human as well as in animal studies that endometrial stroma and glands represent only a minor component of endometriotic lesions. It has been recently emphasized the consistent presence of fibrosis and myofibroblasts in endometriotic lesions and their crucial role in the pathogenesis of the disease [33, 48, 49]. Zhang et al., proposed that endometriotic lesions consequent to the implantation of endometrial tissue are essentially wounds undergoing repeated tissue injury and repair (ReTIAR) ultimately leading to fibrosis [48]. Indeed, endometrial cells present cyclic bleeding under hormonal stimulation causing subsequent tissue repair by recruiting neutrophils and macrophages M2 to the lesions [50, 51]. These events imply the development of "leaky" blood vessels resulting in platelets extravasation, leading to an increased platelet aggregation in endometriotic lesions [52]. Activated platelets contain more than 30 important proteins involved in angiogenesis and, along with macrophages, can induce fibrosis through the release of Transforming Growth Factor beta (TGF-β1) and the induction of the TGF-β1/Smad3 signaling pathway. Recent studies in mice showed that the

STAT3 signaling pathway is a potent inducer of epithelial-mesenchymal transition (EMT), fibroblast-myofibroblast transdifferentiation (FMT), and smooth muscle metaplasia (SMM) in endometriotic epithelial and stromal cells, resulting in increased contractility, collagen deposition and ultimately in fibrosis [53, 54]. The same mechanisms have been also suggested to be involved in DIE fibrosis development. It seems that ovarian endometriosis and DIE both undergo the same cellular changes consistent with EMT, FMT, SMM, and eventually fibrosis [55]. However, recent findings from the immunohisto-chemistry analysis revealed that DIE is character-ized by a higher production of TGF-β1 and a higher fibrotic content, with a more elevated expression of mesenchymal marker (vimentin) and but lower epithelial markers level (E-cadherin), suggesting an EMT process. Less vascularity and less platelet aggregation have been reported in DIE when compared to ovarian endometriosis [55]. Thus, the accelerated fibrosis observed in DIE might require more factors other than platelets to happen [56]. Recently, the role of oxidative stress known to be strongly present in DIE lesions has been associated with the acti-vation of A Disintegrin and Metalloproteases (ADAM17)/Notch signaling pathway. This path-way has been suggested to have a role in the development of endometriosis and, especially, of fibrosis inducing the transcription of fibrosis-related genes and the enhanced fibroblast activa-tion [57].

1.4.2 Histological Appearance of DIE

In accordance with these pathogenetic findings, deep endometriosis nodules (as the rectovaginal endometriotic nodules) have been already con-sidered in the past essentially as proliferating smooth muscle cells with active glandular epithe-lium and scanty stroma, with a consistent similar-ity with adenomyotic nodule [27].

According to Donnez and coworkers this smooth muscle content pre-existed in the corre-spondent normal area and then was invaded by the ectopic endometrium [58]. Subsequently, other authors proposed different theories with regard to the origin of the smooth muscle cells in deep endometriosis. Van Kaam et al. [59], not only showed that all the 20 deep infiltrating endometriotic lesions studied contained fibro-muscular tissue and myofibroblastic cells, but again raised reasonable doubts on the origin of this muscle content. Indeed, they demonstrated that the inoculation of human endometrium into a nude mouse could induce α-SMA expression in the surrounding murine tissue, as a conse-quence of a reaction of the local environment to the presence of ectopic endometrium, rather than representing the stromal differentiation toward smooth muscle cells. Despite the identification of a fibrotic component in DIE, Matsuzaki et al. [60], suggested that in patients with endometrio-sis, the epithelial-to-mesenchymal transition-like processes of endometrial epithelial cells, even in absence of TGF-β, was the real origin of myofibroblasts. These phenomena are probably generated by the increased stiffness (due to increased myofibroblast collagen I production) resulting in a fibrotic environment in deep dis-ease over time [55, 61].

Proliferation of normal fibroblasts is usually tightly regulated by the presence of type I colla-gen. In endometriosis, deep endometriotic stro-mal cells can persist and are not inhibited in their growth by the surrounding fibrotic environment. Matsusaki et al. suggested that this uncontrolled growth is due to the aberrant activation of AKT and ERK pathways [62]. Unlike the other sub-types of endometriosis, DIE lesions are situated in proximity to several nerve plexus and are fre-quently hyperinnervated [63, 64]. Anaf and coworkers observed that deep endometriotic lesions infiltrate the large bowel wall preferen-tially along the nerves, even at a distance from the palpated nodule, while the mucosa is rarely and only focally involved. The most richly innervated layers of the large bowel are the most intensely involved by endometriosis, supporting a close his-tological relationship between endometriotic lesions of large bowel and the nerves of the large bowel wall [65]. The sensory nerves-derived neu-ropeptides Substance P (SP) and Calcitonin gene-related peptide (CGRP) have been suggested to be involved in the development of endometriosis-associated fibrosis. This also provides an answer as why DIE lesions have abundant smooth muscle-like cells and more fibrosis than other lesions [56, 59, 66]. Anyway, regardless of the different hypotheses provided to explain the origin of myofibroblasts and fibrosis in endometriotic lesions, all investigators agree on the importance of this component in DIE lesions particularly and the fibromuscular component of endometriotic deep lesion seems to represent a self-amplifying event of endometriosis.

References

1. Vercellini P, Frontino G, Pietropaolo G, et al. Deep endometriosis: definition, pathogenesis, and clinical management. J Am Assoc Gynecol Laparosc. 2004;11:153–61.
2. Skoog SM, Foxx-Orenstein AE, Levy MJ, Rajan E, Session DR. Intestinal endometriosis: the great masquerader. Curr Gastroenterol Rep. 2004;6:405–9.
3. Katsikogiannis N, Tsaroucha A, Dimakis K, et al. Rectal endometriosis causing colonic obstruction and concurrent endometriosis of the appendix: a case report. J Med Case Rep. 2011;5:320.
4. Macafee CH, Greer HL. Intestinal endometriosis. A report of 29 cases and a survey of the literature. J Obstet Gynaecol Br Emp. 2016;196067:539–55.
5. Seracchioli R, Poggioli G, Pierangeli F, et al. Surgical outcome and long-term follow up after laparoscopic rectosigmoid resection in women with deep infiltrating endometriosis. BJOG. 2007;114:889–95.
6. Ribeiro PA, Rodrigues FC, Kehdi IP, et al. Laparoscopic resection of intestinal endometriosis: a 5-year experience. J Minim Invasive Gynecol. 2006;13:442–6.
7. Iaroshenko VI, Salokhina MB. [Endometriosis of the stomach]. Vestn Khir Im I I Grek. 1979;123:82–3.
8. Hartmann D, Schilling D, Roth SU, et al. [Endometriosis of the transverse colon--a rare localization]. Dtsch Med Wochenschr. 2002;127:2317–20.
9. Chapron C, Chopin N, Borghese B, et al. Deeply infiltrating endometriosis: pathogenetic implications of the anatomical distribution. Hum Reprod. 2006;21:1839–45.
10. Kavallaris A, Köhler C, Kühne-Heid R, Schneider A. Histopathological extent of rectal invasion by rectovaginal endometriosis. Hum Reprod. 2003;18:1323–7.
11. Markham SM, Carpenter SE, Rock JA. Extrapelvic endometriosis. Obstet Gynecol Clin N Am. 1989;16:193–219.
12. Veeraswamy A, Lewis M, Mann A, et al. Extragenital endometriosis. Clin Obstet Gynecol. 2010;53:449–66.
13. Remorgida V, Ragni N, Ferrero S, et al. The involvement of the interstitial Cajal cells and the enteric nervous system in bowel endometriosis. Hum Reprod. 2005;20:264–71.
14. Abrão MS, Petraglia F, Falcone T, et al. Deep endometriosis infiltrating the recto-sigmoid: critical factors to consider before management. Hum Reprod Update. 2015;21:329–39.
15. Chapron C, Bourret A, Chopin N, et al. Surgery for bladder endometriosis: long-term results and concomitant management of associated posterior deep lesions. Hum Reprod. 2010;25:884–9.
16. Rowland R, Langman JM. Endometriosis of the large bowel: a report of 11 cases. Pathology. 1989;2:259–65.
17. Noël JC, Chapron C, Fayt I, et al. Lymph node involvement and lymphovascular invasion in deep infiltrating rectosigmoid endometriosis. Fertil Steril. 2008;89:1069–72.
18. Abrao MS, Podgaec S, Dias JA Jr, et al. Deeply infiltrating endometriosis affecting the rectum and lymph nodes. Fertil Steril. 2006;86:543–7.
19. Mechsner S, Weichbrodt M, Riedlinger WF, et al. Immunohistochemical evaluation of endometriotic lesions and disseminated endometriosis-like cells in incidental lymph nodes of patients with endometriosis. Fertil Steril. 2010;94:457–63.
20. Sampson JA. Peritoneal endometriosis due to the menstrual dissemination of endometrial tissue into the peritoneal cavity. Am J Obstet Gynecol. 1927;14:422–69.
21. Halme J, Hammond MG, Hulka JF, et al. Retrograde menstruation in healthy women and in patients with endometriosis. Obstet Gynecol. 1984;64:151–4.
22. Liu DT, Hitchcock A. Endometriosis: its association with retrograde menstruation, dysmenorrhoea and tubal pathology. Br J Obstet Gynaecol. 1986;93:859–62.
23. Brosens IA, Puttemans P, Deprest J, et al. The endometriosis cycle and its derailments. Hum Reprod. 1994;9:770–1.
24. Vercellini P, Viganò P, Somigliana E, et al. Endometriosis: pathogenesis and treatment. Nat Rev Endocrinol. 2014;10:261–75.
25. Meyer R. Uber den stand der frage der adenomyositis und adenomyoma in algemeinen und insbesondere uber adenomyositis und adenomyometritis sarcomatosa. Zentrlbl Gynäkol. 1919;43:745–50.
26. Gruenwald P. Origin of endometriosis from mesenchyme of the coelomic walls. Am J Obstet Gynecol. 1942;44:470–4.
27. Donnez J, Nisolle M, Casanas-Roux F, et al. Rectovaginal septum, endometriosis or adenomyosis: laparoscopic management in a series of 231 patients. Hum Reprod. 1995;10:630–5.
28. Nisolle M, Donnez J. Peritoneal endometriosis, ovarian endometriosis, and adenomyotic nodules of the rectovaginal septum are three different entities. Fertil Steril. 1997;68:585–96.

29. Nakamura M, Katabuchi H, Tohya TR, et al. Scanning electron microscopic and immunohistochemical studies of pelvic endometriosis. Hum Reprod. 1993;8:2218–26.
30. Martin DC, Batt RE. Retrocervical, retrovaginal pouch, and rectovaginal septum endometriosis. J Am Assoc Gynecol Laparosc. 2001;8:12–7.
31. De Lancey JOL. Surgical anatomy of the female pelvis. In: Rock JA, Thompson JD, editors. The Linde's operative gynecology. 8th ed. Philadelphia, PA: Lippincott-Raven; 1997. p. 63–93.
32. Vercellini P, Aimi G, Panazza S, et al. Deep endometriosis conundrum: evidence in favor of a peritoneal origin. Fertil Steril. 2000;73:1043–6.
33. Anaf V, Simon P, Fayt I, et al. Smooth muscles are frequent components of endometriotic lesions. Hum Reprod. 2000;15:767–71.
34. Somigliana E, Infantino M, Candiani M, et al. Association rate between deep peritoneal endometriosis and other forms of the disease: pathogenetic implications. Hum Reprod. 2004;19:168–71.
35. Bulun SE, Cheng YH, Yin P, et al. Progesterone resistance in endometriosis: link to failure to metabolize estradiol. Mol Cell Endocrinol. 2006;248:94–103.
36. Hapangama DK, Turner MA, Drury JA, et al. Sustained replication in endometrium of women with endometrios is occurs without evoking a DNA damage response. Hum Reprod. 2009;24:687–96.
37. Attia GR, Zeitoun K, Edwards D, et al. Progesterone receptor isoform A but not B is expressed in endometriosis. J Clin Endocrinol Metab. 2000;85:2897–902.
38. Brosens I, Gordts S, Benagiano G. Endometriosis in adolescents is a hidden, progressive and severe disease that deserves attention, not just compassion. Hum Reprod. 2013;28:2026–31.
39. Leyendecker G, Kunz G, Herbertz M, et al. Uterine peristaltic activity and the development of endometriosis. Ann N Y Acad Sci. 2004;1034:338–55.
40. Maruyama T, Masuda H, Ono M, Kajitani T, et al. Stem cell theory for the pathogenesis of endometriosis. Front Biosci. 2012;4:2854–63.
41. Maruyama T, Masuda H, Ono M, et al. Human uterine stem/progenitor cells: their possible role in uterine physiology and pathology. Reproduction. 2010;140:11–22.
42. Santamaria X, Massasa EE, Taylor HS. Migration of cells from experimental endometriosis to the uterine endometrium. Endocrinology. 2012;153:5566–74.
43. Simpson JL, Bischoff F. Heritability and candidate genes for endometriosis. Reprod BioMed Online. 2003;7:162–9.
44. Campbell IG, Thomas EJ. Endometriosis: candidate genes. Hum Reprod Update. 2001;7:15–20.
45. Thomas EJ, Campbell IG. Molecular genetic defects in endometriosis. Gynecol Obstet Investig. 2000;50(suppl 1):44–50.
46. Anglesio MS, Papadopoulos N, Ayhan A, et al. Cancer-associated mutations in endometriosis without cancer. N Engl J Med. 2017;376:1835.
47. Vigano P, Candiani M, Monno A, et al. Time to redefine endometriosis including its pro-fibrotic nature. Hum Reprod. 2018;33:347–52.
48. Zhang Q, Duan J, Olson M, et al. Cellular changes consistent with epithelial-mesenchymal transition and fibroblast-to-myofibroblast transdifferentiation in the progression of experimental endometriosis in baboons. Reprod Sci. 2016;23:1409–21.
49. Barcena de Arellano ML, Gericke J, Reichelt U, et al. Immunohistochemical characterization of endometriosis-associated smooth muscle cells in human peritoneal endometriotic lesions. Hum Reprod. 2011;26:2721–30.
50. Bacci M, Capobianco A, Monno A, et al. Macrophages are alternatively activated in patients with endometriosis and required for growth and vascularization of lesions in a mouse model of disease. Am J Pathol. 2009;175:547–56.
51. Lin YJ, Lai MD, Lei HY, et al. Neutrophils and macrophages promote angiogenesis in the early stage of endometriosis in a mouse model. Endocrinology. 2006;147:1278–86.
52. Guo SW, Ding D, Liu X. Anti-platelet therapy is efficacious in treating endometriosis induced in mouse. Reprod BioMed Online. 2016;33:484–99.
53. Ding D, Liu X, Duan J, et al. Platelets are an unindicted culprit 485 in the development of endometriosis: clinical and experimental evidence. Hum Reprod. 2015;30:812–32.
54. Guo SW, Ding D, Geng JG, et al. P-selectin as a potential therapeutic target 488 for endometriosis. Fertil Steril. 2015;103:990–1000.
55. Liu X, Zhang Q, Guo SW. Histological and immunohistochemical characterization of the similarity and difference between ovarian endometriomas and deep infiltrating endometriosis. Reprod Sci. 2018;25:329–40.
56. Matsuzaki S, Darcha C. Epithelial to mesenchymal transition-like and mesenchymal to epithelial transition-like processes might be involved in the pathogenesis of pelvic endometriosis. Hum Reprod. 2012;27:712–21.
57. González-Foruria I, Santulli P, Chouzenoux S, et al. Dysregulation of the ADAM17/Notch signalling pathways in endometriosis: from oxidative stress to fibrosis. Mol Hum Reprod. 2017;23:488–99.
58. Donnez J, Nisolle M, Casanas-Roux F, et al. Stereometric evaluation of peritoneal endometriosis and endometriotic nodules of the rectovaginal septum. Hum Reprod. 1996;11:224–8.
59. van Kaam KJ, Schouten JP, Nap AW, et al. Fibromuscular differentiation in deeply infiltrating endometriosis is a reaction of resident fibroblasts to the presence of ectopic endometrium. Hum Reprod. 2008;23:2692–700.
60. Matsuzaki S, Darcha C, Pouly JL, et al. Effects of matrix stiffness on epithelial to mesenchymal transition-like processes of endometrial epithelial cells: implications for the pathogenesis of endometriosis. Sci Rep. 2017;7:44616.

61. Itoga T, Matsumoto T, Takeuchi H, et al. Fibrosis and smooth muscle metaplasia in rectovaginal endometriosis. Pathol Int. 2003;53:371–5.
62. Matsuzaki S, Darcha C. Co-operation between the AKT and ERK signaling pathways may support growth of deep endometriosis in a fibrotic microenvironment in vitro. Hum Reprod. 2015;30:1606–16.
63. Wang G, Tokushige N, Markham R, et al. Rich innervation of deep infiltrating endometriosis. Hum Reprod. 2009;24:827–34.
64. Arnold J, Barcena de Arellano ML, Rüster C, et al. Imbalance between sympathetic and sensory innervation in peritoneal endometriosis. Brain Behav Immun. 2012;26:132–41.
65. Anaf V, El Nakadi I, Simon P, et al. Preferential infiltration of large bowel endometriosis along the nerves of the colon. Hum Reprod. 2004;19:996–1002.
66. Yan D, Liu X, Guo SW. The establishment of a mouse model of deep endometriosis. Hum Reprod. 2019;34:235–47.

Simone Ferrero, Fabio Barra, Michele
Altieri, Andrea Orsi, Giancarlo Icardi,
and Giovanni Noberasco

2.1 Introduction

Endometriosis is a disease characterized by the presence of functional endometrial-like tissue outside the uterine cavity [1]. Endometriotic lesions may have various locations: they can be found more frequently on the ovaries, the uterosacral and the large ligaments, the fallopian tubes, the pelvic peritoneum, the pouch of Douglas, the vesicouterine fold, and the bowel. Extraperitoneal locations include the uterine cervix [2–5], the bladder and the ureters [6, 7], the umbilicus [8–10], the abdominal scars after gynecological surgery [11, 12] and cesarian section [13]. Endometriosis rarely affects extra-abdominal organs such as kidneys [14–17], skin [18], central nervous system [19–21], and thoracic cavity including lung [22–24], pleura [25, 26], diaphragm [17, 25–27], and pericardium [25, 26]. The term "bowel endometriosis" is employed for indicating endometrial-like glands and stroma that infiltrate the bowel wall. Bowel endometriosis was originally described by Sampson [28] in 1922. The diagnosis of bowel endometriosis is made when infiltration needs to reach at least the muscularis propria of the bowel wall; superficial endometriotic lesion infiltrating only the intestinal serosa should be considered "peritoneal endometriosis" [29]. Intestinal endometriosis typically involves the serosa and the intestinal muscularis propria, less frequently it infiltrates the submucosa and the mucosa (Figs. 2.1 and 2.2) [30].

S. Ferrero (✉) · F. Barra · M. Altieri
Academic Unit of Obstetrics and Gynecology, IRCCS
Ospedale Policlinico San Martino, Genova, Italy

Department of Neurosciences, Rehabilitation,
Ophthalmology, Genetics, Maternal and Child Health
(DiNOGMI), University of Genova, Genova, Italy
e-mail: simone.ferrero@unige.it

A. Orsi · G. Noberasco
Department of Health Sciences, University of Genoa,
Genoa, Italy
e-mail: andrea.orsi@unige.it

G. Icardi
Department of Health Sciences, University of Genoa,
Genoa, Italy

Academic Unit of Hygiene and Preventive Medicine,
Ospedale San Martino, Genoa, Italy
e-mail: icardi@unige.it

© Springer Nature Switzerland AG 2020
S. Ferrero, M. Ceccaroni (eds.), *Clinical Management of Bowel Endometriosis*,
https://doi.org/10.1007/978-3-030-50446-5_2

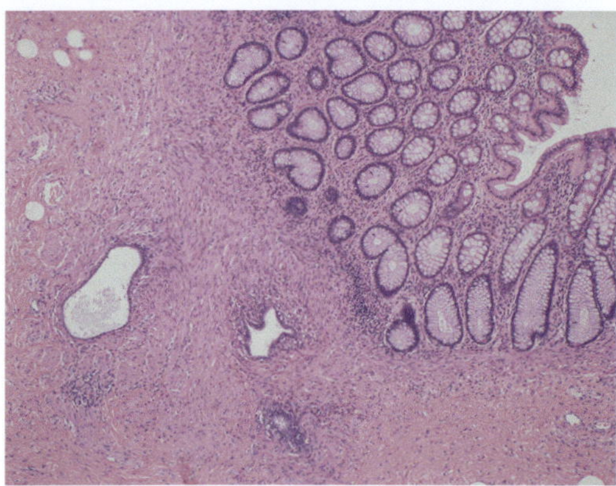

Fig. 2.1 Endometriotic nodule infiltrating the intestinal submucosa

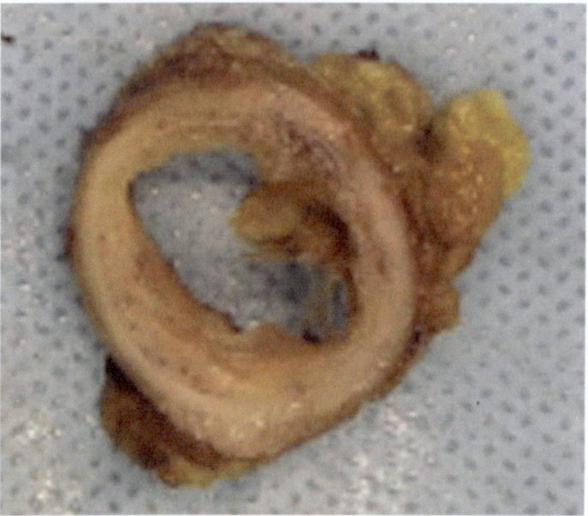

Fig. 2.2 Section of a rectal nodule excised by laparoscopic segmental resection. The nodule infiltrates the muscularis propria of the rectum

2.2 Epidemiology of Endometriosis

Several methodological issues complicate the assessment of the epidemiology of endometriosis: firstly, the need for surgery in order to establish the diagnosis affects the study of prevalence and incidence [31]; additionally, surgical confirmation may also lead to selection bias since the patients with symptomatic disease, high utilization of the medical system and comorbidities are more likely to undergo laparoscopy than the general population. Control selection is another issue: it is important to prevent the inclusion of

undiagnosed cases in the control group in order to decrease the risk of misclassification and to apply to the control group every restriction applied to cases [32]. It is also very difficult to evaluate the incidence of a chronic disease like endometriosis since the delay from symptoms to diagnosis makes impossible to assess the exact onset of the disease [33].

Published studies investigated the epidemiology of endometriosis in different populations. The prevalence of endometriosis was found to be between 2% and 19% among women undergoing tubal ligation [34–41]; between 11% and 47% among those undergoing surgery because of infertility [34, 35, 39, 42–48]; between 14% and 45% among patients undergoing surgery because of pelvic pain [36, 39, 47, 49, 50]; between 50% and 70% among adolescents with severe dysmenorrhea [51], and approximately 4% among patients having routine consultation with the general practitioner [52]. Based on the prevalence of pelvic pain in the general population and the data on endometriosis diagnostic rates, it can be estimated that prevalence endometriosis of any stage in the general population is between 5% and 10% [33]. The prevalence of deep infiltrating endometriosis is estimated to be the 1% of women of reproductive age. In line with this, a recent retrospective population-based study investigated the epidemiology of endometriosis in the databases of the Maccabi Healthcare Services, a two-million-member healthcare provider representing a quarter of the Israeli population [53]. The crude point prevalence of endometriosis was 10.8 per 1000 (95% CI, 10.5–11.0); women aged 40–44 years had the highest prevalence rate (18.6 per 1000; 95% CI, 17.7–19.5); the average annual incidence rate of newly diagnosed endometriosis was 7.2 (95% CI 6.5–8.0) per 10,000 women aged 15–55 years.

A prospective observational study including 1101 patients with laparoscopic diagnosis of endometriosis investigated the distribution of endometriotic lesions [54]. The mean age of patients was 33 years. The ovary was the most frequent site of endometriotic lesions (66.94%) followed by the uterosacral ligaments (45.51%), the ovarian fossa (32.15%), the pouch of Douglas

(29.52%), and the bladder (21.25%). Deep infiltrating endometriosis was diagnosed in 14.4% of the patients and rectosigmoid endometriosis was present in 8.5% of the patients.

2.3 Epidemiology of Bowel Endometriosis

Bowel endometriosis is a rare condition and, therefore, it is impossible to estimate its exact prevalence in the general population due to the lack of major well-designed epidemiological studies. A retrospective review of 3037 patients that underwent laparotomy for endometriosis found histologically confirmed bowel lesions in 163 patients (5.4%) [55]. Another study including 1785 women surgically treated for endometriosis reported histologically confirmed bowel endometriosis in 25.4% of the patients [56].

Bowel endometriosis is estimated to be found in 8–12% women with endometriosis [57] and in 5–37% of patients with diagnosis of deep infiltrating endometriosis [29]. A retrospective study including 688 patients who underwent laparoscopy because of deep infiltrating endometriosis found that 168 women (24.4%) had bowel endometriotic lesions [58]. There are no available data in order to have a meaningful estimation of bowel endometriosis incidence also due to major changes in diagnosis and health-seeking behavior between generations. Moreover, data obtained from surgical groups are affected by referral bias [59] and lack the cohort dimension required for meaningful statistics [60].

2.3.1 Rectosigmoid Endometriosis

Bowel endometriosis develops more frequently on the left side of the abdominal cavity, even though this evidence could be biased by considering rectum involvement part of the left abdominal side whereas it could derive from endometriotic cells from the pouch of Douglas and so should be considered a midline lesion [55, 61, 62]. Due to its proximity to the fallopian tubes, the rectosigmoid is the bowel segment most commonly affected by endometriosis [62]. In fact, the sigmoid and the left tube create a pouch which facilitates implantation of endometriotic cells [61]. Rectum and rectosigmoid junction are the most common localizations, affecting up to three-quarters of the patients (10.6–75%), followed by the sigmoid colon (14.3–65%) [63]. A retrospective study including 168 women with 252 bowel endometriotic lesions found that 11.5% of the intestinal nodules were located in the lower rectum, 23.0% in the middle rectum, 18.3% in the upper rectum, and 24.2% in the sigmoid colon [58].

2.3.2 Endometriosis of the Appendix

Appendicular endometriosis (Fig. 2.3) may be asymptomatic or present as acute or chronic appendicitis, lower gastrointestinal bleeding, intestinal perforation, or intestinal obstruction as a result of intussusception of the appendix in the inferior pole of the cecum [64]. The diagnosis of appendiceal endometriosis tends to histologically do after surgical approach. Appendectomy can be performed in case of gross alterations of the appendix at intraoperative evaluation or preoperative imaging (selective appendectomy) or at the time of procedures unrelated to suspected appendiceal pathology (incidental appendectomy) [65, 66]. In the published series, the prevalence of

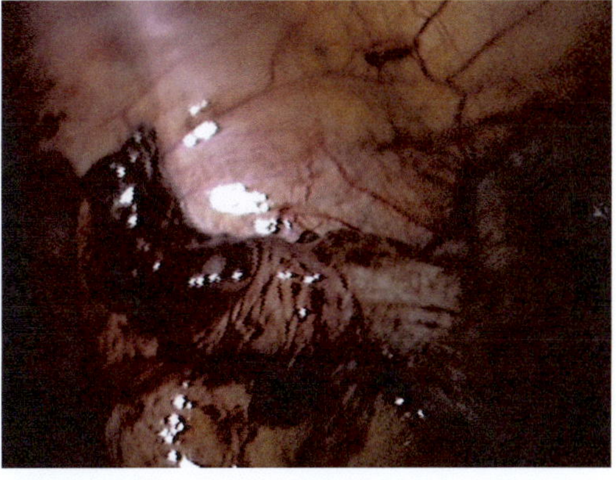

Fig. 2.3 Endometriosis of the appendix. The appendix was adherent to a right endometriotic cyst

appendicular endometriosis is dependent on the characteristics of the study population. It is estimated that appendiceal endometriosis is present in approximately 15% of the patients with bowel endometriosis [67, 68] and it approximately affects 3% of patients with endometriosis and 0.4% of the general population [69]. The prevalence of appendiceal endometriosis in patients with histological diagnosis of endometriosis and in those submitted to surgery for benign gynecological and nongynecological conditions is 2.5% and 1.2%, respectively [65]. However, the available data on the prevalence of appendiceal endometriosis are characterized by wide heterogeneity because of various populations included in the published studies and the differences in the surgical strategies adopted to perform the appendectomy. A retrospective study investigated the prevalence of appendiceal endometriosis in 395 women undergoing benign gynecological surgery [70]. In this population, 38.2% of the women had endometriosis and 54.3% of them had deep infiltrating endometriosis. The prevalence of appendiceal endometriosis was 13.2%; among these, 11.6% of patients had superficial endometriosis, and 39.0% deep infiltrating endometriosis. A retrospective cohort study including 1935 patients who underwent surgery because of symptomatic endometriosis found that appendiceal endometriosis had a prevalence of 2.6% [65]. This latter study also showed that independent risk factors for appendiceal endometriosis are adenomyosis, right endometrioma, bladder endometriosis, pelvic posterior endometriosis, left lateral pelvic endometriosis, and ileocecal involvement. In a case series, it was observed that endometriosis involves the body of the appendix in 56% of the cases, the tip in 44% of the cases while involvement of the base of the appendix does not seem to be present [71]. Endometriosis affects the muscularis of the appendix in two-thirds of cases and the serosa in one-third [72].

2.3.3 Other Intestinal Lesions

Endometriosis of the cecum may present as a mass causing bowel obstruction [73], ileocolic intussusception [74–76] or volvulus [77]. A

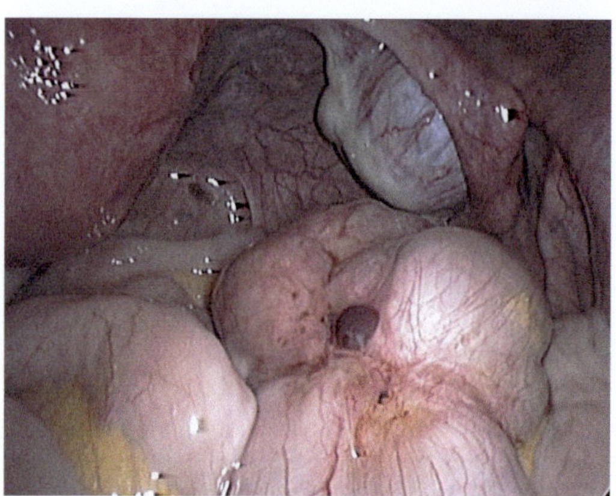

Fig. 2.4 Ileal endometriotic nodule

Brazilian retrospective study including 168 women with bowel endometriotic lesions with 252 intestinal nodules found that three nodules (1.2%) were located on the cecum and five nodules (2%) were in the terminal ileum (Fig. 2.4) [58]. A retrospective study including 241 patients operated for endometriosis found that ileocecal endometriosis has a prevalence of 3.3% [78]. A large multicentric retrospective study including 1135 patients operated because of rectosigmoid endometriosis found that involvement of the cecum was present in 6.6% of the cases [79].

Overall, endometriosis affects the descending colon more frequently than the ascending colon [55]. Case reports showed that endometriosis can also affect the omentum [80–84], the stomach [85, 86], transverse colon [86, 87], the gallbladder [88–90], and the Meckel's diverticulum [91, 92]. In addition, endometriosis of liver [93] and pancreas [94–97] have been described.

2.3.4 Multifocal and Multicentric Endometriosis

Bowel endometriosis can present with multiple lesions in the same bowel segment (multifocal disease) or affecting different bowel segments (multicentric disease). When the rectosigmoid is affected, multifocal bowel lesions tend to be present in more than 40% patients [63, 98]; moreover, rectal endometriosis is reported to be multifocal in 62% of the patients and multicentric in 38% [99].

2.3.5 Endometriosis of the Lymph Nodes

The lymph nodes involvement is considered to be underestimated since it is not routinely assessed in clinical practice; it is likely that this phenomenon is not as rare as we thought. Lymph node involvement is present in 18–20% of women with deep infiltrating endometriosis [100]. Concerning bowel endometriosis, two case series reported lymph node involvement in 42.3% [101] and in 26.3% of the cases, respectively [102].

2.4 Conclusion

Approximately a quarter of patients with deep infiltrating endometriosis have intestinal bowel lesions. Rectosigmoid endometriosis is the most frequent form of bowel endometriosis. However, endometriosis may also affect the appendix, terminal ileum, descending, ascending and transverse colon and stomach. Some patients may have multiple endometriotic nodules in the same bowel segment (multifocal disease) or in different bowel segments (multifocal disease).

References

1. Ferrero S. Endometriosis: modern management of an ancient disease. Eur J Obstet Gynecol Reprod Biol. 2017;209:1–2.
2. Jaiman S, Gundabattula SR, Pochiraju M, Sangireddy JR. Polypoid endometriosis of the cervix: a case report and review of the literature. Arch Gynecol Obstet. 2014;289(4):915–20.
3. Seval MM, Cavkaytar S, Atak Z, Guresci S. Postcoital bleeding due to cervical endometriosis. BMJ Case Rep. 2013;2013:bcr2012008209.
4. Rodolakis A, Akrivos N, Haidopoulos D, Kyritsis N, Sotiropoulou M, Thomakos N, et al. Abdominal radical trachelectomy for treatment of deep infiltrating endometriosis of the cervix. J Obstet Gynaecol Res. 2012;38(4):729–32.
5. Wang S, Li XC, Lang JH. Cervical endometriosis: clinical character and management experience in a 27-year span. Am J Obstet Gynecol. 2011;205(5):452 e1–5.
6. Barra F, Scala C, Biscaldi E, Vellone VG, Ceccaroni M, Terrone C, et al. Ureteral endometriosis: a systematic review of epidemiology, pathogenesis, diagnosis, treatment, risk of malignant transformation and fertility. Hum Reprod Update. 2018;24(6):710–30.
7. Leone Roberti Maggiore U, Ferrero S, Candiani M, Somigliana E, Vigano P, Vercellini P. Bladder endometriosis: a systematic review of pathogenesis, diagnosis, treatment, impact on fertility, and risk of malignant transformation. Eur Urol. 2017;71(5):790–807.
8. Ghosh A, Das S. Primary umbilical endometriosis: a case report and review of literature. Arch Gynecol Obstet. 2014;290(4):807–9.
9. Kyamidis K, Lora V, Kanitakis J. Spontaneous cutaneous umbilical endometriosis: report of a new case with immunohistochemical study and literature review. Dermatol Online J. 2011;17(7):5.
10. Rosina P, Pugliarello S, Colato C, Girolomoni G. Endometriosis of umbilical cicatrix: case report and review of the literature. Acta Dermatovenerol Croat. 2008;16(4):218–21.
11. Emre A, Akbulut S, Yilmaz M, Bozdag Z. Laparoscopic trocar port site endometriosis: a case report and brief literature review. Int Surg. 2012;97(2):135–9.
12. Siddiqui ZA, Husain F, Siddiqui Z, Siddiqui M. Port site endometrioma: a rare cause of abdominal wall pain following laparoscopic surgery. BMJ Case Rep. 2017;2017:bcr2017219291.
13. Zhang P, Sun Y, Zhang C, Yang Y, Zhang L, Wang N, et al. Cesarean scar endometriosis: presentation of 198 cases and literature review. BMC Womens Health. 2019;19(1):14.
14. Badri AV, Jennings R, Patel P, Eun DD. Renal endometriosis: the case of an endometrial implant mimicking a renal mass. J Endourol Case Rep. 2018;4(1):176–8.
15. Cheng CH, Kuo HC, Su B. Endometriosis in a kidney with focal xanthogranulomatous pyelonephritis and a perinephric abscess. BMC Res Notes. 2015;8:591.
16. Gupta K, Rajwanshi A, Srinivasan R. Endometriosis of the kidney: diagnosis by fine-needle aspiration cytology. Diagn Cytopathol. 2005;33(1):60–1.
17. Chinegwundoh FI, Ryan P, Luesley T, Chan SY. Renal and diaphragmatic endometriosis de novo associated with hormone replacement therapy. J Urol. 1995;153(2):380–1.
18. Fernandez-Acenero MJ, Cordova S. Cutaneous endometriosis: review of 15 cases diagnosed at a single institution. Arch Gynecol Obstet. 2011;283(5):1041–4.
19. Maniglio P, Ricciardi E, Meli F, Tomao F, Peiretti M, Caserta D. Complete remission of cerebral endometriosis with dienogest: a case report. Gynecol Endocrinol. 2018;34(10):837–9.
20. Ichida M, Gomi A, Hiranouchi N, Fujimoto K, Suzuki K, Yoshida M, et al. A case of cerebral endometriosis causing catamenial epilepsy. Neurology. 1993;43(12):2708–9.
21. Thibodeau LL, Prioleau GR, Manuelidis EE, Merino MJ, Heafner MD. Cerebral endometriosis. Case report. J Neurosurg. 1987;66(4):609–10.

22. Matsushima K, Ono M, Hayashi S, Sonoda D, Matsui Y, Shiomi K, et al. Resection of intrapulmonary endometriosis by video-assisted thoracoscopic surgery under pre-operative CT-guided marking synchronized with menstrual cycle. Gen Thorac Cardiovasc Surg. 2020;68:549.

23. Gates J, Sharma A, Kumar A. Rare case of thoracic endometriosis presenting with lung nodules and pneumothorax. BMJ Case Rep. 2018;2018:bcr2018224181.

24. Huang H, Li C, Zarogoulidis P, Darwiche K, Machairiotis N, Yang L, et al. Endometriosis of the lung: report of a case and literature review. Eur J Med Res. 2013;18:13.

25. Ceccaroni M, Roviglione G, Rosenberg P, Pesci A, Clarizia R, Bruni F, et al. Pericardial, pleural and diaphragmatic endometriosis in association with pelvic peritoneal and bowel endometriosis: a case report and review of the literature. Wideochir Inne Tech Maloinwazyjne. 2012;7(2):122–31.

26. Ceccaroni M, Clarizia R, Placci A. Pericardial, pleural, and diaphragmatic endometriosis. J Thorac Cardiovasc Surg. 2010;140(5):1189–90.

27. Seidler S, Shabanov S, Andres A, Karenovics W, Wenger JM, Pluchino N. Diaphragmatic endometriosis: multidisciplinary treatment. J Minim Invasive Gynecol. 2019;26(3):404.

28. Sampson JA. Intestinal adenomas of endometrial type: their importance and their relation to ovarian hematomas of endometrial type (perforating hemorrhagic cysts of the ovary). Arch Surg. 1922;5:217–80.

29. Ferrero S, Camerini G, Leone Roberti Maggiore U, Venturini PL, Biscaldi E, Remorgida V. Bowel endometriosis: recent insights and unsolved problems. World J Gastrointest Surg. 2011;3(3):31–8.

30. Veeraswamy A, Lewis M, Mann A, Kotikela S, Hajhosseini B, Nezhat C. Extragenital endometriosis. Clin Obstet Gynecol. 2010;53(2):449–66.

31. Eskenazi B, Warner ML. Epidemiology of endometriosis. Obstet Gynecol Clin N Am. 1997;24(2):235–58.

32. Cramer DW, Missmer SA. The epidemiology of endometriosis. Ann N Y Acad Sci. 2002;955:11–22. Discussion 34–6, 396–406.

33. Zondervan KT, Cardon LR, Kennedy SH. What makes a good case-control study? Design issues for complex traits such as endometriosis. Hum Reprod. 2002;17(6):1415–23.

34. Drake TS, Grunert GM. The unsuspected pelvic factor in the infertility investigation. Fertil Steril. 1980;34(1):27–31.

35. Strathy JH, Molgaard CA, Coulam CB, Melton LJ III. Endometriosis and infertility: a laparoscopic study of endometriosis among fertile and infertile women. Fertil Steril. 1982;38(6):667–72.

36. Kresch AJ, Seifer DB, Sachs LB, Barrese I. Laparoscopy in 100 women with chronic pelvic pain. Obstet Gynecol. 1984;64(5):672–4.

37. Moen MH. Endometriosis in women at interval sterilization. Acta Obstet Gynecol Scand. 1987;66(5):451–4.

38. Kirshon B, Poindexter AN 3rd, Fast J. Endometriosis in multiparous women. J Reprod Med. 1989;34(3):215–7.

39. Mahmood TA, Templeton A. Prevalence and genesis of endometriosis. Hum Reprod. 1991;6(4):544–9.

40. Moen MH, Muus KM. Endometriosis in pregnant and non-pregnant women at tubal sterilization. Hum Reprod. 1991;6(5):699–702.

41. Sangi-Haghpeykar H, Poindexter AN III. Epidemiology of endometriosis among parous women. Obstet Gynecol. 1995;85(6):983–92.

42. Peterson EP, Behrman SJ. Laparoscopy of the infertile patient. Obstet Gynecol. 1970;36(3):363–7.

43. Goldenberg RL, Magendantz HG. Laparoscopy and the infertility evaluation. Obstet Gynecol. 1976;47(4):410–4.

44. Musich JR, Behrman SJ. Infertility laparoscopy in perspective: review of five hundred cases. Am J Obstet Gynecol. 1982;143(3):293–303.

45. Nordenskjold F, Ahlgren M. Laparoscopy in female infertility. Diagnosis and prognosis for subsequent pregnancy. Acta Obstet Gynecol Scand. 1983;62(6):609–15.

46. Matorras R, Rodiquez F, Pijoan JI, Ramon O, Gutierrez de Teran G, Rodriguez-Escudero F. Epidemiology of endometriosis in infertile women. Fertil Steril. 1995;63(1):34–8.

47. Prevalence and anatomical distribution of endometriosis in women with selected gynaecological conditions: results from a multicentric Italian study. Gruppo italiano per lo studio dell'endometriosi. Hum Reprod. 1994;9(6):1158–62.

48. Meuleman C, Vandenabeele B, Fieuws S, Spiessens C, Timmerman D, D'Hooghe T. High prevalence of endometriosis in infertile women with normal ovulation and normospermic partners. Fertil Steril. 2009;92(1):68–74.

49. Lundberg WI, Wall JE, Mathers JE. Laparoscopy in evaluation of pelvic pain. Obstet Gynecol. 1973;42(6):872–6.

50. Talbot HM, Leeton J. The role of laparoscopy in 1,400 patients. Med J Aust. 1974;1(2):36–8.

51. Janssen EB, Rijkers AC, Hoppenbrouwers K, Meuleman C, D'Hooghe TM. Prevalence of endometriosis diagnosed by laparoscopy in adolescents with dysmenorrhea or chronic pelvic pain: a systematic review. Hum Reprod Update. 2013;19(5):570–82.

52. Ferrero S, Arena E, Morando A, Remorgida V. Prevalence of newly diagnosed endometriosis in women attending the general practitioner. Int J Gynaecol Obstet. 2010;110(3):203–7.

53. Eisenberg VH, Weil C, Chodick G, Shalev V. Epidemiology of endometriosis: a large population-based database study from a health-care provider with 2 million members. BJOG. 2018;125(1):55–62.

54. Audebert A, Petousis S, Margioula-Siarkou C, Ravanos K, Prapas N, Prapas Y. Anatomic distribution of endometriosis: a reappraisal based on series of 1101 patients. Eur J Obstet Gynecol Reprod Biol. 2018;230:36–40.

55. Weed JC, Ray JE. Endometriosis of the bowel. Obstet Gynecol. 1987;69(5):727–30.

56. Redwine DB. Endometriosis of the bowel. Surgical management of endometriosis. London: Taylor & Francis; 2004. p. 157–73.

57. Guerriero S, Ajossa S, Orozco R, Perniciano M, Jurado M, Melis GB, et al. Accuracy of transvaginal ultrasound for diagnosis of deep endometriosis in the rectosigmoid: systematic review and meta-analysis. Ultrasound Obstet Gynecol. 2016;47(3):281–9.

58. Pereira RM, Zanatta A, Preti CD, de Paula FJ, da Motta EL, Serafini PC. Should the gynecologist perform laparoscopic bowel resection to treat endometriosis? Results over 7 years in 168 patients. J Minim Invasive Gynecol. 2009;16(4):472–9.

59. Koninckx PR. Biases in the endometriosis literature. Illustrated by 20 years of endometriosis research in Leuven. Eur J Obstet Gynecol Reprod Biol. 1998;81(2):259–71.

60. Koninckx PR, Ussia A, Adamyan L, Wattiez A, Donnez J. Deep endometriosis: definition, diagnosis, and treatment. Fertil Steril. 2012;98(3):564–71.

61. Vercellini P, Chapron C, Fedele L, Gattei U, Daguati R, Crosignani PG. Evidence for asymmetric distribution of lower intestinal tract endometriosis. BJOG. 2004;111(11):1213–7.

62. Markham SM, Carpenter SE, Rock JA. Extrapelvic endometriosis. Obstet Gynecol Clin N Am. 1989;16(1):193–219.

63. Chapron C, Chopin N, Borghese B, Foulot H, Dousset B, Vacher-Lavenu MC, et al. Deeply infiltrating endometriosis: pathogenetic implications of the anatomical distribution. Hum Reprod. 2006;21(7):1839–45.

64. Ardies P, Vanwambeke K, Hanssens M, Knockaert D, Penninckx F, Lauwereyns J, et al. Endometriosis of the cecum and appendix: two case reports. Gastrointest Radiol. 1990;15(3):263–4.

65. Mabrouk M, Raimondo D, Mastronardi M, Raimondo I, Del Forno S, Arena A, et al. Endometriosis of the appendix: when to predict and how to manage-a multivariate analysis of 1935 endometriosis cases. J Minim Invasive Gynecol. 2020;27(1):100–6.

66. Guaitoli E, Gallo G, Cardone E, Conti L, Famularo S, Formisano G, et al. Consensus Statement of the Italian Polispecialistic Society of Young Surgeons (SPIGC): diagnosis and treatment of acute appendicitis. J Investig Surg. 2020:1–15.

67. Abrao MS, Dias JA Jr, Rodini GP, Podgaec S, Bassi MA, Averbach M. Endometriosis at several sites, cyclic bowel symptoms, and the likelihood of the appendix being affected. Fertil Steril. 2010;94(3):1099–101.

68. Nezhat C, Li A, Falik R, Copeland D, Razavi G, Shakib A, et al. Bowel endometriosis: diagnosis and management. Am J Obstet Gynecol. 2018;218(6):549–62.

69. Gustofson RL, Kim N, Liu S, Stratton P. Endometriosis and the appendix: a case series and comprehensive review of the literature. Fertil Steril. 2006;86(2):298–303.

70. Moulder JK, Siedhoff MT, Melvin KL, Jarvis EG, Hobbs KA, Garrett J. Risk of appendiceal endometriosis among women with deep-infiltrating endometriosis. Int J Gynaecol Obstet. 2017;139(2):149–54.

71. Uwaezuoke S, Udoye E, Etebu E. Endometriosis of the appendix presenting as acute appendicitis: a case report and literature review. Ethiop J Health Sci. 2013;23(1):69–72.

72. Gupta R, Singh AK, Farhat W, Ammar H, Azzaza M, Mizouni A, et al. Appendicular endometriosis: a case report and review of literature. Int J Surg Case Rep. 2019;64:94–6.

73. Molina GA, Ramos DR, Yu A, Paute PA, Llerena PS, Alexandra Valencia S, et al. Endometriosis mimicking a cecum mass with complete bowel obstruction: an infrequent cause of acute abdomen. Case Rep Surg. 2019;2019:7024172.

74. Nozari N, Shafiei M, Sarmadi S. An unusual presentation of endometriosis as an ileocolic intussusception with cecal mass: a case report. J Reprod Infertil. 2018;19(4):247–9.

75. Rodriguez-Lopez M, Bailon-Cuadrado M, Tejero-Pintor FJ, Choolani E, Fernandez-Perez G, Tapia-Herrero A. Ileocecal intussusception extending to left colon due to endometriosis. Ann R Coll Surg Engl. 2018;100(3):e62–e3.

76. Katagiri H, Lefor AK, Nakata T, Matsuo T, Shimokawa I. Intussusception secondary to endometriosis of the cecum. Int J Surg Case Rep. 2014;5(12):890–2.

77. Ito D, Kaneko S, Morita K, Seiichiro S, Teruya M, Kaminishi M. Cecal volvulus caused by endometriosis in a young woman. BMC Surg. 2015; 15:77.

78. Fedele L, Berlanda N, Corsi C, Gazzano G, Morini M, Vercellini P. Ileocecal endometriosis: clinical and pathogenetic implications of an underdiagnosed condition. Fertil Steril. 2014;101(3):750–3.

79. Roman H, Group F. A national snapshot of the surgical management of deep infiltrating endometriosis of the rectum and colon in France in 2015: a multicenter series of 1135 cases. J Gynecol Obstet Hum Reprod. 2017;46(2):159–65.

80. Haeri S, Cosin JA. Endometriosis mimicking ovarian cancer in the setting of acquired immune deficiency syndrome. Obstet Gynecol. 2009;114(2, Pt 2):425–6.

81. Santeusanio G, Ventura L, Partenzi A, Spagnoli LG, Kraus FT. Omental endosalpingiosis with endometrial-type stroma in a woman with extensive hemorrhagic pelvic endometriosis. Am J Clin Pathol. 1999;111(2):248–51.

82. Grouls V, Berndt R. Endometrioid adenoma (polypoid endometriosis) of the omentum maius. Pathol Res Pract. 1995;191(10):1049–52.

83. Rorat E, Wallach RC. Endometriosis of the omentum and borderline ovarian malignancy. Eur J Gynaecol Oncol. 1986;7(1):12–5.

84. Naraynsingh V, Raju GC, Ratan P, Wong J. Massive ascites due to omental endometriosis. Postgrad Med J. 1985;61(716):539–40.

85. Iaroshenko VI, Salokhina MB. [Endometriosis of the stomach]. Vestn Khir Im I I Grek. 1979;123(8):82–3.
86. Anaf V, Buggenhout A, Franchimont D, Noel JC. Gastric endometriosis associated with transverse colon endometriosis: a case report of a very rare event. Arch Gynecol Obstet. 2014;290(6):1275–7.
87. Hartmann D, Schilling D, Roth SU, Bohrer MH, Riemann JF. [Endometriosis of the transverse colon--a rare localization]. Dtsch Med Wochenschr. 2002;127(44):2317–20.
88. Iafrate F, Ciolina M, Iannitti M, Baldassari P, Pichi A, Rengo M, et al. Gallbladder and muscular endometriosis: a case report. Abdom Imaging. 2013;38(1):120–4.
89. Saldana DG, de Acosta DA, Aleman HP, Gebrehiwot D, Torres E. Gallbladder endometrioma associated with obstructive jaundice and a serous ovarian cystic adenoma. South Med J. 2010;103(12):1250–2.
90. Saadat-Gilani K, Bechmann L, Frilling A, Gerken G, Canbay A. Gallbladder endometriosis as a cause of occult bleeding. World J Gastroenterol. 2007;13(33):4517–9.
91. Honore LH. Endometriosis of Meckel's diverticulum associated with intestinal obstruction--a case report. Am J Proctol. 1980;31(2):11–2.
92. Frey GH, Scott CM. Incidental Meckel's diverticulum associated with endometriosis. Am J Surg. 1956;91(5):861–2.
93. Prodromidou A, Machairas N, Paspala A, Hasemaki N, Sotiropoulos GC. Diagnosis, surgical treatment and postoperative outcomes of hepatic endometriosis: a systematic review. Ann Hepatol. 2020;19(1):17–23.
94. Yamamoto R, Konagaya K, Iijima H, Kashiwagi H, Hashimoto M, Shindo A, et al. A rare case of pancreatic endometrial cyst and review of the literature. Intern Med. 2019;58(8):1097–101.
95. Mederos MA, Villafane N, Dhingra S, Farinas C, McElhany A, Fisher WE, et al. Pancreatic endometrial cyst mimics mucinous cystic neoplasm of the pancreas. World J Gastroenterol. 2017;23(6): 1113–8.
96. Plodeck V, Sommer U, Baretton GB, Aust DE, Laniado M, Hoffmann RT, et al. A rare case of pancreatic endometriosis in a postmenopausal woman and review of the literature. Acta Radiol Open. 2016;5(9):2058460116669385.
97. Monrad-Hansen PW, Buanes T, Young VS, Langebrekke A, Qvigstad E. Endometriosis of the pancreas. J Minim Invasive Gynecol. 2012;19(4):521–3.
98. Remorgida V, Ragni N, Ferrero S, Anserini P, Torelli P, Fulcheri E. How complete is full thickness disc resection of bowel endometriotic lesions? A prospective surgical and histological study. Hum Reprod. 2005;20(8):2317–20.
99. Kavallaris A, Kohler C, Kuhne-Heid R, Schneider A. Histopathological extent of rectal invasion by rectovaginal endometriosis. Hum Reprod. 2003;18(6):1323–7.
100. Mechsner S, Weichbrodt M, Riedlinger WF, Kaufmann AM, Schneider A, Kohler C. Immunohistochemical evaluation of endometriotic lesions and disseminated endometriosis-like cells in incidental lymph nodes of patients with endometriosis. Fertil Steril. 2010;94(2):457–63.
101. Anaf V, El Nakadi I, Simon P, Van de Stadt J, Fayt I, Simonart T, et al. Preferential infiltration of large bowel endometriosis along the nerves of the colon. Hum Reprod. 2004;19(4):996–1002.
102. Abrao MS, Podgaec S, Dias JA Jr, Averbach M, Garry R, Ferraz Silva LF, et al. Deeply infiltrating endometriosis affecting the rectum and lymph nodes. Fertil Steril. 2006;86(3):543–7.

Pathologic Characteristics of Bowel Endometriosis

3

Valerio Gaetano Vellone, Chiara Maria Biatta, Michele Paudice, Fabio Barra, Simone Ferrero, and Giulia Scaglione

3.1 Introduction

Endometriosis is a widespread disease, affecting at least 4% of women of reproductive age [1]. It is characterized by the presence of endometrial tissue (glands and/or stroma) outside the uterine wall. Its histological diagnosis can be challenging due to unusual sites, especially on small biopsies. Intestinal endometriosis has been a well-known disorder since Dr. John Sampson's crucial contribution on the topic in 1922 [2]. The term "bowel endometriosis" should be used when endometrial-like glands and stroma infiltrate the bowel wall reaching at least the muscular layer of the bowel wall. As initially suggested by Chapron et al., endometriotic foci located on the bowel serosa should be considered peritoneal and not bowel endometriosis [3].

Gastrointestinal (GI) tract involvement is found in 15–37% of patients with pelvic endometriosis and it may be focal [4]. The most common locations in the pelvic GI tract are sigmoid colon and rectum, while typical extra-pelvic GI locations are ileum, cecum, and appendix [5]. Intestinal endometriosis tends to affect the subserous fat tissue and external bowel wall, while only 10% of GI cases show mucosal involvement [6, 7].

Endometriosis of the intestinal tract may mimic a number of diseases both clinically and pathologically. Bowel endometriosis is typically associated with genital endometriosis and hence its management is usually referred to the gynecologist, often untrained in bowel disease. Although GI endometriosis may cause severe intestinal symptoms and pain, frequently these manifestations are not adequately investigated at the time of gynecologic evaluation. In some cases, especially when symptoms are not clearly associated with the menstrual cycle (approximately 40%), differential diagnosis between inflammatory bowel diseases (IBD) and intestinal endometriosis may be clinically challenging as both conditions are associated with abdominal pain and bloody stools [8]. Other differential diagnosis includes diverticulitis, appendicitis, tubo-ovarian abscess, irritable bowel syndrome [9, 10], and neoplastic conditions.

V. G. Vellone (✉)
Department of Integrated Surgical and Diagnostic Sciences (DISC), University of Genoa, Genoa, Italy

Pathology Academic Unit, IRCCS Ospedale Policlinico San Martino, Genoa, Italy
e-mail: valerio.vellone@unige.it

C. M. Biatta · M. Paudice · G. Scaglione
Department of Integrated Surgical and Diagnostic Sciences (DISC), University of Genoa, Genoa, Italy

F. Barra · S. Ferrero
Academic Unit of Obstetrics and Gynecology, IRCCS Ospedale Policlinico San Martino, Genova, Italy

Department of Neurosciences, Rehabilitation, Ophthalmology, Genetics, Maternal and Child Health (DiNOGMI), University of Genova, Genova, Italy

© Springer Nature Switzerland AG 2020
S. Ferrero, M. Ceccaroni (eds.), *Clinical Management of Bowel Endometriosis*,
https://doi.org/10.1007/978-3-030-50446-5_3

During the past decades, many therapeutic protocols have been proposed for IE. There is solid evidence that hormonal therapy improves pain and intestinal symptoms of patients with IE, but obviously it does not cure the disease [11–13]. Bowel resection has been performed to treat bowel endometriosis since the early 1900s [14]. Although over a century has passed, the surgical approach is non-standardized. Some surgeons still routinely perform segmental resection for bowel endometriosis. In an effort to decrease postoperative morbidity, conservative approaches (including shaving excision and disc resection have been developed). Hence the pathologist is called to examine different surgical specimens seeking endometriotic lesions and sometimes dealing with diagnostic pitfalls.

3.2 Macroscopic Findings

Adhesions and serosal fibrosis are often a prominent feature of bowel endometriosis causing obstructive symptoms. In a minority of cases, gray-brown discoloration of the serosal surface ("powder burns") similar to that commonly observed on other visceral sites is a prominent feature [15]. More frequently, bowel endometriosis causes a wall thickening associated to luminal stenosis, due to the fibrosis present within the muscularis propria. The length of the strictures may vary a lot (ranging from 1 to 10 cm). Endometriosis-associated smooth muscle hyperplasia and fibrosis may result in the formation of mural masses even of several centimeters, cystic at times; multiple small nodules can be detected adjacent to the largest nodule. Endometriosis can seldom produce pseudopolyps bulging into the visceral lumen [16, 17], with central ulceration and induration of the overlying mucosa. Bowel endometriotic foci may develop as one single main mass with small satellite lesions ("multifocal disease") it or as multiple isolated nodules located in different bowel segments (i.e., the sigmoid and cecum, "multicentric disease"). Although the former pattern is more common [6], multicentric disease is observed in 15–35% of the cases. Redwine observed at least two intestinal

lesions in 154 (34%) out of 453 women with histologically proven bowel endometriosis [18]. In a series of more than 200 patients, Keckstein and Wiesinger observed multifocal involvement of the bowel wall in 25% of the cases [19].

3.3 Microscopic Findings

3.3.1 Usual Findings

In most of the cases, the histopathological appearance of bowel endometriosis is similar to that of other sites, although some differences may exist. Typically, endometriosis appears as one or more endometrioid glands surrounded by stromal cells, resembling the endometrial stromal cells of the proliferative phase. The glandular epithelium is one-layer thick with cuboidal or tall cells, ciliated occasionally, with eosinophilic cytoplasm. Nuclei are ovoid with vertical orientation and very rare mitoses (Fig. 3.1). Stromal cells are supported by a fine reticulin network with congested small vessels. The whole picture is usually consistent with inactive or irregular proliferative endometrium, although typical proliferative or secretory changes may be observed. In case of exogenous administration of progestins, cyclically functioning endometriosis or pregnancy, a stromal decidual

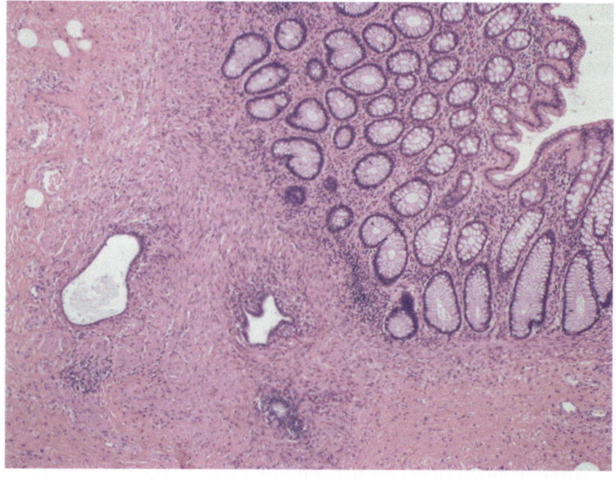

Fig. 3.1 Usual features of intestinal endometriosis. Submucosal endometriotic foci can be observed. The endometrial epithelium is surrounded by endometrial stroma infiltrating the bowel wall. Hematoxylin/eosin; 100×

reaction may be observed. Histiocytes are commonly present, converting the red blood cells into glucolipid and brown pigment (pseudoxanthoma cells). This pigment is usually a ceroid such as lipofuscin and to a lesser extent hemosiderin. Inflammatory cell infiltration may coexist and a small component of smooth muscle cells may be observed.

Abrao et al. attempted to correlate the histologic features of endometriosis with symptoms and clinical behavior [20]. The following classification was proposed. "Well-differentiated glandular pattern," surface epithelium or glandular epithelium indistinguishable from endometrium during different phases of the menstrual cycle. "Pure stromal pattern," stroma morphologically similar to endometrial stroma in any phase of the cycle, without glandular epithelium. "Undifferentiated glandular pattern": surface, glandular, or cyst-lining epithelium consisting of flattened or low cuboidal cells, different from typical endometrial epithelium and resembling peritoneal mesothelial cells. "Glandular pattern with mixed differentiation," epithelium composed of endometrial-like cells, undifferentiated cells, and sometimes cells with other Müllerian differentiation such as serous or mucinous cells. Even when the endometriotic glandular epithelium is indistinguishable from the normal endometrium, isolated flattened or low cuboidal cells can be observed in glands. Well-differentiated and undifferentiated components coexist in mixed pattern.

Endometriotic implants are typically located in the antimesenteric edge of the bowel. Endometrial gland and stroma are seen to invade the bowel wall from the serosa inward. In the muscularis, endometriotic nodules may be surrounded by smooth muscle hyperplasia and fibrosis, which may produce mural thickening and associated luminal stenosis [15, 21]. However, not all deep endometriotic bowel nodules are surrounded by extensive fibrosis. The myenteric Auerbach's plexus and the submucosal Meissner plexus may be disrupted by direct infiltration of endometriotic glands (Fig. 3.2). Not only the enteric nervous system but also the interstitial cells of Cajal are functionally damaged close to bowel endometriotic nodules [22].

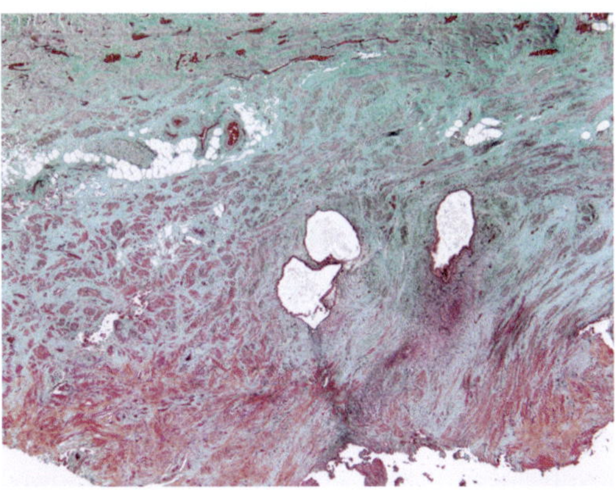

Fig. 3.2 Endometriotic foci surrounded by dense fibrosis (in green) and hyperplastic muscularis propria bundles. Masson Trichrome Stain; 100×

3.3.2 Infiltration of the Mucosal Layer

Intestinal mucosa infiltrated by bowel endometriosis may macroscopically appear as ulceration, fissures, and polypoid masses. In these cases, endometriosis can be a diagnostic challenge as patients may complain inflammatory bowel diseases (IBD)-like symptoms (abdominal pain, diarrhea, rectal bleeding) and associated mucosal inflammatory lesions are present [23, 24]. Guadagno et al. analyzed a series of 100 surgical specimens. In 75 cases there was no evidence of mucosal chronic alterations; in 25 cases there was mucosal involvement presenting mainly as mild architectural distortion with no evidence of inflammation; only in a minority of cases IBD-like mucosal changes were observed. These abnormalities are probably secondary to surface erosions, which permit intestinal microbiota/fecal material to access the submucosa [7]. An epidemiological study from Denmark suggests that women with endometriosis (not only intestinal) are at increased risk of developing IBD over time [25].

In brief, women with mucosal endometriosis may show excessive mucosal reaction and inflammation with ulcers and fissures. In patients with known endometriosis, IBD-like lesions in endoscopic biopsies may represent an epiphenomenon of endometriosis and not a true IBD. Women complaining intestinal IBD-like symptoms who lack a known diagnosis of endometriosis may undergo colonoscopy and a misdiagnosis of IBD [7].

3.3.3 Perineural Infiltration

Very little is known on the infiltration and progression of endometriosis into the bowel wall. Anaf et al. demonstrated that there is a close histological relationship between deep retroperitoneal endometriotic lesions and the subperitoneal nerves, and that this relationship is correlated with pain scores [26]. In addition, Anaf et al. also showed that all large bowel resected specimens, even those of the rectosigmoid tract with an involvement of the rectovaginal septum, showed peritoneal lesions histologically continuous with the underlying deep endometriotic lesions. Such histological continuity between the superficial and the underlying deep lesions strongly suggests a progression/invasion from the serosa into the large bowel wall [27]. Therefore, it is possible to hypothesize that endometriotic lesions follow the nerve pathways and extend longitudinally; in fact, the nerves are the locus minoris resistentiae of the muscularis propria. As a consequence, most large bowel endometriotic localizations present as plaque rather than a nodular lesion, like in the bladder or in the rectovaginal septum [28]. Besides the mechanical barrier represented by the muscularis propria, deep endometriotic lesions are accompanied by smooth muscle hyperplasia.

Perineural infiltration can be easily demonstrated by S100 immunostaining showing endometriotic glands and stroma running alongside and sometimes inside nerves fibers.

Perineural invasion of endometriotic foci may have relevance in the evaluation of the surgical margins even if the exact consequences of positive margins on the resected bowel are still unclear. Positive margins might theoretically be responsible for potential complications such as local recurrence or anastomotic fistulae. Endometriosis is a benign disease and therefore the most conservative surgical approach is to be preferred.

3.3.4 Cajal Cell Depletion

The enteric nervous system (ENS) is responsible for both bowel contractility and pain referral. The ENS is divided into three nervous plexuses: the subserous or perivisceral plexus, the intramuscular or Auerbach plexus, and the submucosal or Meissner plexus. Furthermore, in the bowel, there are specialized myofibroblast cells named interstitial cells of Cajal (ICC). These cells, found throughout the gut from the esophagus to the anus, are gastrointestinal pacemakers that generate and propagate electrical slow waves [29]. They also play other important roles in the control of gut motor activity, acting as neural intermediaries, as spatial coordinators of gut motility, and as stretch receptors [30]. The damage of ICC is associated with the functional loss of the spontaneous electrical slow wave and contractile activity [31]. Previous studies evaluated the relationship between endometriosis and gastrointestinal complaints, reporting, for instance, a characteristic dysfunction of the ENS (ampulla of Vater–duodenal wall spasm) secondary to injury or lack of inhibitory control of the ENS [32].

Anaf et al. demonstrated the strong relationship between nerves and endometriosis demonstrating perineural and endoneural invasion of the large bowel wall [27]. Later, Remorgida et al. observed that women suffering bowel complaints have deep endometriotic lesions infiltrating at least the subserous plexus. The depth of invasion into the bowel wall appeared correlated with severity of symptoms and the surgical resection of lesions improved the symptoms. Moreover, Remorgida et al. demonstrated the disappearance of c-kit reactivity, universally considered a marker of ICC function, around the endometriotic bowel lesions. In conclusion, endometriosis-induced damage of ICC, even before muscular infiltration, may cause bowel symptoms [22].

3.3.5 Sympathetic Nerve Fibers Damage

As previously stated, deep intestinal nodules may cause pain and a variety of intestinal symptoms, which sometimes mimic irritable bowel syndrome and Crohn disease [9]. The precise mechanisms by which endometriosis affects gastrointestinal function remain largely unknown but nerve fibers and their respective neurotransmitters seem to contribute to intestinal inflammation associated with endometriosis [33]. The wall of the human gut is richly innervated by sympathetic nerve fibers and by sensory fibers expressing the neuropeptide substance P (SP). Immune cells express adrenergic receptors; catecholamines at low concentrations bind to α-adrenoceptors and lead to cyclic adenosine monophosphate (cAMP) decrease and production of pro-inflammatory cytokines, whereas catecholamines at high concentrations bind to β-adrenoceptors and lead to cAMP increase and anti-inflammatory effects. Therefore, sympathetic nerve fibers may directly influence the immune response and play different roles depending on neurotransmitter concentration and on the adrenoceptors bound on the cells. In contrast, SP is always pro-inflammatory. In physiologic conditions, there is a balance between the pro-inflammatory effects of SP and the anti-inflammatory effects of sympathetic neurotransmitters. Ferrero et al. demonstrated by immunohistochemistry that sympathetic nerve density is altered only in the area adjacent to the endometriotic lesions and not in the intestinal tract apart [34]. This finding suggests that the alteration in nerve fibers is related only to the local inflammatory reaction caused by the presence of endometriosis (Fig. 3.3).

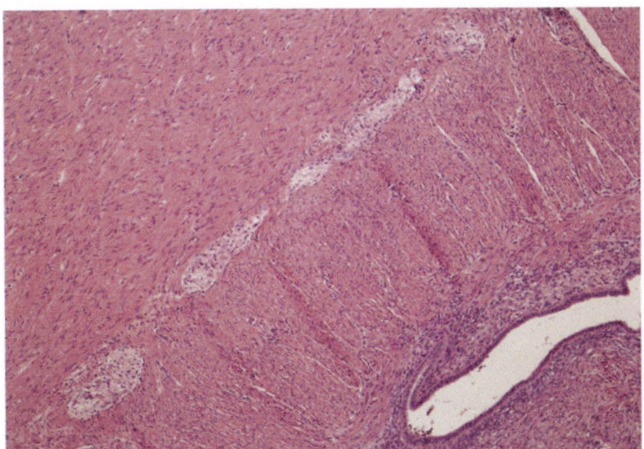

Fig. 3.3 Usual endometriotic cyst infiltrating the bowel muscularis propria close to nerves with signs of reactive hyperplasia and swelling. Hematoxylin and eosin staining; 200×. There is a loss of tyrosine hydroxylase-positive nerve fiber in the area adjacent to the endometriotic foci. An imbalance between sympathetic and sensory nerve fibers may be directly involved in the maintenance of inflammation

3.4 Lymph Nodes Involvement

The presence of endometriotic tissue inside the lymph nodes is a well-covered topic in the literature [35] and it is more often associated to extensive pelvic disease. Endometriosis is a benign disorder mimicking in some features a malignant disease. Like cancer, endometriosis can be both locally and distantly metastatic, it attaches to other tissues, invades and distorts them but does not usually create a consumptive metabolic state [36]. The involvement of lymph nodes is characterized by the presence of endometrial stroma and Müllerian glands with no local reaction. This involvement may be a form of müllerianosis involving the lymph nodes. However, the fact that the presence of endometriosis in nodes is directly proportional to the extent of the lesion may support the hypothesis of a lymphatic dissemination originating from the principal focus located in the rectosigmoid wall [37]. Endometriosis of the large bowel with involvement of regional lymph nodes is quite rare and it may not be evident on routine examination. In fact, this diagnosis requires a multistep procedure with multiple slides cut at different levels [38].

3.5 Small Bowel Involvement

As previously stated, the rectosigmoid is the most common site of GI endometriosis, accounting for 70% of all cases, while small bowel involvement is less frequent (1–7%) and usually confined to the distal ileum. Exclusive ileal localizations are rare [39]. Different incidence rates of endometriosis at different sites may be due to the fact that small bowel endometriosis is still often an incidental finding at surgery. Endometriosis of the distal ileum is an infrequent cause of intestinal obstruction, ranging from 7% to 23% of all cases with intestinal involvement [40].

3.6 Cecal Appendix Involvement

Endometriosis reportedly involves the appendix in up to 2.6% of surgically excised appendices and in 13.6–18% of women with intestinal endometriosis. Infrequently, the disease is limited to the appendix. Many of these cases are asymptomatic but a significant number of patients presents with symptoms of acute appendicitis or abdominal pain that is often localized to the right lower quadrant and may recur with menses. One unusual but well-recognized manifestation of appendiceal endometriosis is intussusception of the appendix into the cecum that can, on occasion, mimic a cecal polyp or carcinoma. Other less common manifestations of appendiceal endometriosis include retention mucocele secondary to luminal obstruction, lower intestinal bleeding and appendiceal perforation. On gross examination, the appendix may show serosal gray-brown discoloration or even small blue-domed cyst. In cases with more extensive involvement, mural thickening and distortion may be evident. Microscopically, endometrial-type glands are embedded in a variable amount of endometrial stroma, similar to endometriosis elsewhere [41].

3.7 The Role of Immunohistochemistry

The histological diagnosis of endometriosis is routinely accomplished on hematoxylin-eosin-stained sections; however, some lesions can be difficult to diagnose without the aid of immuno-histochemistry (IHC). For example, IHC is required when endometriotic foci have undifferentiated glandular pattern or pure stromal pattern. IHS is also useful in "atypical" or "unusual" sites (such as endometrioid adenocarcinoma arising from gut endometriotic foci) [42, 43]. An IHC panel composed of Cytokeratin 7 (CK7), CA 125, CD10, PAX8 and steroid hormones receptors (estrogens and progesterone) is used in clinical practice to confirm the diagnosis of endometriosis in unusual sites (Fig. 3.4). Cytokeratin 7 is an intermediate filament protein of 54 kDa that recognizes the simple epithelium found in most glandular and transitional epithelia; it is expressed in epithelial cells of ovary, lung, breast, and biliopancreatic tract. CA125, called Cancer Antigen 125, reacts with approxi-

mately 80% of epithelial ovarian neoplasia and both normal tissues and neoplasms of fallopian tube, endometrium, endocervix, and mesothelioma. CD10, also known as common acute lymphoblastic leukemia (CALLA), is mainly a hematopoietic marker and it is also expressed in endometrial stromal cells. PAX8 is a member of paired box (PAX) family of transcription factors found immunohistochemically in normal kidney, thyroid, cervix, upper urinary tract, and Müllerian duct system. The steroid hormones receptors are usually intensively expressed by endometrial stroma both in the orthotopic endometrium and in endometriotic foci. Having a lymphocyte-like morphology the positivity for Steroid Hormones Receptors may represent a crucial tool for a differential diagnosis with chronic inflammation especially in pure stromal pattern of endometriosis.

3.8 Complications of Bowel Endometriosis

3.8.1 Perforation

Spontaneous perforation of intestinal endometriosis is a rare complication that generally occurs during pregnancy. As previously stated, transmural bowel wall involvement is uncommon and the intestinal mucosa usually remains intact and, as a result, perforation of the affected intestinal tract is rare. Only few dozens of cases of intestinal perforation related to endometriosis have been reported and among these, almost half, occurred in pregnancy. Sigmoid colon turned out to be the most common site of perforation from endometriosis. In those patients, the entire intestinal wall was replaced by endometriotic tissue. In pregnancy, under the effect of progesterone, the area of ectopic endometrium becomes decidualized with a progressive reduction in size. The shrinking of a transmural endometriotic nodule may lead to perforation, by weakening of the intestinal wall, particularly in the third trimester. Moreover, decidualization causes a severe inflammatory response with an increased number of natural killer cells and decidual changes,

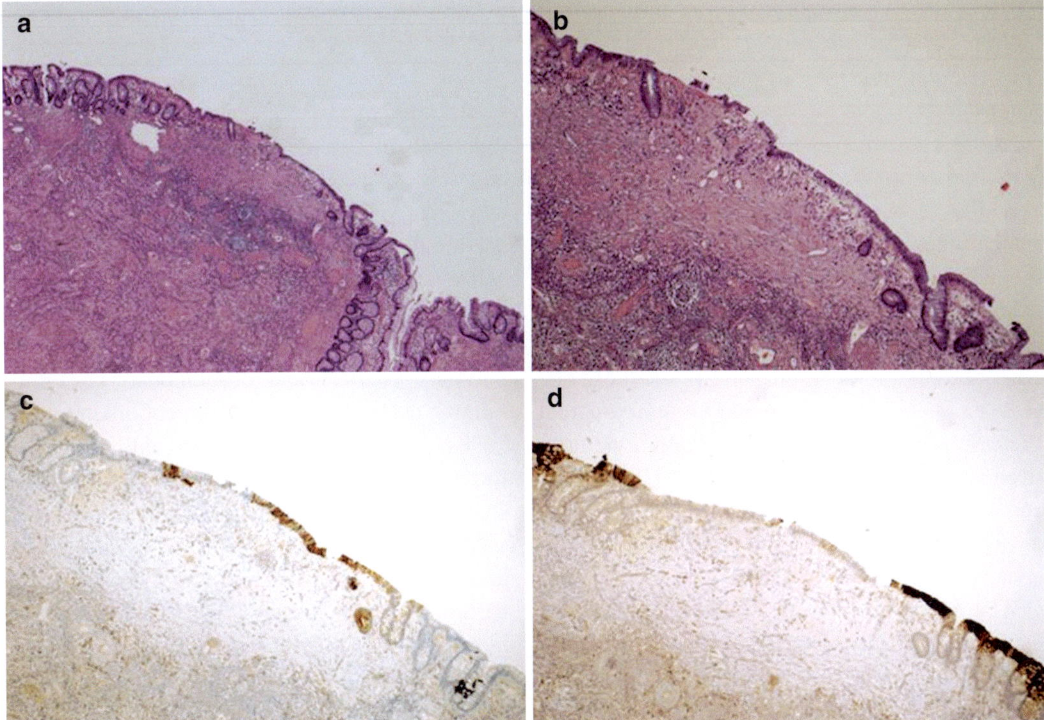

Fig. 3.4 Endometriotic foci infiltrating the bowel mucosa (**a**: hematoxylin and eosin staining 50×; **b**: hematoxylin and eosin staining 100×). The endometriotic epithelial lining confirms its nature showing CK7+/CK20− immuno- phenotype while the surrounding colonic epithelium shows the typical CK7−/CK20+ immunophenotype (**c**: CK7 100×; **d**: CK20 200×)

which are responsible for a higher risk of perforation. Although in the past it has thought that endometriosis improves during pregnancy, the current report shows the potential occurrence of serious and unexpected complications of the disease [44, 45].

3.8.2 Stenosis

Obstructive complications are common in patients with intestinal endometriosis. As described in the previous sections, both functional and anatomical conditions can affect the progression of the stools. In general, bowel endometriosis seems to be an evolutive process causing inflammation and a progressive damage to the autonomic myenteric and submucosal plexa. The subsequent scarring concurs to narrowing the bowel lumen.

3.8.3 Malignant Transformation

The frequency of malignant transformation of endometriosis is unknown, but it is estimated that up to 1% of women with endometriosis will develop endometriosis-associated neoplasm. Almost a quarter of the published cases of malignancy in endometriosis involves extraovarian tissues [46]. The mean age of occurrence of neoplastic transformation of extraovarian endometriosis is reported to be 10–20 years earlier than that of ovarian or endometrial cancer [47]. The most frequent sites of extragonadal involvement are rectovaginal septum, colon, and vagina, accounting for more than 50% of the cases [46].

Several cases of endometriosis-related gastrointestinal (GI) tumors have been reported in the literature, nearly half of them involving primary adenocarcinoma of the rectosigmoid colon [48]. Despite the paucity of data, there is evidence of an increased risk of malignant transformation of intestinal endometriosis in endometrioid or clear cell ovarian carcinoma [49, 50]. In 1925, Sampson reported the first case of malignant transformation of an endometriotic cyst [51]. The author proposed three criteria for the diagnosis of a neoplastic transformation within endometriosis: presence of both cancerous and benign endometrial tissue; histotype compatible with an endometrial origin i.e., consisting of epithelial glands surrounded by endometrial stroma; no other primary tumor sites found. While those criteria are still used and extended to extraovarian sites, Scott considers that additionally a demonstration of a dysplastic phase between the benign endometriosis and the carcinoma may be the most convincing feature and it should be systematically searched [52].

The carcinogenesis of neoplasms arising on endometriosis is similar to that of orthotopic endometrium, with hormonal factors playing a role in their pathogenesis [46].

Konincks et al. suggested that dioxin and polychlorinated biphenyl pollution is a possible cofactor in the etiology and development of deep infiltrating endometriosis, both being known carcinogens and co-carcinogens [53].

Genetic anomalies may also have a role. One-third of endometriotic nodules show a loss of predominant heterozygosity mainly at chromosomes 9p, 11q, or 22q. Loss of heterozygosity on chromosome 5q is also reported to be present in 25% of endometriotic sites synchronously associated with carcinoma, versus 6% of isolated endometriosis [54]. Since most sites of endometriosis remain benign, it is possible that the genetic anomalies only allow the maintenance of endometriosis and that mutations on other genes may promote the precancerous state. Noack et al. revealed a gain of 8q in a endometrioid adenocarcinoma compared to the endometriotic ovarian cyst and concluded that the solitary genomic imbalance chromosome 8 possibly reflects the importance for initiation and/or progression to endometrioid carcinoma, while overexpression of oncoproteins such as bcl-2, c-MYC, cyclin D1, p53, HER-2, and Kit protein occurred subsequently in the malignant transformation of the

ovarian endometriosis [55]. Other alleles such as GSTM1 may predispose to malignant transformation [56].

All types of carcinoma and sarcoma have been described in ectopic endometriosis, but serous and mucinous forms are rare [56, 57]. Bruson noted that 90% are endometrioid tumors and only 5% are clear cell tumors [58]. In contrast, clear cell carcinoma accounts for most malignancies arising in ovarian endometriosis. Although much less common than endometrioid or clear cell tumors, endocervical mucinous borderline tumors, associated with pelvic endometriosis in 30% of cases, can also undergo malignant transformation as reported by Rutgers. He described an endocervical mucinous borderline tumor with microinvasion arisen in polypoid endometriosis in a 43-year-old woman on unopposed estrogen therapy for 17 years after total abdominal hysterectomy with bilateral salpingo-oophorectomy [59].

The term "polypoid endometriosis" was first coined by Mostoufizadeh and Scully for an uncommon and distinctive variant of endometriosis with "histologic features simulating those of an endometrial polyp." They also noted that this type of endometriosis may form large, often multiple, polypoid masses that "not only simulate malignant tumors at operation but may also recur after operative removal" [56]. Although polypoid endometriosis essentially represents a growth pattern variant, several clinicopathologic features distinguish it from typical endometriosis, causing a diagnostic challenge. Polypoid endometriosis can mimic a neoplasm clinically, at the time of surgery and on gross examination. Unlike endometriosis of usual type (which commonly presents as dysmenorrhea, pelvic or back pain, dyspareunia, irregular bleeding, or infertility), in the largest case series by Parker et al. the commonest symptoms were related to the mass effect, especially in the rectosigmoid colon. Large bowel obstruction and other surgical findings were sometimes suspicious for intestinal adenocarcinoma [60].

A number of histologic features distinguish endometrioid carcinoma arising from endometriosis and colorectal cancer. In the case of an endometriosis-associated intestinal tumor, the bulk of the tumor is located in the outer wall of the bowel, and adenomatous glandular mucosal changes do not occur [61]. Endometrioid carcinomas typically form tubular glands with "clean" luminal contents, and their neoplastic cells lack intracellular mucin, usually positive for Alcian blue PAS stain. Immunohistochemistry can help to distinguish grade 3 endometrioid carcinoma from poorly differentiated colonic carcinoma. Endometriosis-associated intestinal tumors can be distinguished from metastases by the presence of endometriosis admixed with or adjacent to the tumor, and a transition from benign to malignant epithelium in the endometriotic tissue [52]. The most challenging issue in the differential diagnosis is probably that with Müllerian (mesodermal) adenosarcoma. Although generally occurs in uterus, adenosarcoma arising from endometriosis is anecdotally reported [46].

References

1. Ferrero S, Arena E, Morando A, Remorgida V. Prevalence of newly diagnosed endometriosis in women attending the general practitioner. Int J Gynaecol Obstet. 2010;110(3):203–7.
2. Sampson JA. Intestinal adenomas of endometrial type: their importance and their relation to ovarian hematomas of endometrial type (perforating hemorrhagic cysts of the ovary). Arch Surg. 1922;5: 217–80.
3. Chapron C, Fauconnier A, Vieira M, Barakat H, Dousset B, Pansini V, et al. Anatomical distribution of deeply infiltrating endometriosis: surgical implications and proposition for a classification. Hum Reprod. 2003;18(1):157–61.
4. Parr NJ, Murphy C, Holt S, Zakhour H, Crosbie RB. Endometriosis and the gut. Gut. 1988;29(8):1112–5.
5. Jerby BL, Kessler H, Falcone T, Milsom JW. Laparoscopic management of colorectal endometriosis. Surg Endosc. 1999;13(11):1125–8.
6. Kavallaris A, Kohler C, Kuhne-Heid R, Schneider A. Histopathological extent of rectal invasion by rectovaginal endometriosis. Hum Reprod. 2003;18(6):1323–7.
7. Guadagno A, Grillo F, Vellone VG, Ferrero S, Fasoli A, Fiocca R, et al. Intestinal endometriosis: mimicker of inflammatory bowel disease? Digestion. 2015;92(1):14–21.
8. Remorgida V, Ferrero S, Fulcheri E, Ragni N, Martin DC. Bowel endometriosis: presentation, diagnosis, and treatment. Obstet Gynecol Surv. 2007;62(7):461–70.
9. Ferrero S, Abbamonte LH, Remorgida V, Ragni N. Irritable bowel syndrome and endometriosis. Eur J Gastroenterol Hepatol. 2005;17(6):687.
10. Ferrero S, Camerini G, Ragni N, Remorgida V. Endometriosis and irritable bowel syndrome: comorbidity or misdiagnosis? BJOG. 2009;116(1):129. Author reply 130.
11. Ferrero S, Camerini G, Ragni N, Venturini PL, Biscaldi E, Remorgida V. Norethisterone acetate in the treatment of colorectal endometriosis: a pilot study. Hum Reprod. 2010;25(1):94–100.
12. Ferrero S, Camerini G, Ragni N, Menada MV, Venturini PL, Remorgida V. Triptorelin improves intestinal symptoms among patients with colorectal endometriosis. Int J Gynaecol Obstet. 2010;108(3):250–1.
13. Ferrero S, Camerini G, Ragni N, Venturini PL, Biscaldi E, Seracchioli R, et al. Letrozole and norethisterone acetate in colorectal endometriosis. Eur J Obstet Gynecol Reprod Biol. 2010;150(2):199–202.
14. Nezhat C, Nezhat F, Nezhat C. Endometriosis: ancient disease, ancient treatments. Fertil Steril. 2012;98(6 Suppl):S1–62.
15. Yantiss RK, Clement PB, Young RH. Endometriosis of the intestinal tract: a study of 44 cases of a disease that may cause diverse challenges in clinical and pathologic evaluation. Am J Surg Pathol. 2001;25(4):445–54.
16. Lopez-Roman O, Cruz-Corea M, Toro DH, Gonzalez-Keelan C. Unintended endoscopic appendectomy of an endometriosis-induced intussuscepted appendix presenting as a sessile cecal polyp. Gastrointest Endosc. 2012;76(3):672–4.
17. Sriram PV, Seitz U, Soehendra N, Schroeder S. Endoscopic appendectomy in a case of appendicular intussusception due to endometriosis, mimicking a cecal polyp. Am J Gastroenterol. 2000;95(6):1594–6.
18. Redwine DB. Ovarian endometriosis: a marker for more extensive pelvic and intestinal disease. Fertil Steril. 1999;72(2):310–5.
19. Keckstein J, Wiesinger H. The laparoscopic treatment of intestinal endometriosis. In: Sutton C, Adamson GD, Jones KD, editors. Modern management of endometriosis. Abington: Taylor & Francis; 2005. p. 177–87.
20. Abrao MS, Neme RM, Carvalho FM, Aldrighi JM, Pinotti JA. Histological classification of endometriosis as a predictor of response to treatment. Int J Gynaecol Obstet. 2003;82(1):31–40.
21. Remorgida V, Ragni N, Ferrero S, Anserini P, Torelli P, Fulcheri E. How complete is full thickness disc resection of bowel endometriotic lesions? A prospective surgical and histological study. Hum Reprod. 2005;20(8):2317–20.
22. Remorgida V, Ragni N, Ferrero S, Anserini P, Torelli P, Fulcheri E. The involvement of the interstitial Cajal cells and the enteric nervous system in bowel endometriosis. Hum Reprod. 2005;20(1):264–71.
23. Langlois NE, Park KG, Keenan RA. Mucosal changes in the large bowel with endometriosis: a possible cause of misdiagnosis of colitis? Hum Pathol. 1994;25(10):1030–4.

24. Rowland R, Langman JM. Endometriosis of the large bowel: a report of 11 cases. Pathology. 1989;21(4):259–65.
25. Jess T, Frisch M, Jorgensen KT, Pedersen BV, Nielsen NM. Increased risk of inflammatory bowel disease in women with endometriosis: a nationwide Danish cohort study. Gut. 2012;61(9):1279–83.
26. Anaf V, Simon P, El Nakadi I, Fayt I, Buxant F, Simonart T, et al. Relationship between endometriotic foci and nerves in rectovaginal endometriotic nodules. Hum Reprod. 2000;15(8):1744–50.
27. Anaf V, El Nakadi I, Simon P, Van de Stadt J, Fayt I, Simonart T, et al. Preferential infiltration of large bowel endometriosis along the nerves of the colon. Hum Reprod. 2004;19(4):996–1002.
28. Koninckx PR, Martin DC. Deep endometriosis: a consequence of infiltration or retraction or possibly adenomyosis externa? Fertil Steril. 1992;58(5):924–8.
29. Huizinga JD, Thuneberg L, Kluppel M, Malysz J, Mikkelsen HB, Bernstein A. W/kit gene required for interstitial cells of Cajal and for intestinal pacemaker activity. Nature. 1995;373(6512):347–9.
30. Faussone-Pellegrini MS. Histogenesis, structure and relationships of interstitial cells of Cajal (ICC): from morphology to functional interpretation. Eur J Morphol. 1992;30(2):137–48.
31. Mikkelsen HB, Malysz J, Huizinga JD, Thuneberg L. Action potential generation, Kit receptor immunohistochemistry and morphology of steel-Dickie (Sl/Sld) mutant mouse small intestine. Neurogastroenterol Motil. 1998;10(1):11–26.
32. Mathias JR, Franklin R, Quast DC, Fraga N, Loftin CA, Yates L, et al. Relation of endometriosis and neuromuscular disease of the gastrointestinal tract: new insights. Fertil Steril. 1998;70(1):81–8.
33. Straub RH, Wiest R, Strauch UG, Harle P, Scholmerich J. The role of the sympathetic nervous system in intestinal inflammation. Gut. 2006;55(11):1640–9.
34. Ferrero S, Haas S, Remorgida V, Camerini G, Fulcheri E, Ragni N, et al. Loss of sympathetic nerve fibers in intestinal endometriosis. Fertil Steril. 2010;94(7):2817–9.
35. Javert CT. Pathogenesis of endometriosis based on endometrial homeoplasia, direct extension, exfoliation and implantation, lymphatic and hematogenous metastasis, including five case reports of endometrial tissue in pelvic lymph nodes. Cancer. 1949;2(3):399–410.
36. Thomas EJ, Campbell IG. Evidence that endometriosis behaves in a malignant manner. Gynecol Obstet Investig. 2000;50(Suppl 1):2–10.
37. Abrao MS, Podgaec S, Dias JA Jr, Averbach M, Garry R, Ferraz Silva LF, et al. Deeply infiltrating endometriosis affecting the rectum and lymph nodes. Fertil Steril. 2006;86(3):543–7.
38. Insabato L, Pettinato G. Endometriosis of the bowel with lymph node involvement. A report of three cases and review of the literature. Pathol Res Pract. 1996;192(9):957–61. Discussion 62.
39. Macafee CH, Greer HL. Intestinal endometriosis. A report of 29 cases and a survey of the literature. J Obstet Gynaecol Br Emp. 1960;67:539–55.
40. De Ceglie A, Bilardi C, Blanchi S, Picasso M, Di Muzio M, Trimarchi A, et al. Acute small bowel obstruction caused by endometriosis: a case report and review of the literature. World J Gastroenterol. 2008;14(21):3430–4.
41. Misdraji J, Graeme-Cook FM. Miscellaneous conditions of the appendix. Semin Diagn Pathol. 2004;21(2):151–63.
42. Carbone A, Prete FP, Sofo L, Alfieri S, Rotondi F, Zannoni GF, et al. Morphological and immunohistochemical characterization of an endometriotic cyst of the liver: diagnostic approach to endometriosis. Histopathology. 2004;45(4):420–2.
43. Ferrero S, Ragni N, Remorgida V, Arena E. CD10 in the cytological diagnosis of endobronchial endometriosis. Pediatr Pulmonol. 2007;42(8):746.
44. Pisanu A, Deplano D, Angioni S, Ambu R, Uccheddu A. Rectal perforation from endometriosis in pregnancy: case report and literature review. World J Gastroenterol. 2010;16(5):648–51.
45. Leone Roberti Maggiore U, Ferrero S, Mangili G, Bergamini A, Inversetti A, Giorgione V, et al. A systematic review on endometriosis during pregnancy: diagnosis, misdiagnosis, complications and outcomes. Hum Reprod Update. 2016;22(1):70–103.
46. Benoit L, Arnould L, Cheynel N, Diane B, Causeret S, Machado A, et al. Malignant extraovarian endometriosis: a review. Eur J Surg Oncol. 2006;32(1):6–11.
47. Modesitt SC, Tortolero-Luna G, Robinson JB, Gershenson DM, Wolf JK. Ovarian and extraovarian endometriosis-associated cancer. Obstet Gynecol. 2002;100(4):788–95.
48. Jones KD, Owen E, Berresford A, Sutton C. Endometrial adenocarcinoma arising from endometriosis of the rectosigmoid colon. Gynecol Oncol. 2002;86(2):220–2.
49. Nezhat FR, Pejovic T, Reis FM, Guo SW. The link between endometriosis and ovarian cancer: clinical implications. Int J Gynecol Cancer. 2014;24(4):623–8.
50. Nezhat FR, Apostol R, Nezhat C, Pejovic T. New insights in the pathophysiology of ovarian cancer and implications for screening and prevention. Am J Obstet Gynecol. 2015;213(3):262–7.
51. Sampson JA. Endometrial carcinoma of the ovary, arising in endometrial tissue of that organ. Arch Surg. 1925;10:1–72.
52. Scott RB. Malignant changes in endometriosis. Obstet Gynecol. 1953;2(3):283–9.
53. Koninckx PR, Braet P, Kennedy SH, Barlow DH. Dioxin pollution and endometriosis in Belgium. Hum Reprod. 1994;9(6):1001–2.
54. Jiang X, Morland SJ, Hitchcock A, Thomas EJ, Campbell IG. Allelotyping of endometriosis with adjacent ovarian carcinoma reveals evidence of a common lineage. Cancer Res. 1998;58(8):1707–12.

55. Noack F, Schmidt H, Buchwcitz O, Malik E, Horny HP. Genomic imbalance and onco-protein expression of ovarian endometrioid adenocarcinoma arisen in an endometriotic cyst. Anticancer Res. 2004;24(1):151–4.

56. Mostoufizadeh M, Scully RE. Malignant tumors arising in endometriosis. Clin Obstet Gynecol. 1980;23(3):951–63.

57. Stern RC, Dash R, Bentley RC, Snyder MJ, Haney AF, Robboy SJ. Malignancy in endometriosis: frequency and comparison of ovarian and extraovarian types. Int J Gynecol Pathol. 2001;20(2):133–9.

58. Brunson GL, Barclay DL, Sanders M, Araoz CA. Malignant extraovarian endometriosis: two case reports and review of the literature. Gynecol Oncol. 1988;30(1):123–30.

59. Rutgers JL, Scully RE. Ovarian mullerian mucinous papillary cystadenomas of borderline malignancy. A clinicopathologic analysis. Cancer. 1988;61(2):340–8.

60. Parker RL, Dadmanesh F, Young RH, Clement PB. Polypoid endometriosis: a clinicopathologic analysis of 24 cases and a review of the literature. Am J Surg Pathol. 2004;28(3):285–97.

61. Slavin RE, Krum R, Van Dinh T. Endometriosis-associated intestinal tumors: a clinical and pathological study of 6 cases with a review of the literature. Hum Pathol. 2000;31(4):456–63.

Simone Ferrero, Melita Moioli, Danilo Dodero, and Fabio Barra

4.1 Introduction

Bowel endometriosis is defined as the presence of endometriotic lesions infiltrating at least the muscular layer of the intestinal wall. Superficial endometriotic lesions infiltrating only the intestinal serosa should not be considered bowel endometriosis and they are usually asymptomatic [1, 2]. Bowel endometriosis is estimated to affect between 5% and 25% of patients with surgical diagnosis of endometriosis [3, 4]. The majority of bowel endometriotic nodules are located on the rectosigmoid junction and rectum (65.7%); however, endometriotic lesions may also be located on the sigmoid colon (17.4%), caecum and ileocecal junction (4.1%), appendix (6.4%), and omentum (1.7%) [5].

Patients affected by bowel endometriosis usually complain pain and intestinal symptoms. Pain may be caused by the intestinal nodules and also by other deep endometriotic nodules (such as those of the rectovaginal septum, uterosacral ligaments, and parametrium) that are usually associated with intestinal lesions. In addition, bowel nodules may cause various intestinal symptoms depending on the location of the nodules, their size and the degree of stenosis of the intestinal lumen.

4.2 Rectosigmoid Endometriosis

Patients with rectosigmoid endometriosis may present a wide range in intestinal symptoms including dyschezia, cyclic bowel alterations, abdominal cramping, feeling incomplete evacuation, stool fragmentation, passage of mucus with the stools and rectal bleeding [1, 6]. A prospective study investigated the frequency of digestive symptoms reported by women with rectal endometriosis who were not using hormonal treatment [7]. Eighty-four percent of the patients enrolled in this study had deep nodules infiltrating the rectum and 12% of the nodules caused a stenosis of the intestinal lumen. Questionnaires were completed during the post-menstrual phase and focused on digestive complaints perceived during the previous 24 h. The most frequent complaints were constipation (40%), feeling incomplete evacuation (36%), and stool fragmentation (52%). The intensity of dyschezia assessed on a

S. Ferrero (✉) · F. Barra
Academic Unit of Obstetrics and Gynecology, IRCCS
Ospedale Policlinico San Martino, Genova, Italy

Department of Neurosciences, Rehabilitation,
Ophthalmology, Genetics, Maternal and Child Health
(DiNOGMI), University of Genova, Genova, Italy
e-mail: simone.ferrero@unige.it

M. Moioli
Academic Unit of Obstetrics and Gynecology, IRCCS
Ospedale Policlinico San Martino, Genoa, Italy

D. Dodero
Piazza della Vittoria 14 S.r.l, Genoa, Italy
e-mail: danilo.dodero@fastwebnet.it

© Springer Nature Switzerland AG 2020
S. Ferrero, M. Ceccaroni (eds.), *Clinical Management of Bowel Endometriosis*,
https://doi.org/10.1007/978-3-030-50446-5_4

10-point visual analogue scale was 7.1. Study patients underwent anorectal manometry, which did not reveal marked motility or sensitive dysfunctions. No alterations of the rectoanal inhibitory reflex were found. Hypertone of the internal anal sphincter was found in 80% of the patients. Almost half of the patients had an increase of the threshold of desire to defecate, and 28% of them had a reduction of the anal sphincter squeeze pressure. Another prospective study investigated the types and frequency of digestive symptoms in patients with three different localization of pelvic endometriosis: superficial implants located on the Douglas pouch peritoneum, deep endometriosis (posterior vagina, rectovaginal space and on uterosacral ligaments) without intestinal infiltration and deep endometriosis infiltrating the rectum [8]. Patients with deep endometriosis infiltrating the rectum were more likely to present cyclic defecation pain (67.9%), cyclic constipation (54.7%), and presented a significantly longer time to evacuate stools. However, these complaints were also frequent in other study groups (38.1% and 33.3% for the superficial endometriosis group and 42.9% and 26.2% for the group with deep endometriosis sparing the rectum, respectively). Women with rectal endometriosis were also more likely to present with appetite disorders. Stenosis of the intestinal lumen was assessed by preoperative computed tomographic colonography and it was observed in 26.4% of women with rectal endometriosis. When compared with other study groups, women with rectal stenosis were significantly more likely to report constipation, defecation pain, and appetite disorders. They also reported increased evacuation time, increased stool consistency without laxatives and had strong tendency toward increased feelings of incomplete evacuation. Notably, unsuccessful evacuatory attempt was the only factor independently related to rectal stenosis. The results of these studies suggest that most of digestive complains reported by patients with rectosigmoid endometriosis may not simply be the consequence of infiltration of endometriosis in the intestinal wall, but they may be caused by the cyclic micro-hemorrhages and inflammation within endometriotic lesions. This hypothesis is supported by the worsening of digestive symptoms during the menstrual cycle and by their improvement during hormonal treatment [9–12]. In addition, the distortion of the anatomy caused by endometriosis may contribute to intestinal symptoms. The fixation of the rectum to the uterine cervix and the vagina (Fig. 4.1) may lead to abnormal angulations of the digestive tract, disturbing stool progression and causing dyschezia and/or constipation [13].

Pain and intestinal symptoms associated with rectosigmoid endometriosis are nonspecific and this may lead to a diagnostic dilemma. In fact, before a concrete diagnosis is made, patients with endometriosis receive several other diagnoses such as irritable bowel syndrome (IBS). An Australian study investigated the intestinal symptoms of patients with endometriosis [14]. The study included 355 consecutive women with suspicion of endometriosis; 84.5% of the patients had surgical confirmation of endometriosis and 7.6% had bowel endometriosis. Ninety percent of women had one or more intestinal symptoms; the overall duration of symptoms exceeded 5 years in 50.3% of the patients. Bloating was the most common symptom (82.8%), but 71.3% also had other bowel symptoms. All intestinal symptoms were similarly predictive of histologically confirmed endometriosis. Seventy-six women (21.4%) had previously been diagnosed with irri-

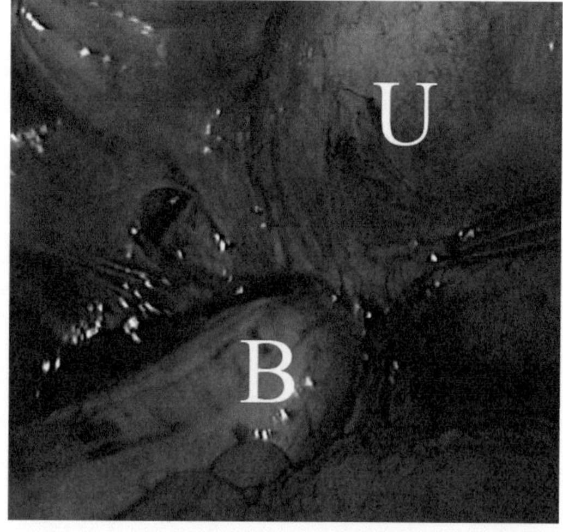

Fig. 4.1 Laparoscopic view of the pelvic. A rectal nodule is adherent to the posterior uterine wall. *U* uterus, *B* bowel

table bowel syndrome and 79% of them had endometriosis confirmed; it is difficult to assess if this was a diagnostic mistake or a genuine comorbidity. However, this study shows that the differential diagnosis between endometriosis-related intestinal symptoms (even in patients without bowel endometriosis) and IBS is challenging [15, 16]. In fact, approximately 20% of women with IBS show an exacerbation of their symptoms during menstruation [17].

Significant narrowing of the intestinal lumen occurs in a minority of patients with rectosigmoid endometriosis and it may cause subocclusive or occlusive symptoms. Bowel obstruction caused by rectosigmoid endometriosis causes symptoms similar to those of other causes of bowel obstruction such as abdominal distention, diffuse or moderate abdominal pain, vomiting, no gas or stool passing [18, 19]. The actual incidence of bowel obstruction in patients with bowel endometriosis is unknown. Although this complication is considered a rare event [20], it is likely that cases of bowel occlusion are underreported in the literature because of a publication bias. In fact, women with bowel occlusion are often managed in local general surgery department rather than by endometriosis centers [21]. A prospective study including 241 patients with rectosigmoid endometriosis reported two cases of occlusion and ten cases of subocclusion (5.0%) during a follow-up of 37 months [22]; the major digestive complaints were bloating, defecation pain, constipation, liquid stools, and a feeling of incomplete stool evacuation. Endometriosis-related bowel occlusion may occur during ovarian stimulation for in vitro fertilization [23] and during pregnancy. The development of colonic ischemia in the upstream dilated bowel may cause perforation with subsequent peritonitis and sepsis. Rectosigmoid perforations have been reported during pregnancy [24–28] and in the postpartum [28].

4.3 Ileocecal Endometriosis

Ileocecal endometriosis may present with intestinal obstruction [29–34], intestinal intussusception [35–39], or ileocecal perforation [40]. Thus, ileo-

cecal endometriosis usually causes intestinal cramps, vomiting, abdominal distention, and catamenial subocclusion. In other patients, ileocecal endometriosis may cause aspecific symptoms similar to those of intestinal malignancies or Crohn's disease. Magnetic resonance imaging and computed tomography may detect an ileocecal mass, but they do not always allow to suspect the diagnosis of endometriosis (Figs. 4.2 and 4.3). Double-contrast barium enema does not detect small extraluminal lesions. Rarely, isolated ileocecal endometriosis may be asymptomatic, and it may appear as submucosal polyp at screening colonoscopy [41]. In a retrospective study performed in a referral center for the treatment of endometriosis, ileocecal endometriosis was observed in 31 women; notably, all patients underwent surgery for deep endometriosis, but the ileocecal involvement was always an incidental finding during surgery although the preoperative

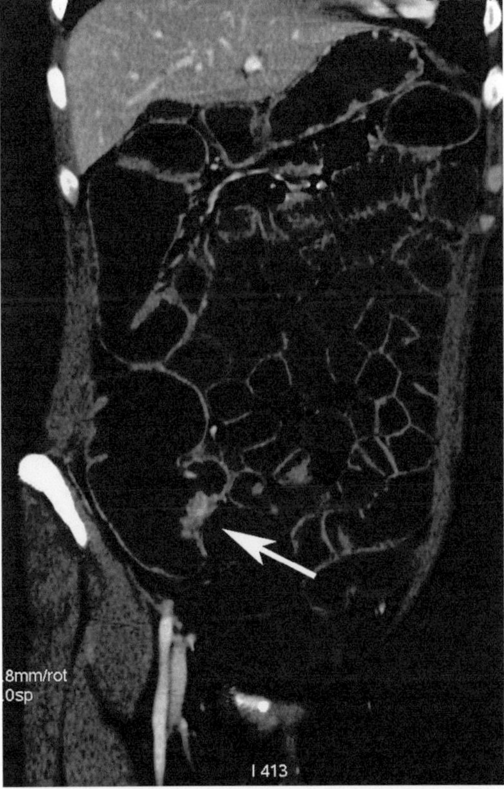

Fig. 4.2 Multidetector computerized enema demonstrating a cecal endometriotic nodule (arrow)

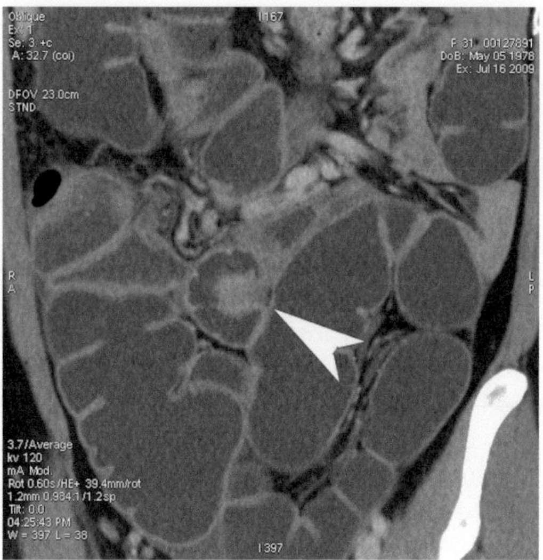

Fig. 4.3 Multidetector computerized enema demonstrating an ileal endometriotic nodule (arrowhead)

workup included barium double-contrast enema [42]. In 29 patients, ileocecal nodules were associated with colorectal endometriosis which was detected at preoperative imaging. In a retrospective study including seven patients with ileocecal endometriosis, the diagnosis was performed preoperatively by magnetic resonance imaging or double-contrast barium enema in four patients (57.1%) [33]. Thus, the diagnosis of ileocecal endometriosis is often performed at surgery or at histological exam.

Cases of endometriosis-related ileocecal perforation during pregnancy [43] and postpartum [44] have been described. Since ectopic endometriotic tissue is highly vascularized, ileocolic perforation may cause massive intraperitoneal hemorrhage during pregnancy [43, 45].

4.4 Endometriosis of the Appendix

Appendiceal endometriosis occurs approximately in 2.6% of patients undergoing surgery for endometriosis [46]. The diagnosis of appendiceal endometriosis is often done during surgery for endometriosis-related pain without preoperative suspicion of localization of endometriosis on the appendix (incidental appendectomy) [47].

However, gross alterations of the appendix may be the indications for surgery in some patients (selective appendectomy) [46].

In fact, appendiceal endometriosis may cause the symptoms (such as fever, right lower quadrant pain, nausea and vomiting) and signs (such as pain at the McBurney's point) of acute appendicitis [48–51]. Some authors reported cases of appendix with endometriosis undergoing perforation [52, 53]. Acute inflammation arises because endometriosis causes partial or complete occlusion of the appendiceal lumen. Rarely, endometriosis may also cause appendiceal intussusception [54, 55].

Several case reports described acute appendicitis and perforation of the appendix in pregnancy secondary to endometriosis, possibly due to the decidual transformation of the endometriotic tissue [56–60]. When appendicitis occurs during pregnancy, several physiologic changes related to the gravid state may make the diagnosis challenging [61]. Anorexia, nausea, and vomiting are very common during pregnancy. The enlarged uterus can displace the appendix upward and, therefore, pregnant women may not have the classical tenderness at the McBurney's point. In addition, there is a physiological elevation of white blood cell count that is considered normal between 8000 and 15,000 cells/mm^3.

4.5 Conclusion

The most common symptoms of bowel endometriosis are pain (dysmenorrhea, non-menstrual pelvic pain, deep dyspareunia), infertility and intestinal complains (such as abdominal bloating, cyclical constipation or diarrhea, tenesmus). These symptoms are not specific and, thus, the diagnosis may be challenging. The complaints of patients without subocclusive symptoms may be misdiagnosed as IBS. Patients with occlusive symptoms may be misdiagnosed with other causes of bowel occlusion (such as malignancies and Crohn's disease). Finally, the diagnosis may be particularly challenging in patients with bowel endometriosis who do not present the typical pain symptoms associated with endometriosis

[29]. These patients are unlikely to undergo diagnostic investigations for deep endometriosis and, thus, they are at higher risk of sudden onset of occlusive or subocclusive symptoms.

References

1. Remorgida V, Ferrero S, Fulcheri E, Ragni N, Martin DC. Bowel endometriosis: presentation, diagnosis, and treatment. Obstet Gynecol Surv. 2007;62(7):461–70.
2. Remorgida V, Ragni N, Ferrero S, Anserini P, Torelli P, Fulcheri E. The involvement of the interstitial Cajal cells and the enteric nervous system in bowel endometriosis. Hum Reprod. 2005;20(1):264–71.
3. Weed JC, Ray JE. Endometriosis of the bowel. Obstet Gynecol. 1987;69(5):727–30.
4. Audebert A, Petousis S, Margioula-Siarkou C, Ravanos K, Prapas N, Prapas Y. Anatomic distribution of endometriosis: a reappraisal based on series of 1101 patients. Eur J Obstet Gynecol Reprod Biol. 2018;230:36–40.
5. Chapron C, Chopin N, Borghese B, Foulot H, Dousset B, Vacher-Lavenu MC, et al. Deeply infiltrating endometriosis: pathogenetic implications of the anatomical distribution. Hum Reprod. 2006;21(7):1839–45.
6. Abrao MS, Petraglia F, Falcone T, Keckstein J, Osuga Y, Chapron C. Deep endometriosis infiltrating the recto-sigmoid: critical factors to consider before management. Hum Reprod Update. 2015;21(3):329–39.
7. Mabrouk M, Ferrini G, Montanari G, Di Donato N, Raimondo D, Stanghellini V, et al. Does colorectal endometriosis alter intestinal functions? A prospective manometric and questionnaire-based study. Fertil Steril. 2012;97(3):652–6.
8. Roman H, Ness J, Suciu N, Bridoux V, Gourcerol G, Leroi AM, et al. Are digestive symptoms in women presenting with pelvic endometriosis specific to lesion localizations? A preliminary prospective study. Hum Reprod. 2012;27(12):3440–9.
9. Barra F, Scala C, Maggiore ULR, Ferrero S. Long-term administration of dienogest for the treatment of pain and intestinal symptoms in patients with recto-sigmoid endometriosis. J Clin Med. 2020;9(1):154.
10. Ferrero S, Camerini G, Ragni N, Venturini PL, Biscaldi E, Seracchioli R, et al. Letrozole and norethisterone acetate in colorectal endometriosis. Eur J Obstet Gynecol Reprod Biol. 2010;150(2):199–202.
11. Ferrero S, Camerini G, Ragni N, Menada MV, Venturini PL, Remorgida V. Triptorelin improves intestinal symptoms among patients with colorectal endometriosis. Int J Gynaecol Obstet. 2010;108(3):250–1.
12. Ferrero S, Camerini G, Ragni N, Venturini PL, Biscaldi E, Remorgida V. Norethisterone acetate in the treatment of colorectal endometriosis: a pilot study. Hum Reprod. 2010;25(1):94–100.
13. Squifflet J, Feger C, Donnez J. Diagnosis and imaging of adenomyotic disease of the retroperitoneal space. Gynecol Obstet Investig. 2002;54(Suppl 1):43–51.
14. Maroun P, Cooper MJ, Reid GD, Keirse MJ. Relevance of gastrointestinal symptoms in endometriosis. Aust N Z J Obstet Gynaecol. 2009;49(4):411–4.
15. Ferrero S, Abbamonte LH, Remorgida V, Ragni N. Irritable bowel syndrome and endometriosis. Eur J Gastroenterol Hepatol. 2005;17(6):687.
16. Ferrero S, Camerini G, Ragni N, Remorgida V. Endometriosis and irritable bowel syndrome: comorbidity or misdiagnosis? BJOG. 2009;116(1):129. Author reply 130.
17. Whitehead WE, Cheskin LJ, Heller BR, Robinson JC, Crowell MD, Benjamin C, et al. Evidence for exacerbation of irritable bowel syndrome during menses. Gastroenterology. 1990;98(6):1485–9.
18. Alexandrino G, Lourenco LC, Carvalho R, Sobrinho C, Horta DV, Reis J. Endometriosis: a rare cause of large bowel obstruction. GE Port J Gastroenterol. 2018;25(2):86–90.
19. de Jong MJ, Mijatovic V, van Waesberghe JH, Cuesta MA, Hompes PG. Surgical outcome and long-term follow-up after segmental colorectal resection in women with a complete obstruction of the rectosigmoid due to endometriosis. Dig Surg. 2009;26(1):50–5.
20. Jubanyik KJ, Comite F. Extrapelvic endometriosis. Obstet Gynecol Clin N Am. 1997;24(2):411–40.
21. Caterino S, Ricca L, Cavallini M, Ciardi A, Camilli A, Ziparo V. [Intestinal endometriosis. Three new cases and review of the literature]. Ann Ital Chir. 2002;73(3):323–9. Discussion 9–30.
22. Roman H, Puscasiu L, Lempicki M, Huet E, Chati R, Bridoux V, et al. Colorectal endometriosis responsible for bowel occlusion or subocclusion in women with pregnancy intention: is the policy of primary in vitro fertilization always safe? J Minim Invasive Gynecol. 2015;22(6):1059–67.
23. Anaf V, El Nakadi I, Simon P, Englert Y, Peny MO, Fayt I, et al. Sigmoid endometriosis and ovarian stimulation. Hum Reprod. 2000;15(4):790–4.
24. Pisanu A, Deplano D, Angioni S, Ambu R, Uccheddu A. Rectal perforation from endometriosis in pregnancy: case report and literature review. World J Gastroenterol. 2010;16(5):648–51.
25. Schweitzer KJ, van Bekkum E, de Groot CJ. Endometriosis with intestinal perforation in term pregnancy. Int J Gynaecol Obstet. 2006;93(2):152–3.
26. Rud B. [Colonic endometriosis with perforation during pregnancy]. Ugeskr Laeger. 1979;141(41):2831–2.
27. Clement PB. Perforation of the sigmoid colon during pregnancy: a rare complication of endometriosis. Case report. Br J Obstet Gynaecol. 1977;84(7):548–50.
28. Setubal A, Sidiropoulou Z, Torgal M, Casal E, Lourenco C, Koninckx P. Bowel complications of deep endometriosis during pregnancy or in vitro fertilization. Fertil Steril. 2014;101(2):442–6.

29. Arata R, Takakura Y, Ikeda S, Itamoto T. A case of ileus caused by ileal endometriosis with lymph node involvement. Int J Surg Case Rep. 2019;54:90–4.
30. Marques Ruiz A, Camara Baeza S, Sanchez Santos Y. A new reported case of ileocecal infiltrative endometriosis, a disease which is probably underdiagnosed. Rev Esp Enferm Dig. 2018;110(12):835.
31. Bacalbasa N, Balescu I, Filipescu A. Ileocecal obstruction due to endometriosis - a case report and literature review. In Vivo. 2017;31(5):999–1002.
32. Imasogie DE, Agbonrofo PI, Momoh MI, Obaseki DE, Obahiagbon I, Azeke AT. Intestinal obstruction secondary to cecal endometriosis. Niger J Clin Pract. 2018;21(8):1081–5.
33. Lopez Carrasco A, Hernandez Gutierrez A, Hidalgo Gutierrez PA, Rodriguez Gonzalez R, Marijuan Martin JL, Zapardiel I, et al. Ileocecal endometriosis: diagnosis and management. Taiwan J Obstet Gynecol. 2017;56(2):243–6.
34. Unalp HR, Akguner T, Yavuzcan A, Ekinci N. Acute small bowel obstruction due to ileal endometriosis: a case report and review of the most recent literature. Vojnosanit Pregl. 2012;69(11):1013–6.
35. Nozari N, Shafiei M, Sarmadi S. An unusual presentation of endometriosis as an ileocolic intussusception with cecal mass: a case report. J Reprod Infertil. 2018;19(4):247–9.
36. Rodriguez-Lopez M, Bailon-Cuadrado M, Tejero-Pintor FJ, Choolani E, Fernandez-Perez G, Tapia-Herrero A. Ileocecal intussusception extending to left colon due to endometriosis. Ann R Coll Surg Engl. 2018;100(3):e62–e3.
37. Guerra Veloz MF, Gomez Rodriguez BJ, Chaaro Benallal D. Ileocecal endometriosis as an infrequent cause of intussusception. Rev Esp Enferm Dig. 2018;110(2):129.
38. Chantalat E, Tuyeras G, Leguevaque P, Delchier MC, Vaysse C, Genre L. Consequences of delayed diagnosis of acute gastrointestinal intussusception, secondary to endometriosis. J Obstet Gynaecol Res. 2017;43(3):595–8.
39. Rivkine E, Emmanuel R, Marciano L, Lea M, Polliand C, Claude P, et al. Ileocolic intussusception due to a cecal endometriosis: case report and review of literature. Diagn Pathol. 2012;7:62.
40. Alborzi S, Rasekhi A, Shomali Z, Madadi G, Alborzi M, Kazemi M, et al. Diagnostic accuracy of magnetic resonance imaging, transvaginal, and transrectal ultrasonography in deep infiltrating endometriosis. Medicine (Baltimore). 2018;97(8):e9536.
41. James O, Williams GL. Prolapsing mass in the caecum: learning point for the colonoscopist. BMJ Case Rep. 2019;12(4):e229811.
42. Ruffo G, Stepniewska A, Crippa S, Serboli G, Zardini C, Steinkasserer M, et al. Laparoscopic ileocecal resection for bowel endometriosis. Surg Endosc. 2011;25(4):1257–62.
43. Nishikawa A, Kondoh E, Hamanishi J, Yamaguchi K, Ueda A, Sato Y, et al. Ileal perforation and massive intestinal haemorrhage from endometriosis in pregnancy: case report and literature review. Eur J Obstet Gynecol Reprod Biol. 2013;170(1):20–4.
44. Beamish RE, Aslam R, Gilbert JM. Postpartum caecal perforation due to endometriosis. JRSM Short Rep. 2010;1(7):61.
45. Bashir RM, Montgomery EA, Gupta PK, Nauta RM, Crockett SA, Collea JV, et al. Massive gastrointestinal hemorrhage during pregnancy caused by ectopic decidua of the terminal ileum and colon. Am J Gastroenterol. 1995;90(8):1325–7.
46. Mabrouk M, Raimondo D, Mastronardi M, Raimondo I, Del Forno S, Arena A, et al. Endometriosis of the appendix: when to predict and how to manage-a multivariate analysis of 1935 endometriosis cases. J Minim Invasive Gynecol. 2020;27(1):100–6.
47. Moulder JK, Siedhoff MT, Melvin KL, Jarvis EG, Hobbs KA, Garrett J. Risk of appendiceal endometriosis among women with deep-infiltrating endometriosis. Int J Gynaecol Obstet. 2017;139(2):149–54.
48. Idetsu A, Ojima H, Saito K, Yamauchi H, Yamaki E, Hosouchi Y, et al. Laparoscopic appendectomy for appendiceal endometriosis presenting as acute appendicitis: report of a case. Surg Today. 2007;37(6):510–3.
49. St John BP, Snider AE, Kellermier H, Minhas S, Nottingham JM. Endometriosis of the appendix presenting as acute appendicitis with unusual appearance. Int J Surg Case Rep. 2018;53:211–3.
50. Lane RE. Endometriosis of the vermiform appendix. Am J Obstet Gynecol. 1960;79:372–7.
51. Adeboye A, Ologun GO, Njoku D, Miner J. Endometriosis of the vermiform appendix presenting as acute appendicitis. Cureus. 2019;11(10):e5816.
52. Akbulut S, Dursun P, Kocbiyik A, Harman A, Sevmis S. Appendiceal endometriosis presenting as perforated appendicitis: report of a case and review of the literature. Arch Gynecol Obstet. 2009;280(3):495–7.
53. Hasegawa T, Yoshida K, Matsui K. Endometriosis of the appendix resulting in perforated appendicitis. Case Rep Gastroenterol. 2007;1(1):27–31.
54. Dickson-Lowe RA, Ibrahim S, Munthali L, Hasan F. Intussusception of the vermiform appendix. BMJ Case Rep. 2015;2015:bcr2014207584.
55. Ijaz S, Lidder S, Mohamid W, Carter M, Thompson H. Intussusception of the appendix secondary to endometriosis: a case report. J Med Case Rep. 2008;2:12.
56. Lam KJ, Tagaloa S. Endometriosis: a rare cause of acute appendicitis in pregnancy. ANZ J Surg. 2020;90:935.
57. Perez CM, Minimo C, Margolin G, Orris J. Appendiceal endometriosis presenting as acute appendicitis during pregnancy. Int J Gynaecol Obstet. 2007;98(2):164–7.
58. Gini PC, Chukudebelu WO, Onuigbo WI. Perforation of the appendix during pregnancy: a rare complication

of endometriosis. Case report. Br J Obstet Gynaecol. 1981;88(4):456–8.

59. Nakatani Y, Hara M, Misugi K, Korehisa H. Appendiceal endometriosis in pregnancy. Report of a case with perforation and review of the literature. Acta Pathol Jpn. 1987;37(10):1685–90.

60. Stefanidis K, Kontostolis S, Pappa L, Kontostolis E. Endometriosis of the appendix with symptoms of acute appendicitis in pregnancy. Obstet Gynecol. 1999;93(5 Pt 2):850.

61. Guaitoli E, Gallo G, Cardone E, Conti L, Famularo S, Formisano G, et al. Consensus Statement of the Italian Polispecialistic Society of Young Surgeons (SPIGC): diagnosis and treatment of acute appendicitis. J Investig Surg. 2020:1–15.

Part II

Diagnosis

Non-enhanced Transvaginal Ultrasonography

5

Stefano Guerriero, Silvia Ajossa, Alba Piras,
Eleonora Musa, Maria Angela Pascual,
Ignacio Rodriguez, Luca Saba, Valerio Mais,
Juan Luis Alcazar, and Anna Maria Paoletti

Transvaginal ultrasound (TVS) is currently considered a fundamental noninvasive diagnostic method to evaluate the extent of rectosigmoid deep infiltrating endometriosis (DIE), when presenting alone or in association with other localizations and able to facilitate the choice of a safe and adequate surgical or medical treatment [1]. Regarding in particular the preoperative evaluation, TVS is crucial to provide a correct informed consent, select the appropriate surgical team and complexity at surgery [2].

Electronic Supplementary Material The online version of this chapter (https://doi.org/10.1007/978-3-030-50446-5_5) contains supplementary material, which is available to authorized users.

5.1 The Diagnosis of Rectosigmoid DIE Using Ultrasound

After the pioneering study of Bazot et al. [3] on rectosigmoid involvement of DIE, other authors have evaluated the presence of endometriosis at this site [4–7]. The ultrasonographic findings of rectosigmoid endometriosis are the presence of an irregular hypoechoic nodule, with or without hypoechoic or, rarely, hyperechoic foci in the anterior wall of rectosigma (Figs. 5.1, 5.2, and 5.3) (Videos 5.1 and 5.2). As stated in the consensus opinion from the International Deep Endometriosis Analysis (IDEA) group [8] several different appearances are possible for these

S. Guerriero (✉)
Department of Obstetrics and Gynecology,
Policlinico Universitario Duilio Casula,
University of Cagliari, Cagliari, Italy

Department of Obstetrics and Gynecology, Blocco Q,
Azienda Ospedaliero Universitaria-Policlinico Duilio
Casula, Monserrato, Italy
e-mail: gineca.sguerriero@tiscali.it

S. Ajossa · A. Piras · E. Musa · V. Mais
A. M. Paoletti
Department of Obstetrics and Gynecology,
Policlinico Universitario Duilio Casula,
University of Cagliari, Cagliari, Italy
e-mail: gineca.sajossa@tiscali.it; gineca.vmais@
tiscali.it; gineca.annapaoletti@tiscali.it

M. A. Pascual
Department of Obstetrics, Gynecology, and
Reproduction, Hospital Universitari Dexeus,
Barcelona, Spain
e-mail: MARPAS@dexeus.com

I. Rodriguez
Unidad Epidemiología y Estadística, Departamento
de Obstetricia, Ginecología y Reproducción, Hospital
Universitario Quirón Dexeus, Barcelona, Spain
e-mail: NACROD@dexeus.com

L. Saba
Department of Radiology, Azienda Ospedaliero
Universitaria di Cagliari, Cagliari, Italy

J. L. Alcazar
Department of Obstetrics and Gynecology, Clínica
Universidad de Navarra, School of Medicine,
University of Navarra, Pamplona, Spain

© Springer Nature Switzerland AG 2020
S. Ferrero, M. Ceccaroni (eds.), *Clinical Management of Bowel Endometriosis*,
https://doi.org/10.1007/978-3-030-50446-5_5

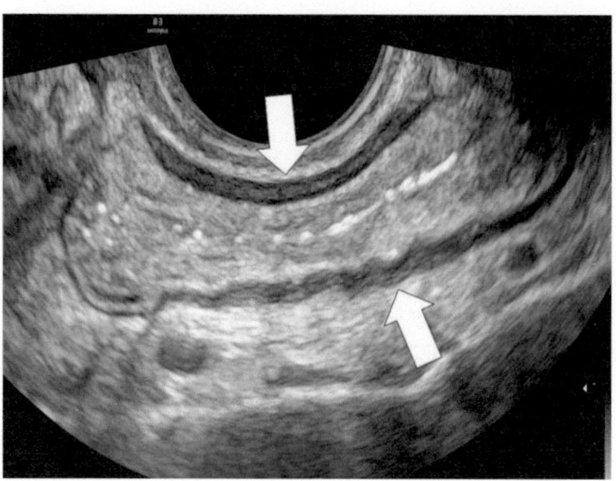

Fig. 5.1 The normal appearance of the muscularis propria of the rectum sigma (straight arrows)

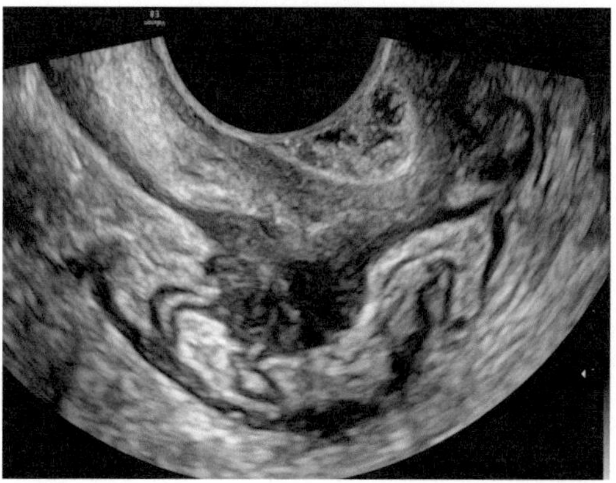

Fig. 5.2 A huge nodule of DIE in the anterior wall of rectosigma

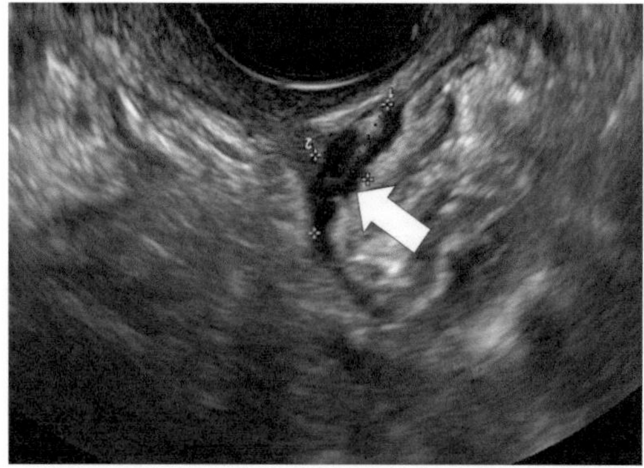

Fig. 5.3 A small nodule of DIE in the anterior wall of rectosigma

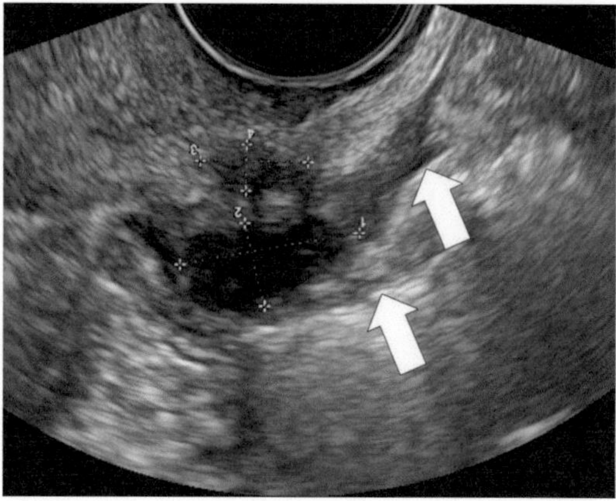

Fig. 5.4 A nodule of abnormal tissue, with visible retraction and adhesions in some cases resulting in the so-called "Indian headdress" (straight arrows)

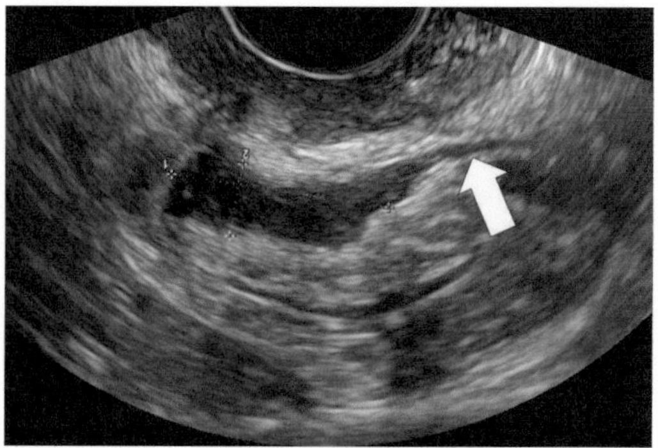

Fig. 5.5 A nodule with a thinner section or a "tail" is noted at one end, resembling a "comet" (straight arrows)

locations. The normal appearance of the muscularis propria of the rectum sigma is replaced with a nodule of abnormal tissue, with visible retraction and adhesions in some cases [4–23] resulting in the so-called "Indian headdress" [9] (Fig. 5.4). In other case, a thinner section or a "tail" is noted at one end, resembling a "comet" [24] (Fig. 5.5); the size of these lesions can vary ranging from few millimeters to some centimeters.

The consensus opinion from the IDEA group [8] proposes that bowel DIE lesions noted on TVS should be described according to the segment of the rectum or sigmoid colon in which they occur, with DIE lesions located below the level of the insertion of the uterosacral ligaments on the cervix being denoted as lower (retroperitoneal) anterior rectal DIE lesions. On the contrary those above this level being denoted as upper (visible at laparoscopy) anterior rectal DIE lesions, those at the level of the uterine fundus being denoted as rectosigmoid junction DIE lesions and those above the level of the uterine fundus being denoted as anterior sigmoid DIE lesions. Following the IDEA consensus [8] the dimensions of the rectal and/or rectosigmoid DIE nodules should be recorded in three orthogonal planes and the distance between the lower margin of the most caudal lesion and the anal verge should be measured using TVS.

Bowel DIE can take the form of an isolated lesion or can be multifocal (multiple lesions affecting the same segment) and/or multicentric (multiple lesions affecting several bowel segments, i.e., small bowel, large bowel, cecum, ileocecal junction, and/or appendix) [25]. In case of multifocal lesions all the interested segment should be measured. Moreover the association with other nodularities in other locations as uterosacral ligaments and forniceal (the so-called diabolo-like nodule) must be noted and described (Figs. 5.6 and 5.7).

Hudelist et al. [26] in 2011 conducted a meta-analysis including 1106 patients and found that the pooled estimates of sensitivity and specificity of TVS in detecting rectosigmoid endometriosis were 91% and 98%, respectively. In a recent meta-analysis Guerriero et al. [27] in 2639 cases found that the pooled sensitivity and specificity of TVS in detecting DIE in the rectosigmoid were 91% and 97%, respectively. The same authors did not find statistical differences, in term of sensitiv-

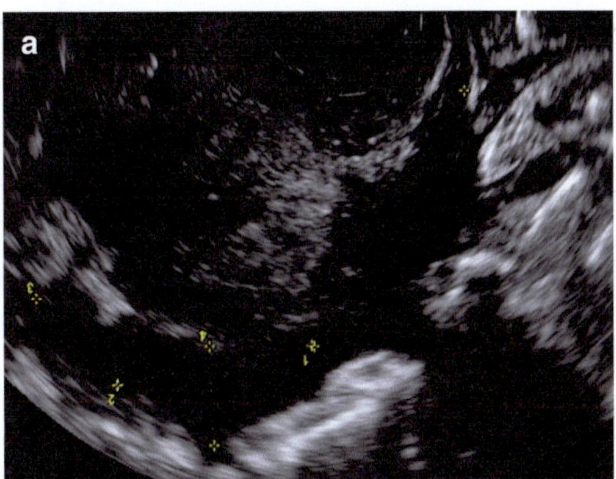
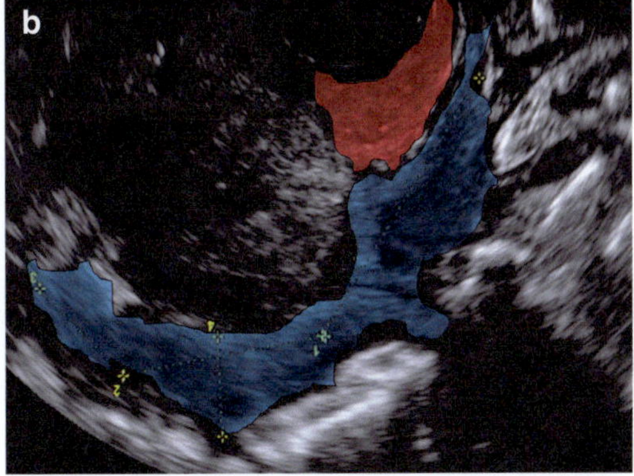

Fig. 5.7 (a, b) A diabolo-like nodule due to the association of a forniceal nodule (in red) with a rectosigmoid lesion (in blue)

ity and specificity, comparing non-enhanced and enhanced (E-TVS) (defined as methods using free fluid, saline, water, or gel in the rectum or vagina) TVS. This may be because of these techniques may be more suitable as second step investigations to ascertain the presence of mucosal involvement or rectal stenosis (see next chapter).

Unfortunately Guerriero et al. [27] found a significant heterogeneity for sensitivity and specificity in the published studies. The major cause of heterogeneity, as shown by the meta-regression performed, is due to the wide prevalence reported in this meta-analysis with values of >50% in some cases but also of <5% in others, probably mainly due to the motivation for surgery in some studies, such as that of Exacoustos et al. [21] which excluded patients with no ultrasonographic appearance of DIE.

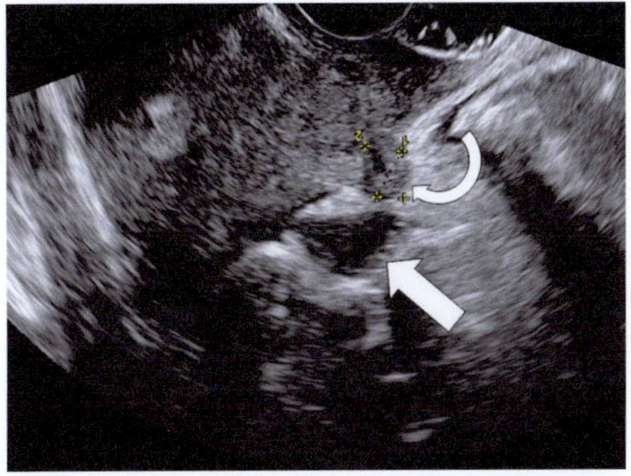

Fig. 5.6 the association between a rectosigmoid nodule (straight arrow) with a nodule of uterosacral ligament (curved arrows)

5.2 Learning Curve for TVS in the Diagnosis of Rectosigmoid DIE

For many years, doubts about operator dependency of TVS have been reported, but it has recently been suggested that an examiner who is familiar with TVS can achieve proficiency in the diagnosis of DIE after performing about 40 examinations [28], and reproducibility seems good among experienced sonographers or gynecologists [29]. Several authors previously evaluated the learning curve for this disease [30–33]. In particular Tammaa et al. [28] reported a similar number of evaluations helpful to the trainees to reach the requested competence for detection of rectosigmoid lesions. However, competency can be achieved within 40 procedures, enabling diagnosis of DIE with similar diagnostic accuracy as reported by centers of excellence after only 1 week of DIE-TVUS training [31]. Other authors [32] also shows that a sonographer trained in general gynecologic ultrasonography, who has invested time to learn TVUS for DIE mapping, can achieve proficiency for diagnosing the major types of DIE lesions after examining less than 50 patients.

Obviously experience is an essential requirement to a good performance in ultrasonographic diagnosis of DIE. Guerriero et al. [34] suggested that the combined use of real-time TVS and offline 3D volumes virtual navigation could be helpful to adequate training, in a short period of time (2 weeks), for ultrasound assessment of DIE. In the suggested learning program, concentrating of cases during the training period, for the rectosigmoid locations competence was reached after only 39 evaluations, but with a wide range between trainees (ranging from 30 to 60 evaluations). The accuracy for each trainee was high ranging from 80% to 94% after the training. The other advantage of a learning program organized in this way was the possibility of carrying out this intensive course without creating discomfort to the patients with such a usually painful disease [34].

5.3 The Role of "Soft Markers" in the Diagnosis of Rectosigmoid DIE

The so-called "soft markers" are indirect sign of presence of DIE. The consensus IDEA proposes four basic sonographic steps when examining women with suspected or known endometriosis. First step is to examine the uterus and the adnexa. The mobility of the uterus should be evaluated: normal, reduced, or fixed ("question mark sign") [35]. Sonographic signs of adenomyosis should be searched for and described using the terms and definitions reported in the Morphological Uterus Sonographic Assessment (MUSA) [36] consensus opinion for the high rate of association between adenomyosis and DIE. Also ovarian endometriomas are frequently associated with other endometriotic lesions, such as adhesions and DIE [37]. Also the position of the ovary containing the endometrioma is important. An ovary stacked to the uterus is suggestive of presence of adhesions. The "kissing" ovaries sign (defined as both ovaries joined together behind the uterus in the cul-de-sac) (Fig. 5.8) suggests [38] an increased risk of bowel endometriosis (18.5% vs. 2.5% without kissing ovaries).

The second step is to search for sonographic "soft markers" as site-specific tenderness and fixed ovaries (Figs. 5.9 and 5.10). The presence

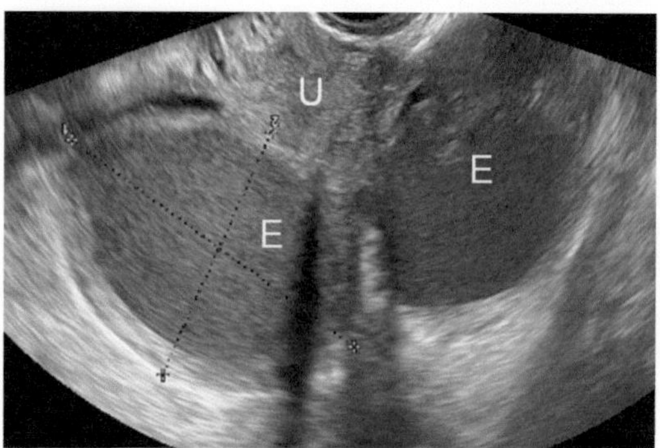

Fig. 5.8 The "kissing" ovaries sign (defined as both ovaries joined together behind the uterus in the cul-de-sac); Endometrioma (E), Uterus (U)

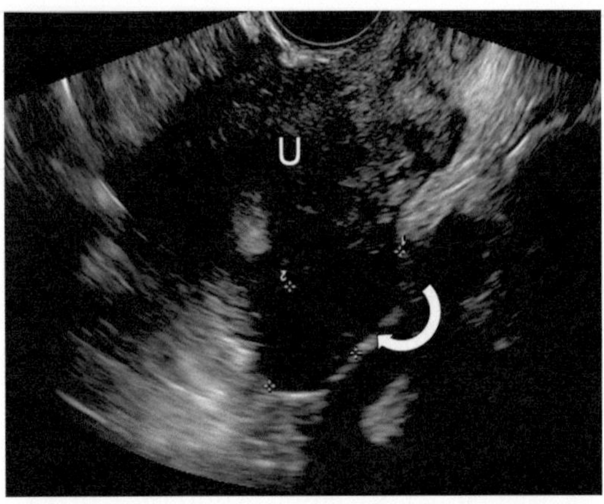

Fig. 5.9 An ovary (curved arrow) fixed to the uterus (U)

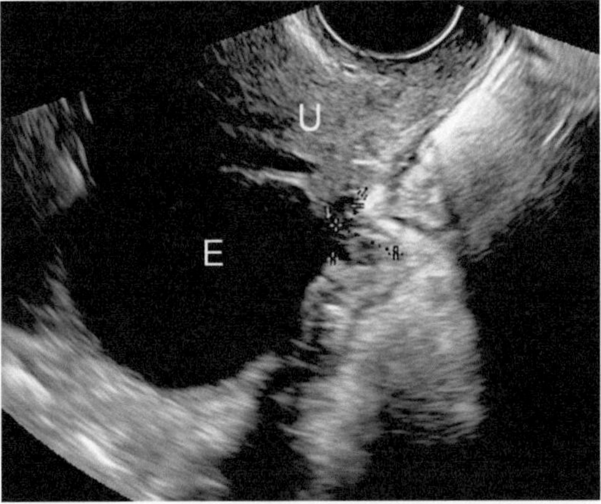

Fig. 5.10 An endometrioma (E) fixed to the uterus (U)

of soft markers increases also the likelihood of superficial endometriosis and adhesions [39, 40].

The third step is to assess the status of the Pouch of Douglas (POD) using the real-time TVS-based "sliding sign" (Videos 5.2 and 5.3). In order to assess the sliding sign when the uterus is anteverted, gentle pressure is placed against the cervix using the transvaginal probe, to establish whether the anterior rectum glides freely across the posterior aspect of the cervix (retrocervical region) and posterior vaginal wall. If the anterior rectal wall does so, the "sliding sign" is considered positive for this location.

Hudelist et al. suggest that this sign is not only related of POD occlusion [41]. For these authors a negative sliding sign on TVS predicted DIE of

rectum with a sensitivity of 85% and specificity of 96%. This sign is reproducible and easy to learn [29, 42].

Recently, some authors suggest the possibility to use transvaginal ultrasound "soft markers" to predict the presence of rectosigmoid endometriosis lesions [43]. Guerriero S et al. in a prospective observational study of [43], evaluated the use of ultrasonographic "soft markers" (presence of US signs of uterine adenomyosis, presence of an endometrioma, adhesions of the ovary to the uterus, presence of "kissing ovaries," absence of sliding sign) for the prediction of rectosigmoid endometriosis. The absence of sliding sign with an odd ratio (OR) of 13.95 and, the presence of "kissing ovaries" with an OR of 22.5 were the only significant variables found. Where the sliding sign was negative (Video 5.2) or kissing ovaries was present (Fig. 5.8), transvaginal US showed a specificity of 75% and a sensitivity of 82% for the detection of rectosigmoid endometriosis. In these patients the pretest probability of rectosigmoid endometriosis was 32%, and this probability increased to 61% when at least one of these features was present and fell to 10% when these TVS "soft markers" were absent. Although larger studies are needed to better estimate the usefulness of "soft markers," these authors suggest that absence of the sliding sign and/or the presence of kissing ovaries can be to accurately screen patients with clinical suspicion of rectosigmoid endometriosis to be referred to dedicated to DIE ultrasonographic operator with a low rate of false negatives [43].

5.4 Comparison with Other Imaging Techniques

The use of three-dimensional (3D) image rendering has been suggested to allow a good analysis of the endometriotic nodule; this reconstruction seems to clearly show the irregular shapes and borders of the lesions [23, 44–46] (Figs. 5.11 and 5.12). This technique allows unrestricted access to an infinite number of viewing planes, which can be very useful for correctly locating lesions within the pelvis and evaluating the relationship with other organs. In addition, the stored 3D vol-

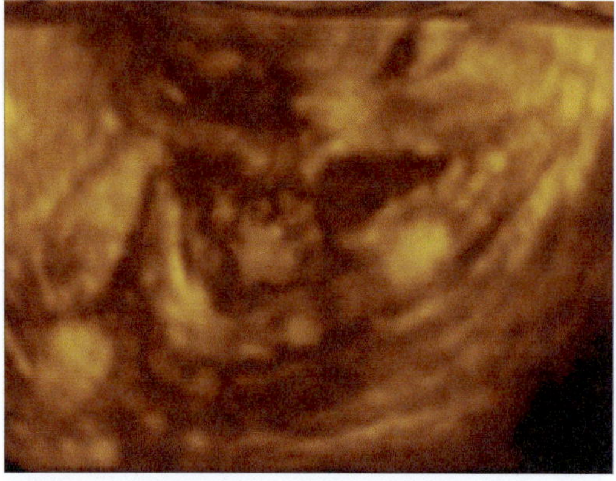

Fig. 5.11 The irregular shapes and borders of a rectosigmoid nodule

umes can be reassessed and compared by the same or different examiners over time and also used for teaching purpose as previously described in the subheading about learning curve. Unfortunately, Guerriero et al. [23] not found a significant difference between two-dimensional ultrasound and 3D for the intestinal involvement with a specificity and sensitivity of 93%, 95%, respectively, for 2D ultrasound and 97% and 91%, respectively, for 3D ultrasound.

Magnetic resonance imaging (MRI) has also been used in the diagnosis of DIE. In this particular location the diagnostic performance of TVS and MRI is similar for detecting DIE involving rectosigmoid when including only studies in which patients underwent both techniques [47]. In a recent meta-analysis of six studies (for a total 424 patients) MRI in the detection of DIE in the

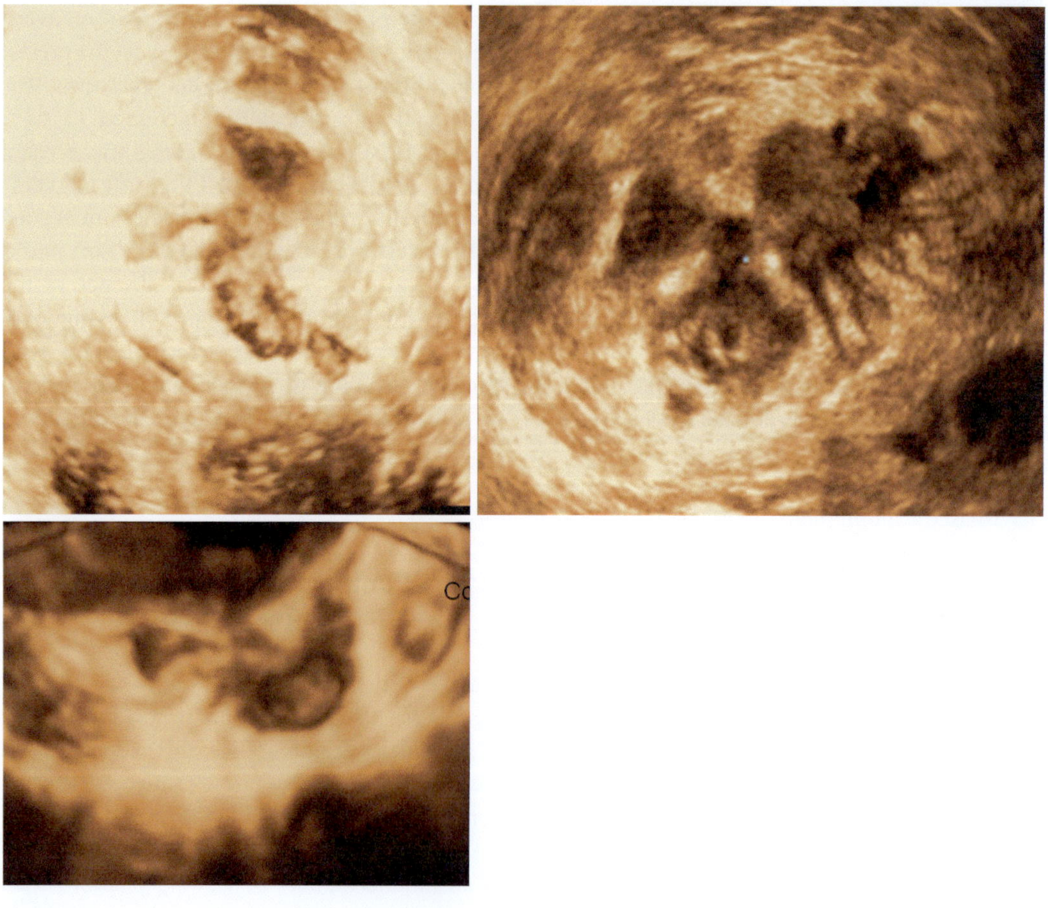

Fig. 5.12 The irregular shapes and borders of some rectosigmoid nodules in different planes

Fig. 5.13 Two rectosigmoid nodules visualized using three-dimensional ultrasonography (**a**) missed using magnetic resonance (**b**)

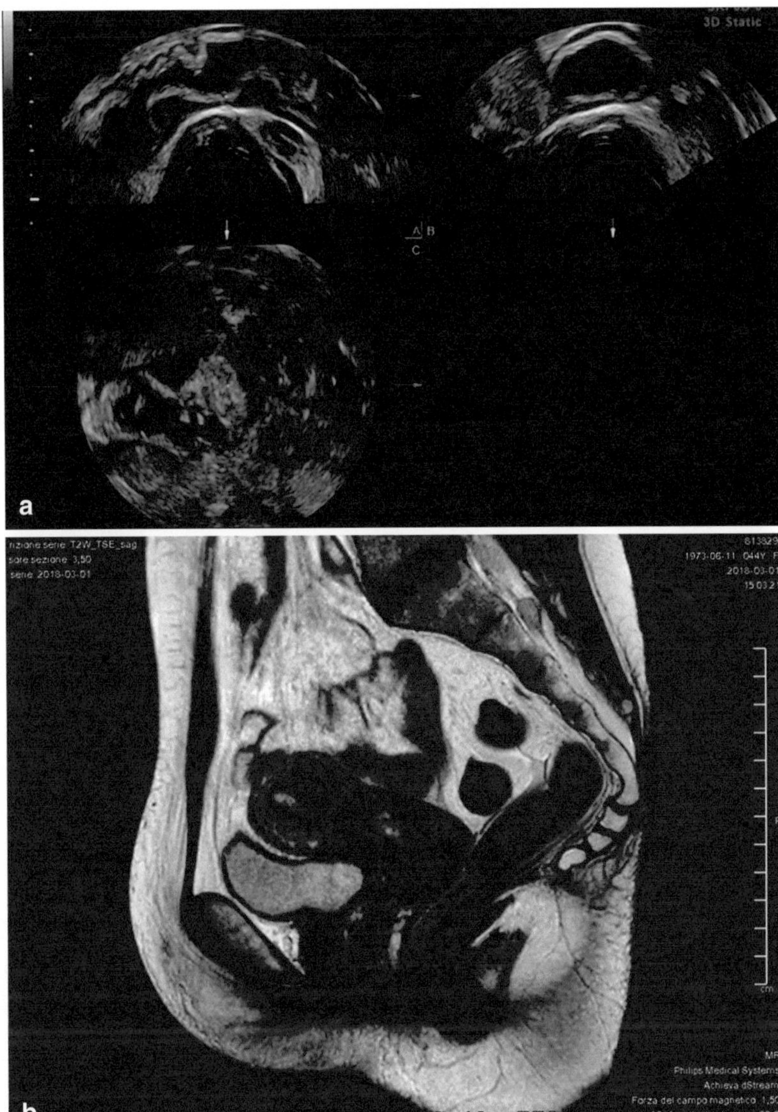

rectosigmoid, showed a pooled sensitivity of 85% and a specificity of 95% while TVS showed a pooled sensitivity of 85% and a specificity of 96% [47] (Fig. 5.13). Another meta-analysis with more cases included showed similar results [48]. Regarding the necessity of a bowel preparation before TVS examination a recent paper suggests that it can be avoided without the reduction of the accuracy but with a sure improvement of the compliance of the patient [49].

5.5 Conclusion

In the last years there are some evidences regarding the change to less laparoscopy-oriented approach to the diagnosis of rectosigmoid DIE. As stated by Bazot [50] TVS and MRI exhibited at least similar sensitivities and specificities to laparoscopy supporting their use as a replacement option. For this pioneer in the diagnosis of DIE, in the light of recent advances in imaging techniques, both the definition of DIE and the use of laparoscopy as the gold standard in the diagnosis of DE, deserve to be revised.

In an editorial Dr Piessens [51] from Australia suggests that it's difficult to understand why despite good test characteristics and an acceptable learning curve, even after 12 years, the ultrasound assessment of DE is still considered a specialist assessment. Even though a "PCO assessment," a "polyp assessment," a "fibroid assessment" and an "ovarian cyst assessment" are all part of a routine examination, this is not the case for an "endometriosis assessment" [52].

Regarding the algorithm for the clinical diagnosis of endometriosis, recently a group of North-American experts of DIE [52] finally suggest to perform or order imaging to evaluate the presence of endometrioma, the presence of adenomyosis, the presence of soft markers, and the presence of nodules and masses. This approach is defined as a fundamental step to reduce the delay in this chronic and invalidating disease.

References

1. Exacoustos C, Manganaro L, Zupi E. Imaging for the evaluation of endometriosis and adenomyosis. Best Pract Res Clin Obstet Gynaecol. 2014;28:655–81.
2. Abrão MS, Petraglia F, Falcone T, Keckstein J, Osuga Y, Chapron C. Deep endometriosis infiltrating the recto-sigmoid: critical factors to consider before management. Hum Reprod Update. 2015;21:329–39.
3. Bazot M, Thomassin I, Hourani R, Cortez A, Darai E. Diagnostic accuracy of transvaginal sonography for deep pelvic endometriosis. Ultrasound Obstet Gynecol. 2004;24:180–5.
4. Hudelist G, Oberwinkler KH, Singer CF, Tuttlies F, Rauter G, Ritter O, Keckstein J. Combination of transvaginal sonography and clinical examination for preoperative diagnosis of pelvic endometriosis. Hum Reprod. 2009;24:1018–24.
5. Guerriero S, Ajossa S, Gerada M, D'Aquila M, Piras B, Melis GB. Tenderness-guided transvaginal ultrasonography: a new method for the detection of deep endometriosis in patients with chronic pelvic pain. Fertil Steril. 2007;88:1293–7.
6. Holland TK, Yazbek J, Cutner A, Saridogan E, Hoo WL, Jurkovic D. Value of transvaginal ultrasound in assessing the severity of pelvic endometriosis. Ultrasound Obstet Gynecol. 2010;36:241–8.
7. Abrao MS, Goncalves MO, Dias JA, Podgaec S, Chamie LP, Blasbalg R. Comparison between clinical examination, transvaginal sonography and magnetic resonance imaging for the diagnosis of deep endometriosis. Hum Reprod. 2007;22:3092–7.
8. Guerriero S, Condous G, van den Bosch T, Valentin L, Leone FP, Van Schoubroeck D, et al. Systematic approach to sonographic evaluation of the pelvis in women with suspected endometriosis, including terms, definitions and measurements: a consensus opinion from the International Deep Endometriosis Analysis (IDEA) group. Ultrasound Obstet Gynecol. 2016;48:318–32.
9. Guerriero S, Ajossa S, Gerada M, Virgilio B, Angioni S, Melis GB. Diagnostic value of transvaginal 'tenderness guided' ultrasonography for the prediction of location of deep endometriosis. Hum Reprod. 2008;23:2452–7.
10. Piketty M, Chopin N, Dousset B, Millischer-Bellaische AE, Roseau G, Leconte M, Borghese B, Chapron C. Preoperative work-up for patients with deeply infiltrating endometriosis: transvaginal ultrasonography must definitely be the first-line imaging examination. Hum Reprod. 2009;24:602–7.
11. Hudelist G, Tuttlies F, Rauter G, Pucher S, Keckstein J. Can transvaginal sonography predict infiltration depth in patients with deep infiltrating endometriosis of the rectum? Hum Reprod. 2009;24:1012–7.
12. Bazot M, Lafont C, Rouzier R, Roseau G, Thomassin-Naggara I, Darai E. Diagnostic accuracy of physical examination, transvaginal sonography, rectal endoscopic sonography, and magnetic resonance imaging to diagnose deep infiltrating endometriosis. Fertil Steril. 2009;92:1825–33.
13. Bazot M, Malzy P, Cortez A, Roseau G, Amouyal P, Darai E. Accuracy of transvaginal sonography and rectal endoscopic sonography in the diagnosis of deep infiltrating endometriosis. Ultrasound Obstet Gynecol. 2007;30:994–1001.
14. Goncalves MO, Podgaec S, Dias JA, Gonzalez M, Abrao MS. Transvaginal ultrasonography with bowel preparation is able to predict the number of lesions and rectosigmoid layers affected in cases of deep endometriosis, defining surgical strategy. Hum Reprod. 2010;25:665–71.
15. Ferrero S, Biscaldi E, Morotti M, Venturini PL, Remorgida V, Rollandi GA, Valenzano Menada M. Multidetector computerized tomography enteroclysis vs. rectal water contrast transvaginal ultrasonography in determining the presence and extent of bowel endometriosis. Ultrasound Obstet Gynecol. 2011;37:603–13.
16. Hudelist G, Ballard K, English J, Wright J, Banerjee S, Mastoroudes H, Thomas A, Singer CF, Keckstein J. Transvaginal sonography vs. clinical examination in the preoperative diagnosis of deep infiltrating endometriosis. Ultrasound Obstet Gynecol. 2011;37:480–7.
17. Savelli L, Manuzzi L, Coe M, Mabrouk M, Di Donato N, Venturoli S, Seracchioli R. Comparison of transvaginal sonography and double-contrast barium enema for diagnosing deep infiltrating endometriosis

of the posterior compartment. Ultrasound Obstet Gynecol. 2011;38:466–71.

18. Saccardi C, Cosmi E, Borghero A, Tregnaghi A, Dessole S, Litta P. Comparison between transvaginal sonography, saline contrast sonovaginography and magnetic resonance imaging in the diagnosis of posterior deep infiltrating endometriosis. Ultrasound Obstet Gynecol. 2012;40:464–9.

19. Holland TK, Cutner A, Saridogan E, Mavrelos D, Pateman K, Jurkovic D. Ultrasound mapping of pelvic endometriosis: does the location and number of lesions affect the diagnostic accuracy? A multicentre diagnostic accuracy study. BMC Womens Health. 2013;13:43.

20. Fratelli N, Scioscia M, Bassi E, Musola M, Minelli L, Trivella G. Transvaginal sonography for preoperative assessment of deep endometriosis. J Clin Ultrasound. 2013;41:69–75.

21. Exacoustos C, Malzoni M, Di Giovanni A, Lazzeri L, Tosti C, Petraglia F, Zupi E. Ultrasound mapping system for the surgical management of deep infiltrating endometriosis. Fertil Steril. 2014;102:143–50.

22. León M, Vaccaro H, Alcázar JL, Martinez J, Gutierrez J, Amor F, Iturra A, Sovino H. Extended transvaginal sonography in deep infiltrating endometriosis: use of bowel preparation and an acoustic window with intra-vaginal gel: preliminary results. J Ultrasound Med. 2014;33:315–21.

23. Guerriero S, Saba L, Ajossa S, Peddes C, Angiolucci M, Perniciano M, Melis GB, Alcázar JL. Three-dimensional ultrasonography in the diagnosis of deep endometriosis. Hum Reprod. 2014;29:1189–98.

24. Benacerraf BR, Groszmann Y, Hornstein MD, Bromley B. Deep infiltrating endometriosis of the bowel wall: the comet sign. J Ultrasound Med. 2015;34:537–42.

25. Belghiti J, Thomassin-Naggara I, Zacharopoulou C, Zilberman S, Jarboui L, Bazot M, Ballester M, Darai E. Contribution of computed tomography enema and magnetic resonance imaging to diagnose multifocal and multicentric bowel lesions in patients with colorectal endometriosis. J Minim Invasive Gynecol. 2015;22:776–84.

26. Hudelist G, English J, Thomas AE, Tinelli A, Singer CF, Keckstein J. Diagnostic accuracy of transvaginal ultrasound for non-invasive diagnosis of bowel endometriosis: systematic review and meta-analysis. Ultrasound Obstet Gynecol. 2011;37:257–63.

27. Guerriero S, Ajossa S, Orozco R, Perniciano M, Jurado M, Melis GB, Alcazar JL. Accuracy of transvaginal ultrasound for diagnosis of deep endometriosis in the rectosigmoid: systematic review and meta-analysis. Ultrasound Obstet Gynecol. 2016;47:281–9.

28. Tammaa A, Fritzer N, Strunk G, Krell A, Salzer H, Hudelist G. Learning curve for the detection of pouch of Douglas obliteration and deep infiltrating endometriosis of the rectum. Hum Reprod. 2014;29:1199–204.

29. Bazot M, Daraï E, Biau DJ, Ballester M, Dessolle L. Learning curve of transvaginal ultrasound for the diagnosis of endometriomas assessed by the cumulative summation test (LC-CUSUM). Fertil Steril. 2011;95:301–3.

30. Fraser MA, Agarwal S, Chen I, Singh SS. Routine vs. expert-guided transvaginal ultrasound in the diagnosis of endometriosis: a retrospective review. Abdom Imaging. 2015;40:587–94.

31. Piessens S, Healey M, Maher P, Tsaltas J, Rombauts L. Can anyone screen for deep infiltrating endometriosis with transvaginal ultrasound? Aust N Z J Obstet Gynaecol. 2014;54:462–8.

32. Eisenberg VH, Alcazar JL, Arbib N, Schiff E, Achiron R, Goldenberg M, et al. Applying a statistical method in transvaginal ultrasound training: lessons from the learning curve cumulative summation test (LC-CUSUM) for endometriosis mapping. Gynecol Surg. 2017;14:19.

33. Young SW, Dahiya N, Patel MD, Abrao MS, Magrina JF, Temkit M, Kho RM. Initial accuracy of and learning curve for transvaginal ultrasound with bowel preparation for deep endometriosis in a US Tertiary Care Center. J Minim Invasive Gynecol. 2017;24:1170–6.

34. Guerriero S, Pascual MA, Ajossa S, Rodriguez I, Zajicek M, Rolla M, Rams NL, Yulzari V, Bardin R, Buonomo F, Comparetto O, Perniciano M, Saba L, Mais V, Alcazar JL. Learning curve for the ultrasonographic diagnosis of deep endometriosis using a structured off-line training program. Ultrasound Obstet Gynecol. 2019;54:262. https://doi.org/10.1002/uog.20176.

35. Di Donato N, Bertoldo V, Montanari G, Zannoni L, Caprara G, Seracchioli R. Question mark form of uterus: a simple sonographic sign associated with the presence of adenomyosis. Ultrasound Obstet Gynecol. 2015;46:126–7.

36. Van den Bosch T, Dueholm M, Leone FP, Valentin L, Rasmussen CK, Votino A, Van Schoubroeck D, Landolfo C, Installe AJ, Guerriero S, Exacoustos C, Gordts S, Benacerraf B, D'Hooghe T, De Moor B, Brolmann H, Goldstein S, Epstein E, Bourne T, Timmerman D. Terms, definitions and measurements to describe sonographic features of myometrium and uterine masses: a consensus opinion from the Morphological Uterus Sonographic Assessment (MUSA) group. Ultrasound Obstet Gynecol. 2015;46:284–98.

37. Chapron C, Pietin-Vialle C, Borghese B, Davy C, Foulot H, Chopin N. Associated ovarian endometrioma is a marker for greater severity of deeply infiltrating endometriosis. Fertil Steril. 2009;92:453–7.

38. Ghezzi F, Raio L, Cromi A, Duwe DG, Beretta P, Buttarelli M, Mueller MD. "Kissing ovaries": a sonographic sign of moderate to severe endometriosis. Fertil Steril. 2005;83:143–7.

39. Guerriero S, Ajossa S, Lai MP, Mais V, Paoletti AM, Melis GB. Transvaginal ultrasonography in the diagnosis of pelvic adhesions. Hum Reprod. 1997;12:2649–53.

40. Okaro E, Condous G, Khalid A, Timmerman D, Ameye L, Huffel SV, Bourne T. The use of ultrasound-based

'soft markers' for the prediction of pelvic pathology in women with chronic pelvic pain--can we reduce the need for laparoscopy? BJOG. 2006;113:251–6.

41. Hudelist G, Fritzer N, Staettner S, Tammaa A, Tinelli A, Sparic R, Keckstein J. Uterine sliding sign: a simple sonographic predictor for presence of deep infiltrating endometriosis of the rectum. Ultrasound Obstet Gynecol. 2013;41:692–5.

42. Menakaya U, Infante F, Lu C, Phua C, Model A, Messyne F, et al. Interpreting the real-time dynamic 'sliding sign' and predicting pouch of Douglas obliteration: an interobserver, intraobserver, diagnostic-accuracy and learning-curve study. Ultrasound Obstet Gynecol. 2016;48:113–20.

43. Guerriero S, Ajossa S, Pascual MA, Rodriguez I, Piras A, Perniciano M, Saba L, Paoletti AM, Mais V, Alcazar JL. Ultrasonographic 'soft' markers for the detection of rectosigmoid endometriosis. Ultrasound Obstet Gynecol. 2020;55:269. https://doi.org/10.1002/uog.20289.

44. Guerriero S, Alcázar JL, Ajossa S, Pilloni M, Melis GB. Three-dimensional sonographic characteristics of deep endometriosis. J Ultrasound Med. 2009;28:1061–6.

45. Pascual MA, Guerriero S, Hereter L, Barri-Soldevila P, Ajossa S, Graupera B, Rodriguez I. Diagnosis of endometriosis of the rectovaginal septum using introital three-dimensional ultrasonography. Fertil Steril. 2010;94:2761–5.

46. Pascual MA, Guerriero S, Hereter L, Barri-Soldevila P, Ajossa S, Graupera B, Rodriguez I. Three-dimensional sonography for diagnosis of rectovaginal septum endometriosis: interobserver agreement. J Ultrasound Med. 2013;32:931–5.

47. Guerriero S, Saba L, Pascual MA, Ajossa S, Rodriguez I, Mais V, Alcazar JL. Transvaginal ultrasound vs magnetic resonance imaging for diagnosing deep infiltrating endometriosis: systematic review and meta-analysis. Ultrasound Obstet Gynecol. 2018;51:586–95.

48. Moura APC, Ribeiro HSAA, Bernardo WM, Simões R, Torres US, D'Ippolito G, Bazot M, Ribeiro PAAG. Accuracy of transvaginal sonography versus magnetic resonance imaging in the diagnosis of rectosigmoid endometriosis: systematic review and meta-analysis. PLoS One. 2019;14:e0214842.

49. Ferrero S, Scala C, Stabilini C, Vellone VG, Barra F, Leone Roberti Maggiore U. Transvaginal sonography with vs without bowel preparation in diagnosis of rectosigmoid endometriosis: prospective study. Ultrasound Obstet Gynecol. 2019;53:402–9.

50. Bazot M, Daraï E. Diagnosis of deep endometriosis: clinical examination, ultrasonography, magnetic resonance imaging, and other techniques. Fertil Steril. 2017;108:886–94.

51. Piessens S. Is it time to include assessment of the most common gynaecological condition in the routine ultrasound evaluation of the pelvis? Australias J Ultrasound Med. 2019;22:83–5.

52. Agarwal SK, Chapron C, Giudice LC, Laufer MR, Leyland N, Missmer SA, Singh SS, Taylor HS. Clinical diagnosis of endometriosis: a call to action. Am J Obstet Gynecol. 2019;220:354.e1–354.e12.

Enhanced Ultrasonographic Techniques

Simone Ferrero, Fabio Barra, Carolina Scala, Martino Rolla, and Mauricio León

6.1 Introduction

Endometriosis affects at least 4% of reproductive age women [1]. Since the diagnosis of endometriosis cannot be reliably be performed on the basis of symptoms and clinical examination [2], imaging techniques have a pivotal role in the noninvasive diagnosis of endometriosis. Nowadays, is well known that transvaginal ultrasonography (TVS) is the first line investigation in patients with suspicion of deep pelvic endometriosis [3]. Compared with other imaging techniques (such as magnetic resonance imaging, MRI), TVS has the advantage of being relatively inexpensive, it is performed by the gynecologists that usually manage patients with endometriosis, it allows a dynamic evaluation of pelvic structures and the identification of deep endometriotic lesions by pain mapping, it is well tolerated by the patients and, in general, it has good diagnostic performance. However, the performance of TVS in diagnosing deep endometriosis is strongly dependent on the experience of the examiner [4].

Over the last 10 years several ultrasonographic techniques based on the distention of the vagina and/or rectosigmoid with saline solution and/or ultrasonographic gel have been proposed with the aim to improve the diagnosis of deep infiltrating endometriosis. These distention media create acoustic windows in the vagina, rectum, or both of them. These procedures may facilitate the diagnosis of deep endometriosis by delineating the margins of pelvic spaces and organs. These techniques are named "enhanced" or "modified" transvaginal ultrasonography [5] and they include: rectal water-contrast transvaginal ultrasonography (RWC-TVS), sonovaginography (SVG), and tenderness-guided transvaginal ultrasonography (tg-TVS).

S. Ferrero (✉) · F. Barra
Academic Unit of Obstetrics and Gynecology, IRCCS Ospedale Policlinico San Martino, Genova, Italy

Department of Neurosciences, Rehabilitation, Ophthalmology, Genetics, Maternal and Child Health (DiNOGMI), University of Genova, Genova, Italy
e-mail: simone.ferrero@unige.it

C. Scala
Obstetrics and Gynecology Unit, Istituto Giannina Gaslini, Genoa, Italy

M. Rolla
Unità Operativa Complessa di Ostetricia e Ginecologia, Azienda Ospedaliero – Universitaria di Parma, Parma, Italy

M. León
Ultrasound Unit, Department of Gynecology and Obstetrics, Clinica INDISA, Santiago, Chile

© Springer Nature Switzerland AG 2020
S. Ferrero, M. Ceccaroni (eds.), *Clinical Management of Bowel Endometriosis*,
https://doi.org/10.1007/978-3-030-50446-5_6

6.2 Rectal Water-Contrast Transvaginal Ultrasonography

RWC-TVS primarily aims to improve the diagnosis of rectosigmoid endometriosis but it may also facilitate the identification of all endometriotic lesions of the posterior compartment. It represents a transvaginal ultrasonographic exam performed after distention of the rectosigmoid with saline solution.

Bowel cleansing is usually performed before RWC-TVS. Some authors recommend the use of bowel purgation in the day before the exam and polyethylene glycol is one of the most commonly employed laxative [6, 7]. Other authors suggest a low-fiber diet (daily fiber intake less than 10 g) in the 3 days before the exam [8]. A rectal enema is usually recommended few hours before the procedure [8–12]. However, a recent prospective study demonstrated that bowel preparation does not improve the performance of RWC-TVS in diagnosing rectosigmoid endometriosis and in assessing the characteristics of these nodules [13]. A flexible catheter (with caliber of approximately 6 mm, 18 Ch) is inserted through the anal canal into the rectosigmoid (up to a 15–20 cm from the anal verge) [6–8, 10, 14]. A gel containing lidocaine may be used to facilitate the passage of the catheter [8, 10, 14]. A 50–100 mL siring with conical tip connected to the catheter is used to inject room temperature or warm saline solution into the rectosigmoid. The volume of the injected saline solution varies between 100 and 350 mL [8, 9, 12, 14]. The distention can be performed under ultrasonographic control [10, 14] or before starting the ultrasonography. When the ultrasonographic control is used, 100 mL are injected continuously at the beginning of the procedure whereas the rest of the solution is injected if requested by the examiner [10, 14]. During the ultrasound, when the solution is not being injected, a Klemmer or ring forceps can be attached to the catheter in order to prevent the backflow of the fluid [8, 10, 14] (Fig. 6.1). By using this technique, most of the studies did not report significant saline solution

leakage in the space between the catheter and the anus [8, 10, 14].

In patients with rectovaginal endometriotic nodules, intestinal infiltration is diagnosed when the hypoechoic endometriotic nodule penetrates the rectal wall thickening the muscularis mucosa [6–8]. Higher intestinal endometriotic nodules appear as solid, hypoechoic, nodular lesions, adjacent or penetrating the intestinal wall [8, 10, 14]; hypoechoic or hyperechoic foci are sometimes present, whereas retraction and adhesions are often present (Fig. 6.2).

Intestinal distension facilitates the identification of the limits of the intestinal nodules [8, 14]. Furthermore, following intestinal distention it is easier to visualize the layers of the rectosigmoid wall [8, 14]. The intestinal serosa is hyperechoic. The two layers in muscularis propria appear as hypoechoic strips (longitudinal smooth muscle and circular smooth muscle) divided by a thin hyperechoic line. The submucosa is hyperechoic, whereas the muscularis mucosa is hypoechoic. The interface between the lumen and the intestinal mucosa is hyperechoic [8–10].

The virtual organ computer-aided analysis (VOCAL) may be used to estimate the volume of intestinal nodules [11, 15]. The tomographic ultrasound imaging (TUI) may be used to better appreciate intestinal wall infiltration (Fig. 6.3) [11]. In the tridimensional ultrasonography, the surface mode may be used to reconstruct the endometriotic nodule in a similar way to what occurs in virtual colonoscopy [11] (Figs. 6.4 and 6.5). This technique allows to estimate the degree of stenosis caused by the nodule.

Published studies report that the time required to perform RWC-TVS ranges between 16 and 18 min [9, 10]. RWC-TVS is usually well tolerated by the patients [6]. Some authors investigated the discomfort caused by RWC-TVS using a 10 cm visual analogue scale (VAS) [7–10, 14], reporting an intensity of pain ranging between 3.9 and 4.1 cm [7, 8, 10, 14]. However, in these previously published studies, no patient required to interrupt the exam because of pain [7, 10, 14].

RWC-TVS is less painful than double-contrast barium enema (DCBE) [14], multidetector com-

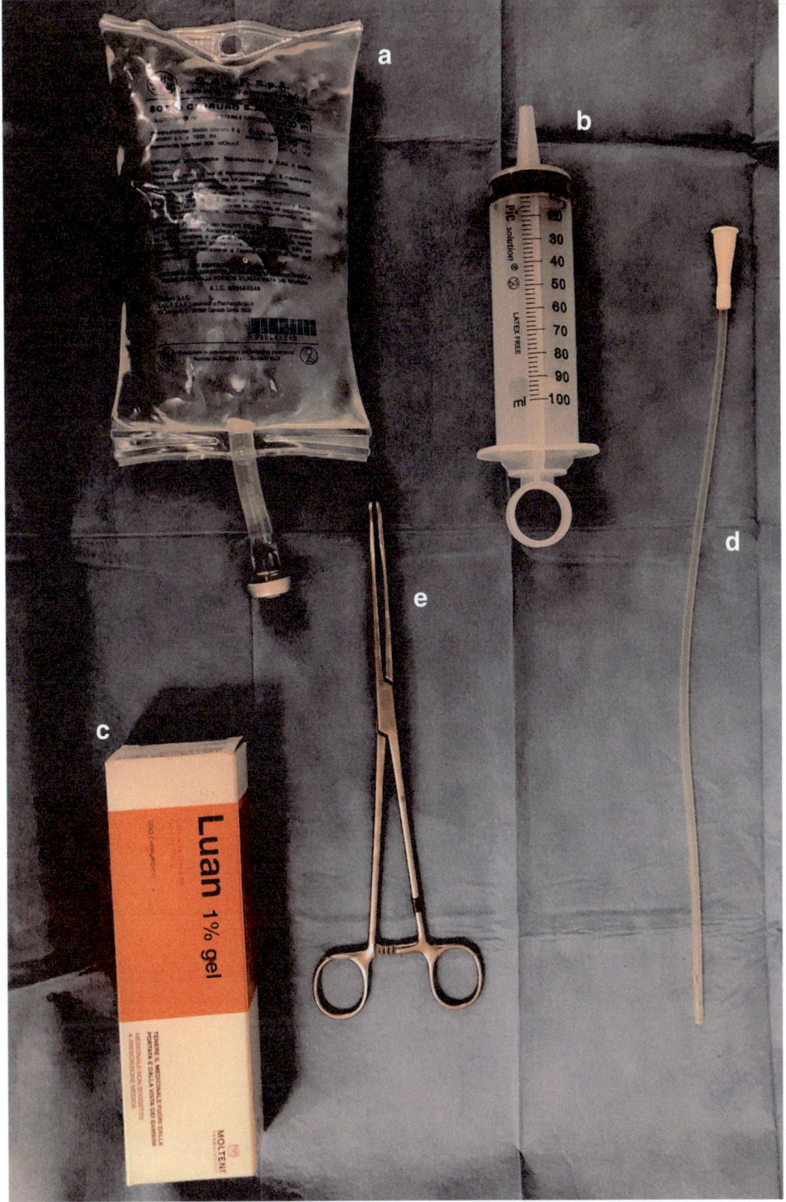

Fig. 6.1 Material required to performed rectal water-contrast transvaginal ultrasonography. (**a**) saline solution; (**b**) syringe; (**c**) gel containing lidocaine; (**d**): catheter; (**e**): ring forceps

puterized tomography enema (MDCT-e) [8], and computed tomographic colonography (CTC) [9].

However, RWC-TVS causes significantly higher intensity of pain in women with rectovaginal nodules infiltrating the rectum than in those with only rectovaginal endometriosis and in those without endometriosis [7].

In 2008 an Italian prospective study proposed the use of RWC-TVS in the diagnosis of rectal infiltration in 35 women with rectovaginal endometriosis [6]. The sensitivity of RWC-TVS in identifying rectal infiltration reaching at least the muscular layer was 100% and the specificity was 85.7% (Table 6.1). RWC-TVS underestimated the depth of infiltration in nodules reaching the submucosa at histopathology but it reliably estimated the largest diameter of the nodules. Subsequently, a prospective study compared the performance of TVS and RWC-TVS in diagnosing rectal infiltration of patients with rectovaginal endometriosis [7]. Two ultrasonographers independently performed the exams. One operator performed TVS; after the completion of this exam, a second examiner performed RWC-TVS; laparoscopic findings were used as the gold standard. Out of 90 patients included in the study, 69 had rectovaginal endometriotic nodules of which 29 had rectal infiltration. There was no significant difference in the accuracy of TVS and RWC-TVS in diagnosing rectovaginal endometriosis. In contrast, RWC-TVS was significantly more accurate than TVS in determining the presence of endometriotic nodules infiltrating the rectal wall. However, combining the results of the two techniques did not increase the sensitivity of RWC-TVS in diagnosing rectal infiltration. Both TVS and RWC-TVS agreed with histology on the largest diameter of the endometriotic nodule.

Several studies compared RWC-TVS with other imaging techniques used for the diagnosis of bowel endometriosis. A prospective study compared the performance of RWC-TVS, DCBE,

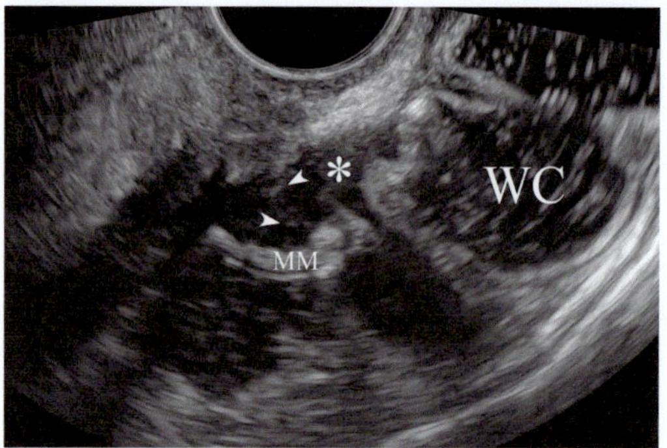

Fig. 6.2 Rectal water-contrast transvaginal ultrasonography. Hypoechoic endometriotic nodule infiltrating the muscularis mucosa (MM) of the rectum (asterisk). Some hyperechoic foci can be observed (arrowheads). The nodule does not cause a significant stenosis of the intestinal lumen (estimated stenosis: 15%). The main diameter of the nodule is 3.2 cm. WC: water contrast

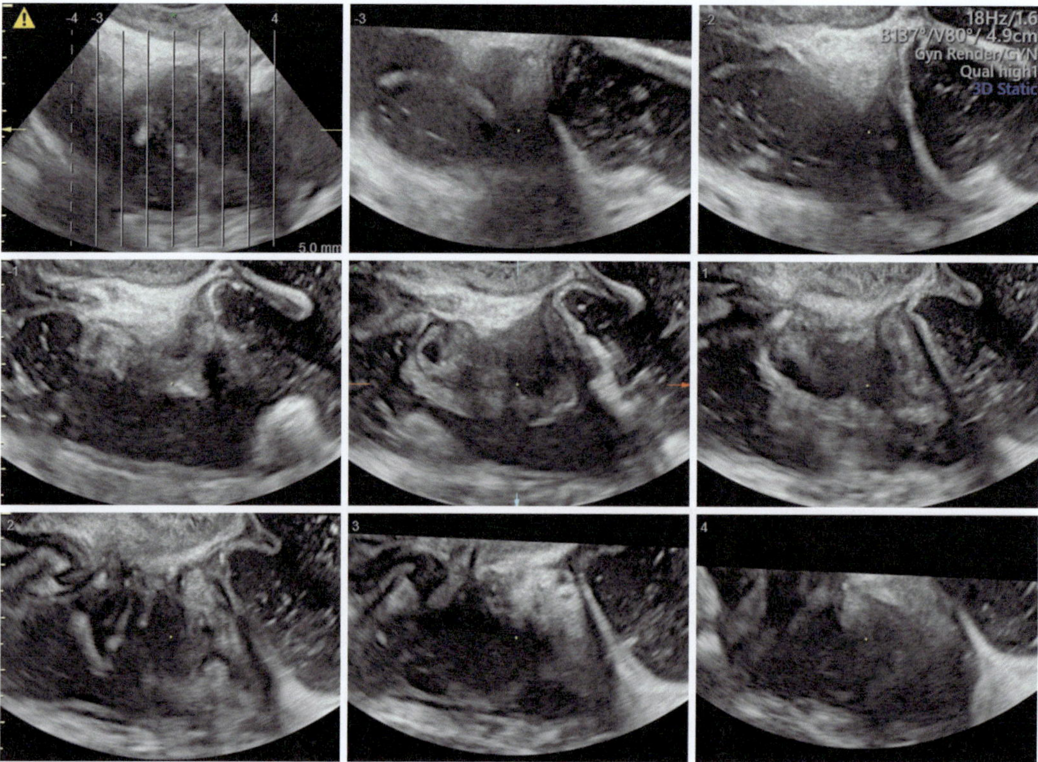

Fig. 6.3 Rectal water-contrast transvaginal ultrasonography. The tomographic ultrasound imaging allows to evaluate several sections of a rectal endometriotic nodule

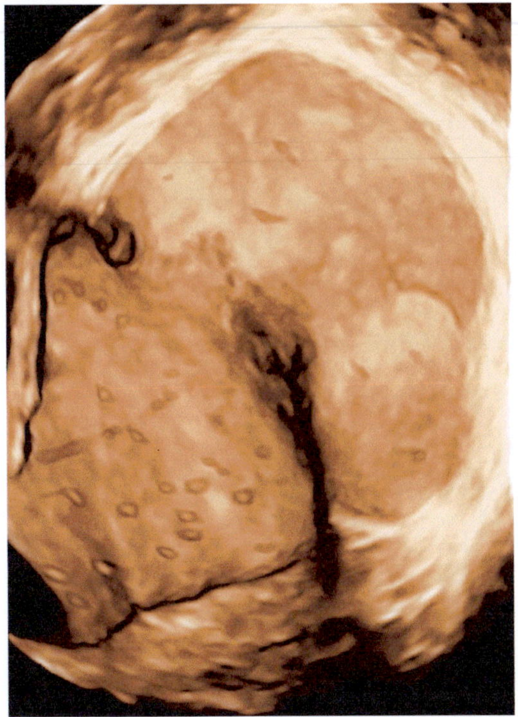

Fig. 6.4 Tridimensional rectal water-contrast transvaginal ultrasonography. Surface mode reconstruction. Normal rectum, no endometriotic lesion in observed

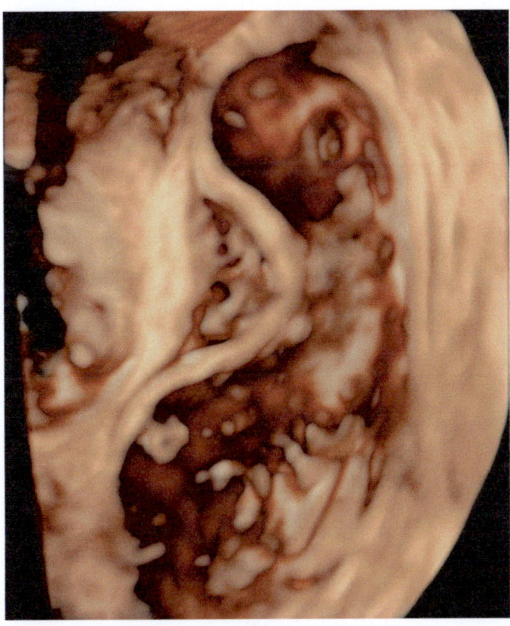

Fig. 6.5 Tridimensional rectal water-contrast transvaginal ultrasonography. Surface mode reconstruction. A rectal endometriotic nodule is observed

and transrectal sonography (TRS) in the assessment of intestinal endometriosis [12]. The study included 61 consecutive patients with clinical suspicion of deep infiltrating endometriosis. Fifty-one patients had rectosigmoid endometriosis at surgery. RWC-TVS identified 49 cases of rectosigmoid endometriosis. Out of 16 patients that required intestinal segmental resection due to a stenosis confirmed at histopathology, a ≥50% lumen restriction was preoperatively detected by RWC-TVS in 14 women. RWC-TVS and TRS were similarly accurate in the diagnosis of rectosigmoid endometriosis and in identifying a significant stenosis of the intestinal lumen (Fig. 6.6). An Italian prospective study (96 patients, 51 with bowel endometriosis) compared the accuracy of RWC-TVS and MDCT-e in diagnosing bowel endometriosis [8]. Obviously, two ileal lesions and one cecal lesion were not detected by RWC-TVS. Overall, the two techniques had similar accuracy in diagnosing bowel endometriosis; moreover, there was no significant difference in the performance of RWC-TVS and MDCT-e in estimating the depth of infiltration of endometriosis in the intestinal wall. Both MDCT-e and RWC-TVS underestimated the largest diameter of the endometriotic nodules; however, the underestimation was greater for RWC-TVS than for MDCT-e; in both imaging techniques the underestimation was greater for nodules with diameter ≥30 mm. The two techniques had similar performance in identifying multifocal disease. More recently, a prospective study including 70 women with suspicion of rectosigmoid endometriosis compared the performance of RWC-TVS and computer tomographic colonography (CTC) in the assessment of rectosigmoid endometriosis [9]. The two techniques had similar performance in diagnosing rectosigmoid endometriosis and in estimating the length of the endometriotic nodules. Nevertheless, CTC was more precise than RWC-TVS in estimating the distance between the lower margin of the endometriotic nodule and the anal verge; RWC-TVS was more accurate than CTC in the diagnosis of multifocal rectosigmoid endometriosis. A Chinese prospective study including 198 patients compared the accuracy of RWC-TVS and DCBE in assessing the presence

Table 6.1 Diagnostic performance of rectal water-contrast transvaginal ultrasonography in the diagnosis of rectosigmoid endometriosis

	Study population	Sensitivity	Specificity	PPV	NPV	Accuracy	LR+	LR−
Valenzano Menada et al. [6]	35 women with rectovaginal endometriosis	100.0%	85.7%	91.3%	100.0%	–	–	–
Valenzano Menada et al. [7]	90 women with suspicion of rectovaginal endometriosis	95.7%	100%	100.0%	98.5%	98.9%	–[a]	0.04
Bergamini et al. [12]	61 women with suspicion of posterior deep infiltrating endometriosis	96.1%	90.0%	98.0%	81.8%	–	–	–
Ferrero et al. [8]	96 women with suspicion of bowel endometriosis	93.8%	97.9%	97.8%	94.0%	95.8%	45.00	0.06
Leone Roberti Maggiore et al. [10]	286 women with suspicion of rectosigmoid endometriosis	92.7%	97.0%	97.2%	92.3%	94.8%	31.29	0.08
Ferrero et al. [9]	70 women with suspicion of intestinal endometriosis	92.5%	96.7%	97.4%	90.6%	94.3%	27.8	0.08
Jiang et al. [14]	198 patients with clinical suspicion of intestinal endometriosis	88.2%	97.3%	98.0%	88.0%	92.4%	41.67	0.13
Barra et al. [17]	36 women with clinical suspicion of rectosigmoid endometriosis	90.1%	78.6%	87.0%	84.6%	86.1%	42.0	0.11

PPV positive predictive value, *NPV* negative predictive value, *LR+* positive likelihood ratio, *LR−* negative likelihood ratio
[a]LR+ could not be calculated because of the absence of false positive cases

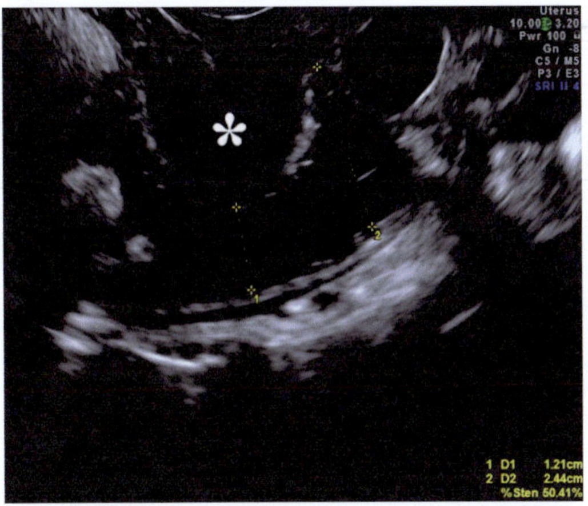

Fig. 6.6 Rectal water-contrast transvaginal ultrasonography. Hypoechoic rectosigmoid endometriotic (asterisk). The estimated stenosis of the intestinal lumen is approximately 50%. The intestinal lumen is measured at the level of the nodule (1.2 cm) and distally to the nodule (2.4 cm)

and characteristics of bowel endometriosis [14]. The two techniques had comparable accuracy in diagnosing bowel endometriosis. RWC-TVS did not identify four ileal lesions and two cecal lesions. There was no significant difference in the performance of the two techniques in assessing the depth of infiltration of endometriosis in the intestinal wall; DCBE correctly defined the infiltration depth in 50.9% of the patients and RWC-TVS correctly defined the infiltration depth in 37.7% of the patients. Both techniques underestimated the largest diameter of the endometriotic nodules; nevertheless, the underestimation was smaller for DCBE than for RWC-TVS. In both techniques, the underestimation was larger for the nodules with the diameter ≥30 mm. A large Italian prospective study compared the performance of RWC-TVS and magnetic resonance enema (MR-e) in the assessment of rectosigmoid endometriosis [10]. Two hundred and eighty six patients with clinical suspicion of rectosigmoid endometriosis were included in the study; 51 of them had bowel endometriosis at surgery. Overall, the two techniques had similar performance in the diagnosis of rectosigmoid endometriosis. RWC-TVS was more accurate than MR-e in the detection of infiltration of the mucosal layer. Both techniques underestimated the size of the endometriotic nodules; the underestimation

was greater for nodules with diameter ≥30 mm for both imaging techniques.

Quite recently, some authors proposed the use of tridimensional ultrasonography during RWC-TVS (3D-RWC-TVS) [16]. These authors suggested that 3D-RWC-TVS compared with 2D-RWC-TVS may provide a better characterization of the lesions (such as measurement of the diameter in three planes, estimation of the volume of the nodule and of the stenosis of the bowel lumen). In a prospective study including 50 women with clinical suspicion of endometriosis, 3D-RWC-TVS was compared with MRI combined with vaginal opacification [11]. Unfortunately, the imaging findings were not compared with surgical results. There was a concordance rate of 96% between the two techniques. Using MRI as the reference technique, 3D-RWC-TVS had sensitivity of 95%, specificity of 97%, positive predictive value (PPV) of 95%, negative predictive value (NPV) of 97%, positive likelihood ratio (LR+) of 30.3, and negative likelihood ratio (LR−) of 0.05. However, a recent prospective pilot study published in the abstract form suggested that tridimensional acquisition does not improve the performance of RWC-TVS in the diagnosis of rectosigmoid endometriosis [17]. In this small trial, 36 women with symptoms suggestive of rectosigmoid endometriosis underwent 2D- and 3D-RWC-TVS, which were independently performed by different examiners. The two techniques had similar performance in the diagnosis of rectosigmoid endometriosis, in estimating the volume of the largest intestinal nodule, and in estimating the distance between the lower endometriotic nodule and the anal verge (Fig. 6.7a, b). Future studies should compare the performance of the two techniques in estimating the stenosis of the intestinal lumen (Fig. 6.8a, b).

In conclusion, the above-mentioned studies show that RWC-TVS is accurate in the diagnosis of rectosigmoid endometriosis (Table 6.1). Furthermore, it allows to estimate the depth of infiltration of endometriosis in the intestinal wall (particularly, the infiltration of the submucosa) and the largest diameter of the nodules; nevertheless, other techniques (such as CTC)

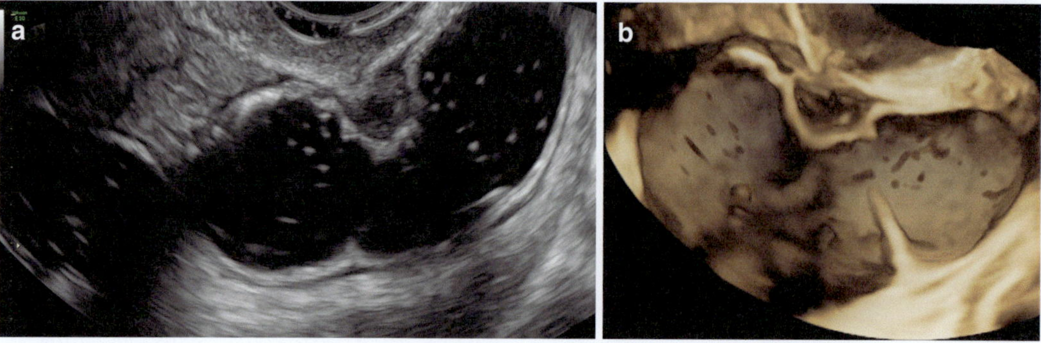

Fig. 6.7 (a) Bidimensional rectal water-contrast transvaginal ultrasonography demonstrating a hypoechoic endometriotic nodule infiltrating the muscularis mucosa of the rectum. (b) Tridimensional rectal water-contrast transvaginal ultrasonography. The surface mode reconstruction demonstrated the endometriotic nodule shown in (a)

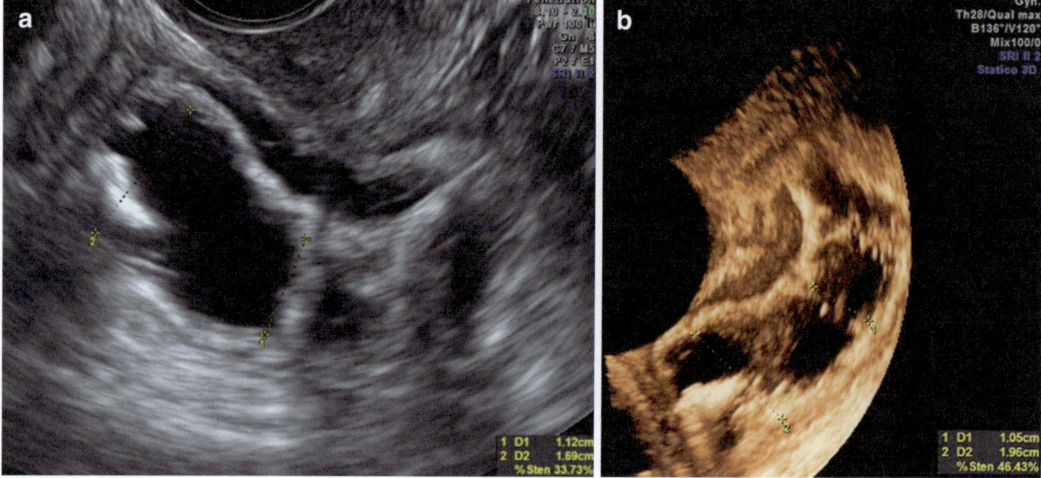

Fig. 6.8 (a) Bowel stenosis estimated at bidimensional rectal water-contrast transvaginal ultrasonography. (b) Bowel stenosis estimated at three-dimensional rectal water-contrast transvaginal ultrasonography

may be more precise in estimating the distance between the more distal endometriotic nodule and the anal verge.

6.3 Tenderness-Guided Transvaginal Ultrasonography

Ten years ago, this ultrasound technique was proposed to improve the diagnosis of posterior deep infiltrating endometriosis. tg-TVS consists in the introduction of 12 mL of ultrasound gel (instead of the usual 3–4 mL) into the probe cover (usually a finger of a latex glove) to create a stand-off to visualize the near-field area. The probe must be gently inserted into the vagina to avoid the risk of squeezing out the gel. The exam is performed with a sliding up-and-down movement of the probe [18, 19]. tg-TVS is considered a dynamic technique; in fact, during the exam the patient is requested to inform the examiner about the onset and site of any tenderness experienced during probe's gentle pressure in the posterior vaginal fornix; when tenderness is evoked, attention should be given to the painful site in order to detect endometriotic lesions [18, 19].

An Italian single-center prospective study including 50 women scheduled for laparoscopy because of chronic pelvic pain investigated the accuracy of tg-TVS in the diagnosis of deep infiltrating endometriosis. Seven patients had rectal infiltration at laparoscopy; all these nodules were identified by tg-TVS [18]. In another single-center prospective study including 88 women with clinically suspected endometriosis (39 with rectosigmoid endometriosis), tg-TVS had good specificity and quite low sensitivity in identifying rectosigmoid involvement (specificity 91.8%, sensitivity 66.7%, LR+ 8.17, LR− 0.36). More recently, a prospective study compared the diagnostic performance of tg-TVS and MRI in the diagnosis of rectosigmoid endometriosis [20]. Out of 59 patients included in the study, 30 had rectosigmoid endometriosis. tg-TVS identified rectosigmoid endometriosis in 22 patients. Therefore, in eight patients the nodules were not identified by tg-TVS; one lesion was located in the midrectum, three in the rectosigmoid junction, and the remaining four in the sigmoid; moreover, tg-TVS gave false positive results in four patients. Overall, there was no significant difference in the specificity and sensitivity of both exams in diagnosing rectosigmoid endometriosis. Specifically, tg-TVS obtained a specificity of 86%, a sensitivity of 73%, a LR+ of 5.317 and a LR− of 0.309 for the diagnosis of rectosigmoid endometriosis was:

6.4 Sonovaginography

SVG was introduced almost 20 years ago for the assessment of rectovaginal endometriosis [21].

Some authors perform a bowel preparation before this exam, such as an oral laxative administered on the night before the exam and/or a rectal enema administered few hours before the exam [22].

The original description of SVG consists in a transvaginal ultrasonographic exam combined with the introduction of saline solution in the vagina [21]. During the exam, the seat is slightly tilted in anti-Trendelenburg position to avoid saline solution reflux from the vagina [21, 23].

Some authors prefer to have a partially empty bladder during the exam as a small amount of urine may enhance the visualization of the anterior vaginal wall and the vesiscovaginal septum [21]. In contrast, other authors prefer emptying the bladder before the exam [23]. In the original description, a 24-mm Foley catheter is introduced into the vagina and its balloon is inflated using 5–6 mL of saline solution. An examiner and an assistant are required to perform each exam. The examiner inserts the transvaginal probe into the vagina using the right hand and closes the vaginal channel with the left hand, narrowing the minor labia with the dorsal surface of the forefinger and the middle finger. This procedure prevents the reflux of saline solution from the vagina. The assistant injects 200–400 mL of saline solution through a Foley catheter and operates the ultrasound machine. Notably, during the exam the transvaginal probe should not be in contact with the uterine cervix [21]. Other techniques of saline solution-based SVG have been proposed: in particular, some authors insert in the posterior vaginal fornix a condom attached to a saline giving set; then, the transvaginal probe is inserted into the vagina superior to the condom that rests against the posterior vaginal wall; when the transvaginal probe is in situ, the condom is filled with 200–400 mL of saline solution [23]. Other authors performed SVG using a purpose-designed hydraulic ring (Colpo-Pneumo Occluder, Cooper Surgical, Berlin, Germany) located at the base of the transvaginal probe; approximately 40 mL of saline solution are injected into the ring in order to prevent the escape of the saline solution (60–120 mL) that is subsequently injected into the vagina using a Foley catheter [24].

A modified SVG consist in the use of ultrasound gel instead of saline solution: in particular, a 20-mL syringe is filled with ultrasound gel with minimal air bubbles within [25]. The syringe is then introduced in the vagina and gently pushed as deeply as possible inside along the posterior vaginal wall. Approximately 20–60 mL of ultrasound gel is thus placed in the upper vagina mainly in the posterior fornix (Fig. 6.9) [22, 25–29]. Too many air bubbles accidentally introduced in the ultrasound gel may hamper proper

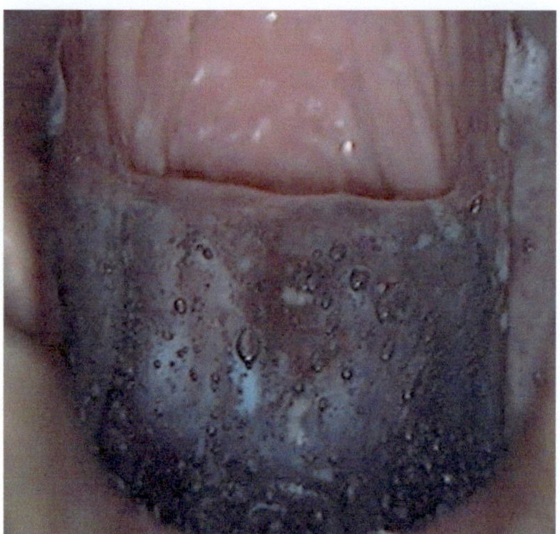

Fig. 6.9 Sonovaginography with ultrasound gel. The ultrasonographic gel in injected along the posterior vaginal wall, mainly in the posterior vaginal fornix

evaluation. In these cases, repeating the procedure in the same sitting is usually not helpful in dismissing the air bubbles. Therefore, it is necessary to repeat the exam on the following day.

The saline solution or ultrasonographic gel introduced in the vagina creates an acoustic window between the probe and the surrounding structures. In addition, it exerts a pressure that is able to distend the vaginal walls [21, 24, 26].

SVG is well tolerated by the patients. Some authors used a VAS scale to estimate the intensity of pain caused by SVG demonstrating that this exam causes an intensity of pain of approximately 2.1 cm [24].

In the study proposing for the first time the use of SVG with saline solution in the diagnosis of deep infiltrating endometriosis, only three patients (out of 46 included in the study) had rectal endometriosis. Bowel infiltration was diagnosed preoperatively by SVG in two patients (66.6%) [21]. Other studies investigating the performance of SVG in the diagnosis of deep endometriosis did not assess the performance of SVG in diagnosing intestinal infiltration [23]. An Italian single-center prospective study including 102 women (six patients with rectosigmoid endometriosis) compared the performance of TVS, SVG with saline solution and MRI in the diagnosis of posterior deep infiltrating endometriosis

[24]. Overall, SVG had modest sensitivity and good specificity in diagnosing rectosigmoid endometriosis (sensitivity 66.7%, specificity 93.8%, PPV 57.1%, NPV 95.7%, LR+ 10.66 and LR− 0.355). A multicenter prospective study investigated the performance of SVG with gel in the diagnosis of posterior deep infiltrating endometriosis [29]. Two hundred and twenty consecutive women with clinical suspicion of deep endometriosis were recruited for the study; laparoscopic findings were used as the gold standard. Definitive data were available for 189 women; 43 of them had rectosigmoid endometriosis at surgery. The sensitivity of SVG in diagnosing rectosigmoid endometriosis was 88.4%, the specificity 93.2%, the PPV 79.2%, the NPV 96.5%, the LR+ 12.9%, and the LR− 0.12%. In this study, the accuracy of SVG was higher in the diagnosis of rectosigmoid endometriosis compared with the diagnosis of anterior rectal endometriosis. Another prospective study including 51 women with suspected deep infiltrating endometriosis (13 with surgical diagnosis of rectosigmoid endometriosis) showed that SVG has sensitivity of 100%, specificity of 93%, and LR+ of 14.0 in detecting rectosigmoid involvement (Fig. 6.10) [22]. A Romanian multicenter prospective study compared the accuracy of TVS and SVG with gel in the diagnosis of deep endometriosis [26]. The study included 193 women with symptoms highly suggestive for endometriosis. SVG was more accurate than TVS in diagnosing rectosigmoid endometriosis. The sensitivity of SVG was 94.0%, the specificity 95.5%, the PPV 91.0%,

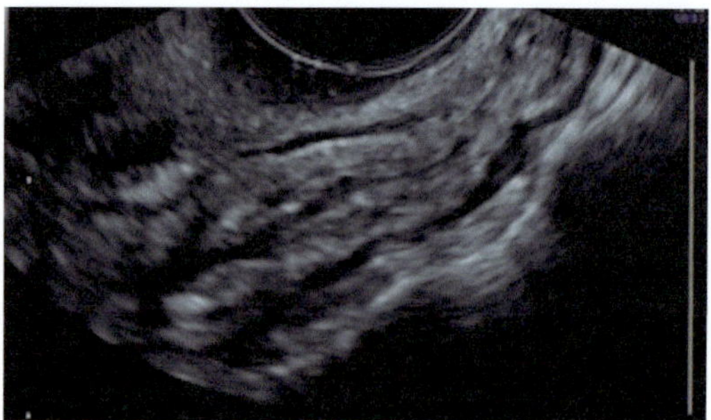

Fig. 6.10 Sonovaginography with ultrasound gel and bowel preparation. The vaginal wall and both rectal walls can be visualized

and the NPV 97.2%. More recently, a Portuguese single-center prospective study including 59 women (eight with rectosigmoid endometriosis) investigated the performance of SVG with gel in the diagnosis of deep infiltrating endometriosis [28]. The sensitivity of SVG in diagnosing rectosigmoid endometriosis was 50%, the specificity 82%, the LR+ 2.75, and the LR− 0.61.

In conclusion, SVG is accurate in the diagnosis of rectosigmoid endometriosis. However, the experience of the examiner is relevant for the diagnosis; in fact, some examiners reported high sensitivity [29] while other reported poor sensitivity [28]. Moreover, no study compared saline solution-based and ultrasound-based SVG in the diagnosis of rectosigmoid endometriosis; therefore, there is no evidence that one technique is superior to the other. However, the use of ultrasound gel may facilitate the exam. In fact, the ultrasound gel is less likely to reflux from the vagina compared with the saline solution. As a consequence, there is no need to narrow the minor labia during the exam which can be performed by a single operator.

6.5 Conclusion

Enhanced TVS techniques are easy to perform and they are cheap. Nevertheless, these techniques may cause some pain because of the distention of the rectosigmoid in RWC-TVS or the compression of the nodules in tg-TVS. However, these exams are generally well tolerated so that they can be routinely performed without anesthesia. An obvious limitation of enhanced TVS techniques is that they cannot diagnose endometriotic nodules located above the rectosigmoid as they are beyond the field of view of ultrasonography. Therefore, when multicentric disease (endometriotic nodules in different bowel segments) is suspected, additional techniques (such as computed tomographic colonoscopy or DCBE) should be used in order to investigate the whole colon [9].

The studies described in this chapter confirm that enhanced TVS techniques (in particular, RWC-TVS) have good performance in the diagnosis of rectosigmoid endometriosis. A recent meta-analysis showed that TVS and enhanced TVS techniques have similar accuracy in diagnosing rectosigmoid endometriosis; however, enhanced techniques seem to add useful information in the preoperative evaluation of patients with deep infiltrating endometriosis (such as the estimation of bowel stenosis) [30]. Surprisingly, no study compared the performance of different enhanced techniques in the diagnosis of rectosigmoid endometriosis. In the near future, a study comparing RWC-TVS and SVG would be advisable.

References

1. Ferrero S, Arena E, Morando A, Remorgida V. Prevalence of newly diagnosed endometriosis in women attending the general practitioner. Int J Gynaecol Obstet. 2010;110(3):203–7.
2. Chapron C, Dubuisson JB, Pansini V, Vieira M, Fauconnier A, Barakat H, et al. Routine clinical examination is not sufficient for diagnosing and locating deeply infiltrating endometriosis. J Am Assoc Gynecol Laparosc. 2002;9(2):115–9.
3. Guerriero S, Condous G, Van den Bosch T, Valentin L, Leone FP, Van Schoubroeck D, et al. Systematic approach to sonographic evaluation of the pelvis in women with suspected endometriosis, including terms, definitions and measurements: a consensus opinion from the International Deep Endometriosis Analysis (IDEA) group. Ultrasound Obstet Gynecol. 2016;48:318.
4. Guerriero S, Pascual MA, Ajossa S, Rodriguez I, Zajicek M, Rolla M, et al. Learning curve for ultrasonographic diagnosis of deep infiltrating endometriosis using structured offline training program. Ultrasound Obstet Gynecol. 2019;54(2):262–9.
5. Ferrero S, Leone Roberti Maggiore U, Barra F, Scala C. Modified ultrasonographic techniques. In: Guerriero S, Condous G, Alcazar JL, editors. How to perform ultrasonography in endometriosis. New York, NY: Springer; 2018. p. 133–45.
6. Menada MV, Remorgida V, Abbamonte LH, Fulcheri E, Ragni N, Ferrero S. Transvaginal ultrasonography combined with water-contrast in the rectum in the diagnosis of rectovaginal endometriosis infiltrating the bowel. Fertil Steril. 2008;89(3):699–700.
7. Valenzano Menada M, Remorgida V, Abbamonte LH, Nicoletti A, Ragni N, Ferrero S. Does transvaginal ultrasonography combined with water-contrast in the rectum aid in the diagnosis of rectovaginal endometriosis infiltrating the bowel? Hum Reprod. 2008;23(5):1069–75.
8. Ferrero S, Biscaldi E, Morotti M, Venturini PL, Remorgida V, Rollandi GA, et al. Multidetector computerized tomography enteroclysis vs. rectal water

contrast transvaginal ultrasonography in determining the presence and extent of bowel endometriosis. Ultrasound Obstet Gynecol. 2011;37(5):603–13.

9. Ferrero S, Biscaldi E, Vellone VG, Venturini PL, Leone Roberti Maggiore U. Computed tomographic colonography vs rectal water- contrast transvaginal sonography in diagnosis of rectosigmoid endometriosis: a pilot study. Ultrasound Obstet Gynecol. 2017;49(4):515–23.

10. Leone Roberti Maggiore U, Biscaldi E, Vellone VG, Venturini PL, Ferrero S. Magnetic resonance enema vs rectal water-contrast transvaginal sonography in diagnosis of rectosigmoid endometriosis. Ultrasound Obstet Gynecol. 2017;49(4):524–32.

11. Philip CA, Bisch C, Coulon A, de Saint-Hilaire P, Rudigoz RC, Dubernard G. Correlation between three-dimensional rectosonography and magnetic resonance imaging in the diagnosis of rectosigmoid endometriosis: a preliminary study on the first fifty cases. Eur J Obstet Gynecol Reprod Biol. 2015;187:35–40.

12. Bergamini V, Ghezzi F, Scarperi S, Raffaelli R, Cromi A, Franchi M. Preoperative assessment of intestinal endometriosis: a comparison of transvaginal sonography with water-contrast in the rectum, transrectal sonography, and barium enema. Abdom Imaging. 2010;35(6):732–6.

13. Ferrero S, Barra F, Stabilini C, Vellone VG, Leone Roberti Maggiore U, Scala C. Does bowel preparation improve the performance of rectal water contrast transvaginal ultrasonography in diagnosing rectosigmoid endometriosis? J Ultrasound Med. 2019;38:1017.

14. Jiang J, Liu Y, Wang K, Wu X, Tang Y. Rectal water contrast transvaginal ultrasound versus double-contrast barium enema in the diagnosis of bowel endometriosis. BMJ Open. 2017;7(9):e017216.

15. Ferrero S, Leone Roberti Maggiore U, Scala C, Di Luca M, Venturini PL, Remorgida V. Changes in the size of rectovaginal endometriotic nodules infiltrating the rectum during hormonal therapies. Arch Gynecol Obstet. 2013;287(3):447–53.

16. Philip CA, Bisch C, Coulon A, Maissiat E, de Saint-Hilaire P, Huissoud C, et al. Three-dimensional sonorectography: a new transvaginal ultrasound technique with intrarectal contrast to assess colorectal endometriosis. Ultrasound Obstet Gynecol. 2015;45(2):233–5.

17. Barra F, Scala C, Vellone GV, Ferrero S. Bidimensional rectal-water contrast-transvaginal ultrasonography (2D-RWC-TVS) versus 3D-RWC-TVS in the diagnosis of rectosigmoid endometriosis: a pilot prospective comparative study. Hum Reprod. 2019;34(Suppl):i61.

18. Guerriero S, Ajossa S, Gerada M, D'Aquila M, Piras B, Melis GB. "Tenderness-guided" transvaginal ultrasonography: a new method for the detection of deep endometriosis in patients with chronic pelvic pain. Fertil Steril. 2007;88(5):1293–7.

19. Guerriero S, Ajossa S, Gerada M, Virgilio B, Angioni S, Melis GB. Diagnostic value of transvaginal 'tenderness-guided' ultrasonography for the prediction of location of deep endometriosis. Hum Reprod. 2008;23(11):2452–7.

20. Saba L, Guerriero S, Sulcis R, Pilloni M, Ajossa S, Melis G, et al. MRI and "tenderness guided" transvaginal ultrasonography in the diagnosis of rectosigmoid endometriosis. J Magn Reson Imaging. 2012;35(2):352–60.

21. Dessole S, Farina M, Rubattu G, Cosmi E, Ambrosini G, Nardelli GB. Sonovaginography is a new technique for assessing rectovaginal endometriosis. Fertil Steril. 2003;79(4):1023–7.

22. Leon M, Vaccaro H, Alcazar JL, Martinez J, Gutierrez J, Amor F, et al. Extended transvaginal sonography in deep infiltrating endometriosis: use of bowel preparation and an acoustic window with intravaginal gel: preliminary results. J Ultrasound Med. 2014;33(2):315–21.

23. Reid S, Bignardi T, Lu C, Lam A, Condous G. The use of intra-operative saline sonovaginography to define the rectovaginal septum in women with suspected rectovaginal endometriosis: a pilot study. Australias J Ultrasound Med. 2011;14(3):4–9.

24. Saccardi C, Cosmi E, Borghero A, Tregnaghi A, Dessole S, Litta P. Comparison between transvaginal sonography, saline contrast sonovaginography and magnetic resonance imaging in the diagnosis of posterior deep infiltrating endometriosis. Ultrasound Obstet Gynecol. 2012;40(4):464–9.

25. Sibal M. Gel sonovaginography: a new way of evaluating a variety of local vaginal and cervical disorders. J Ultrasound Med. 2016;35(12):2699–715.

26. Bratila E, Comandasu DE, Coroleuca C, Cirstoiu MM, Berceanu C, Mehedintu C, et al. Diagnosis of endometriotic lesions by sonovaginography with ultrasound gel. Med Ultrason. 2016;18:469–74.

27. Goncalves MO, Dias JA Jr, Podgaec S, Averbach M, Abrao MS. Transvaginal ultrasound for diagnosis of deeply infiltrating endometriosis. Int J Gynaecol Obstet. 2009;104(2):156–60.

28. Cruz J, Moreira C, Cunha R, Ferreira J, Martinho M, Beires J. Diagnostic accuracy of sonovaginography for deep infiltrating endometriosis. Acta Obstet Ginecol Port. 2018;12(3):190–4.

29. Reid S, Lu C, Hardy N, Casikar I, Reid G, Cario G, et al. Office gel sonovaginography for the prediction of posterior deep infiltrating endometriosis: a multicenter prospective observational study. Ultrasound Obstet Gynecol. 2014;44(6):710–8.

30. Guerriero S, Ajossa S, Orozco R, Perniciano M, Jurado M, Melis GB, et al. Accuracy of transvaginal ultrasound for diagnosis of deep endometriosis in the rectosigmoid: systematic review and meta-analysis. Ultrasound Obstet Gynecol. 2016;47(3): 281–9.

Magnetic Resonance Imaging

7

Cendos Abdel-Wahab, Cyril Touboul, Edwige Pottier,
Edith Kermarrec, Audrey Milon, Asma Bekhouche,
and Isabelle Thomassin-Naggara

7.1 Introduction

Pelvic endometriosis is defined by the presence of endometrial tissue outside the endometrium and myometrium [1]. This phenomenon affects around 10% [1] of women of reproductive age, increasing to 35–50% in symptomatic patients [2, 3]. Pelvic endometriosis can be split into three main entities: peritoneal, ovarian, or deep endometriosis.

The most common locations of endometriosis are the ovaries and the pelvic peritoneum, fol-

lowed in order of decreasing frequency by deep lesions of the pelvic subperitoneal space, the intestinal system, and the urinary system. Deep pelvic endometriosis, or deep infiltrating endometriosis, is defined as infiltration of the implant of endometriosis more than 5 mm under the surface of the peritoneum [4]. Peritoneal endometriosis can be asymptomatic, but in most of cases, deep pelvic endometriosis is symptomatic including chronic pelvic pain, dysmenorrhea, dyspareunia, dyschezia, and urinary symptoms and is associated with infertility [5]. Around 20% of women with pelvic endometriosis are affected by deep endometriosis.

Deep pelvic endometriosis is mainly characterized by fibromuscular hyperplasia that surrounds foci of endometriosis, and the foci sometimes contain small cavities [4] on histologic findings. Diagnosis of the extension of deep pelvic endometriosis can be made by clinical examination and laparoscopic exploration. Among the different locations of deep infiltrating endometriosis, bowel endometriosis is one of the most severe forms [5] and is the most common site of extragenital endometriosis [6]. In women with deep infiltrating endometriosis [7, 8], bowel endometriosis affects between 12% and 37% [7] of women. The most frequent bowel locations of deep infiltrating endometriosis are the rectum and the rectosigmoid junction (52.0–65.7%), followed by the sigmoid colon (17.4–19.4%), ileum (4.1–16.9%), caecum (4.7–6.2%), and

C. Abdel-Wahab · E. Kermarrec · A. Milon
A. Bekhouche
Department of Radiology, APHP, Hôpital Tenon,
Paris, France
e-mail: cendos.abdelwahab@aphp.fr; edith.
kermarrec@aphp.fr; audrey.milon@aphp.fr; asma.
bekhouche@aphp.fr

C. Touboul
Department of Gynecology and Obstetrics, APHP
Sorbonne Université, Hopital Tenon, Paris, France
e-mail: cyril.touboul@aphp.fr

E. Pottier
Department of Radiology, APHP, Hôpital Tenon,
Paris, France

Departement of Radiology, Centre Hospitalier
Intercommunal de Créteil, Créteil, France
e-mail: edwige.pottier@chicreteil.fr

I. Thomassin-Naggara (✉)
Department of Radiology, APHP, Hôpital Tenon,
Paris, France

Department of Radiology, APHP Sorbonne Université,
Site Tenon, Paris, France
e-mail: isabelle.thomassin@aphp.fr

© Springer Nature Switzerland AG 2020
S. Ferrero, M. Ceccaroni (eds.), *Clinical Management of Bowel Endometriosis*,
https://doi.org/10.1007/978-3-030-50446-5_7

appendix (5.0–6.4%) [6, 9]. Up to 55% of patients with rectal endometriosis [8, 10] have bowel deep infiltrating endometriosis multifocal lesions. Around 28% of the rectal and sigmoid lesions are associated with right-sided bowel endometriosis [9] involvement of the appendix, cecum, and ileum. During laparoscopy, additional lesions are detected in up to 20% of patients representing either multifocal (i.e., multiple endometriotic lesions affecting the same segment) or multicentric (i.e., endometriotic lesions affecting several digestive segments) bowel endometriosis [11].

7.2 Clinical Challenges

Symptomatic patients with or without suggestive clinical examination, require additional routine investigations to make the diagnosis and determine the optimal therapeutic strategy. During the two last decades, many papers demonstrated the value of diagnostic imaging including transvaginal sonography (TVS) and MR imaging (MRI), to assess deep endometriosis locations [12–16]. Recent advances in imaging techniques may replace the gold standard of diagnostic laparoscopy for some locations of deep endometriosis.

For patient with endometriosis requiring surgical management, the success in providing long-term symptomatic relief, good quality of life, and fertility is correlated with the radicality of deep infiltrating endometriosis excision for all lesions [17, 18]. It is a challenge to diagnose bowel endometriosis because the patient may be asymptomatic or because the symptoms may not be specific to the lesion locations, particularly lesions located above the rectosigmoid junction [19]. Thus, for gynecologic surgeons, complete preoperative imaging workup is crucial to identify all sites when bowel endometriosis is suspected. Moreover, the preoperative mapping of lesions is crucial for adequate preoperative information of patients. It can determine the risk of multiple bowel resection (detect multifocal bowel endometriosis) and the potential need for a protective defunctioning stoma, and thus guide surgical management [20]. Laterally, further involvement of the deep parametrium or vagina are at risk of postoperative urinary dysfunction [21]. It will serve to inform the patient of the risks of undergoing a one-step pelvis and bowel procedure [22].

For focal rectal or rectosigmoid junction deep infiltrating endometriosis lesions, the first treatment for a superficial infiltration into the muscularis propria may be a shaving of the wall or discoid anterior resection. Alternatively, for deeper infiltrations and other deep infiltrating endometriosis bowel locations, bowel resection is typically performed [9, 22].

The extent of indications for conservative surgery (rectal shaving or discoid resection) is a major point as several retrospective studies have demonstrated the advantages of this surgery including: a shorter operating time, fewer postoperative complications, less postoperative voiding dysfunction, and improved digestive functional outcomes [23].

Multifocal colorectal endometriosis renders conservative surgery less feasible and segmental resection is often required [24]. Several authors have advocated conservative surgery only if the lesions are under 30 mm [23, 25]. A combined technique associating rectal shaving of the serosal component and discoid resection of the remaining infiltrating bowel component with automatic endoscopic stapling and the possibility of two consecutive discoid resections on the same lesion, is an option to remove colorectal endometriosis lesions over 30 mm [26].

Multicentric lesions also represent a surgical challenge especially for patients with ileocecal lesions. This diagnosis may lead to multiple resections with a higher risk of postoperative complications, alterations in digestive function, and the need for a defunctioning stoma [20].

7.3 MRI

In patients with previous equivocal transvaginal sonography, MRI is recommended as a second-line technique in the preoperative workup of deep endometriosis (Grade A) [27].

Bazot and al. [12] obtained for diagnosis deep pelvic endometriosis on MRI a sensitivity, a specificity, a positive predictive value, a negative predictive value, and an accuracy, respectively, of 90.3%, 91%, 92.1%, 89%, and 90.8%.

Rectal and rectosigmoid junction lesions can be thoroughly explored with pelvic magnetic resonance (MR) imaging, which is typically performed to diagnose pelvic deep infiltrating endometriosis [7, 12, 28].

The sensitivity, specificity, positive and negative predictive values, and accuracy of MR imaging for the diagnosis of intestinal involvement compared with pathologic findings were 95%, 100%, 100%, 98.7%, and 99.0%, respectively [12].

7.3.1 Standard MRI

7.3.1.1 MRI Protocol

European Society of Urogenital Radiology (ESUR) [27], experts in gynecological imaging and a gynecologist expert in methodology. The group discussed indications for MRI, technical requirements, patient preparation, MRI protocols, and criteria for the diagnosis of pelvic endometriosis on MRI. The expert panel proposed a final recommendation for each criterion using Oxford Centre for Evidence Based Medicine (OCEBM) 2011 levels of evidence (Table 7.1).

Recommendations for technical requirements:

- **1.5 and 3.0 T systems** seem valuable for the evaluation of deep pelvic endometriosis; however, studies comparing the systems are lacking. Therefore, no recommendation can be made for the use of a specific device and further work is necessary to perform this comparison.
- **Array type:** Pelvic phased array coils are recommended in the evaluation of deep pelvic endometriosis at both 1.5 and 3.0 T (grade C).
- **Timing of MRI examination:** No recommendation can be proposed for timing of MRI in relation to the menstrual cycle in the evaluation of deep pelvic endometriosis.
- **Patient preparation:** There is no consensus regarding patient preparation before MRI. The committee feels that the protocol should be tailored to the main indication for pelvic MRI

Table 7.1 Optimal magnetic resonance imaging protocol in the diagnosis of pelvis endometriosis [12]

MRI protocol	Recommendation (grade)
Technical requirements	
Device: 1.5 or 3.0 T	No recommendation
Phased-array coil	Standard (C)
Timing of MRI examination	No recommendation
Fasting	Standard (B)
Moderately full bladder	Standard (C)
Bowel enema	"Best pratice" (GPP)
Supine position	Standard (B)
Abdominal strapping	Standard (C)
Antiperistaltic agent	Standard (C)
Vaginal opacification (gel)	Option (GPP)
Rectal opacification (water, gel)	Option (GPP)
MR sequences	
2DT2-weighted MRI (sagittal, axial, oblique)	Standard (B)
3DT2-weighted MRI	Option (C)
T1-weighted MRI without/with fat suppression	Standard (B)
Dixon technique (alternative to T1-weighted)	Standard (C)
Intravenous contrast-enhanced MRI	No recommendation
Diffusion-weighted MRI	No recommendation
Susceptibility-weighted MRI	No recommendation
Half-Fourier acquisition single shot turbo spin echo	Standard (C)

GPP good practice point, *MRI* magnetic resonance imaging

(diagnosis/staging of deep pelvic endometriosis, indeterminate adnexal mass).
- **Fasting:** Fasting is recommended in the evaluation of deep pelvic endometriosis (grade B).
- **Bowel preparation:** Bowel preparation is advocated as "best practice" for the detection of deep pelvic endometriosis (Good Practice Point (GPP)).
- **Bladder emptying:** A moderately full bladder is recommended in the evaluation of deep pelvic endometriosis (grade C).
- **Patient position:** The supine position is recommended in the evaluation of pelvic endo-

metriosis (GPP). The prone position is an "option" in claustrophobia (grade B).

- **Abdominal strapping:** Abdominal strapping is recommended in the evaluation of pelvic endometriosis (grade C).
- **Anti-peristaltic agent:** An anti-peristaltic agent is recommended in the evaluation of deep pelvic endometriosis (grade C).
- **Vaginal opacification:** Vaginal opacification with sonographic gel is considered as an "option" in the evaluation of deep pelvic endometriosis (GPP).
- **Rectal opacification:** Rectal opacification is suggested as an "option" in the evaluation of pelvic endometriosis (GPP).

Recommendations for MRI protocol:

- **T2-weighted MRI:** Three 2D-T2W MRI sequences (sagittal, axial, oblique) are recommended in the evaluation of DPE (grade B). The addition of 3D-T2W MRI sequence is proposed as an "option" (grade C).
- **T1-weighted MRI:** T1W MRI sequences without and with fat suppression are recommended in the evaluation of adnexal endometriosis (grade B). The "Dixon technique" may be used as an alternative to standard T1W sequence (grade C).
- **Intravenous contrast-enhanced MRI:** No recommendation can be achieved regarding the use of gadolinium in the evaluation of DPE. The use of gadolinium is recommended as an "option" in the evaluation of indeterminate adnexal endometriosis (grade C).
- **Diffusion-weighted MRI (DWI):** No recommendation can be achieved for the use of DWI in the evaluation of DPE.
- **Susceptibility-weighted MRI (SWI):** No recommendation can be proposed for the use of susceptibility-weighted MR imaging in the evaluation of deep endometriosis.
- **Half-Fourier acquisition single shot turbo spin echo (SSFSE, HASTE):** Half-Fourier acquisition single shot turbo spin echo is recommended for the evaluation of uterine peristalsis (grade C).

7.3.1.2 MRI Features

The diagnosis of deep pelvic endometriosis [12] is based on the combination of signal intensity and morphologic abnormalities (18):

- *Signal intensity abnormalities*: Signal intensity abnormalities include hyperintense foci that corresponded to hemorrhagic foci on T1-weighted and/or fat-suppressed T1-weighted MR images. Other abnormalities include small hyperintense cavities observed on T2-weighted MR images. Still other irregularities include tissue areas that correspond to fibrosis, with signal intensity close to that of pelvic muscle on T1- and T2-weighted MR images. These latter irregularities are observed with or without foci or cavities and with or without contrast enhancement after gadolinium-based contrast material injection.
- *Morphologic abnormalities*: Morphologic abnormalities with regular or irregular stellate margins are searched at each site of posterior or anterior deep pelvic endometriosis, including in intestinal tract involvement.

Intestinal tract involvement This includes abnormalities observed at intraperitoneal locations such as the sigmoid colon, the lower part of the sigmoid colon with rectal involvement and with or without adhesions to the posterior wall of the uterine body, and the presence of posterior wall endometriosis.

Three MR imaging patterns are observed for **bowel endometriosis** according to the site of the lesions [12]:

- The most frequent location is the **rectosigmoid junction**. In most cases the rectum is attracted forward, converged on the torus uterinus with disappearance of the fat tissue plane lying between the uterus and the rectum and sigmoid colon, and obliterates the cul-de-sac associated with USL involvement. Fluid is sometimes visualized lateral to the rectum or hanging above the fibrotic area.

The lesion itself is visualized as a thickening of the rectal wall, with disappearance of the hypointense signal of the anterior wall of the rectum and sigmoid colon on T2-weighted MR images and forms an obtuse angle with the normal wall. On transverse T2-weighted MR images, the lesion of the anterior wall of the rectum is usually located between the 10- and 2-o'clock positions; it yielded a triangular aspect, with the tip of the triangle pointing anteriorly. The aspect of the lesion is mainly fibromuscular and sometimes contains hyperintense foci on T1-weighted or fat-suppressed MR images. Gadolinium-based contrast material injection is used to prevent a false-positive diagnosis of rectal wall invasion, and to help the radiologist to clearly distinguish between the lesion and the rectal wall. The degree of extension, and particularly the dis-

tance between the lower limit of the fibrotic mass and the rectal-anal junction must be noted (Figs. 7.1 and 7.2).

- The intestinal involvement can be restricted to the **sigmoid colon**. The involvement is always located on the lower surface of the colon (Fig. 7.3). Involvement at these locations is difficult to diagnose with standard MR imaging sequences. Opacification with a water enema is very helpful in the confirmation of this diagnosis.
- The lesion can be involved in the lower part of the pouch of Douglas, and it extends downward to the anterolateral wall of **the rectum** and to the rectovaginal septum.

Less frequently, bowel involvement may interest the cecum (Fig. 7.4), ileocecal junction, or loops.

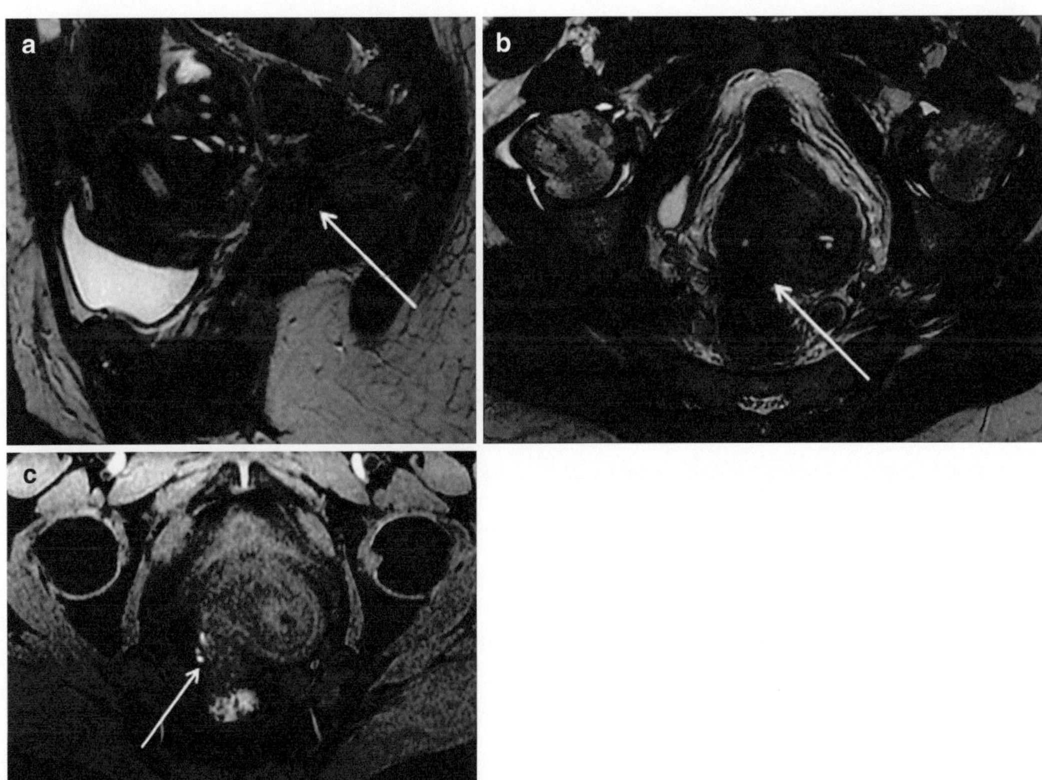

Fig. 7.1 A 26-year-old woman with deep pelvic endometriosis with involvement of posterior and lateral compartments. MRI showed in sagittal T2-weighted (**a**) lesion involved right parametrium (arrow). Axial T2-weighted (**b**) showed spotted nodule on low T2 signal intensity with rectosigmoid junction involvement and hemorrhagic foci on axial T1-weighted (arrow) (**c**)

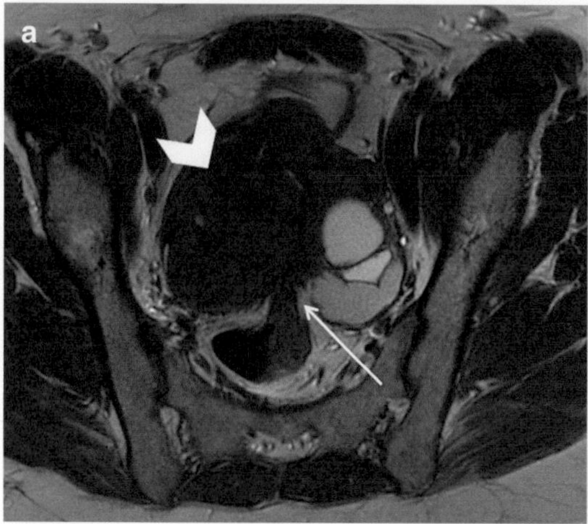

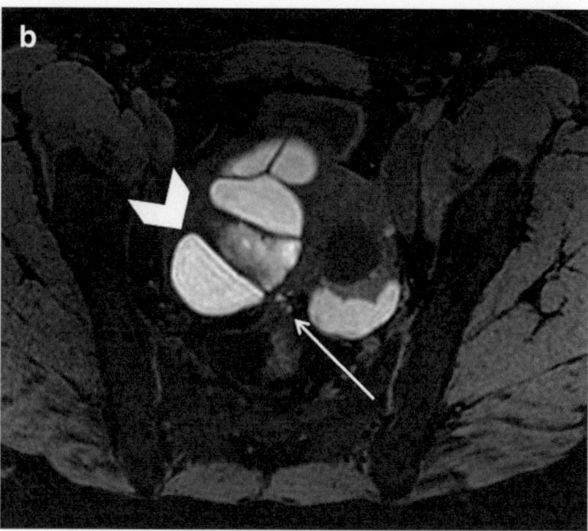

Fig. 7.2 A 25-year-old woman with deep pelvic endometriosis associated with adnexal endometriosis. MRI showed in axial T2-weighted (**a**) typical endometrioma (arrowhead) and rectosigmoid involvement (arrow). Axial T1-weighted (**b**) showed hemorrhagic foci (arrow) and typical high T1-weighted signal intensity on endometrioma (arrowhead)

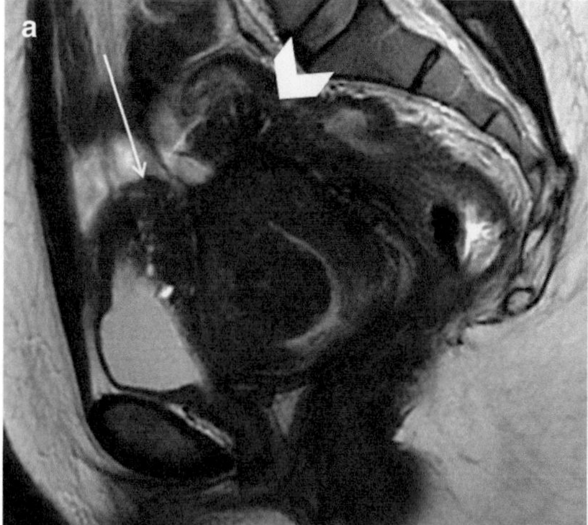

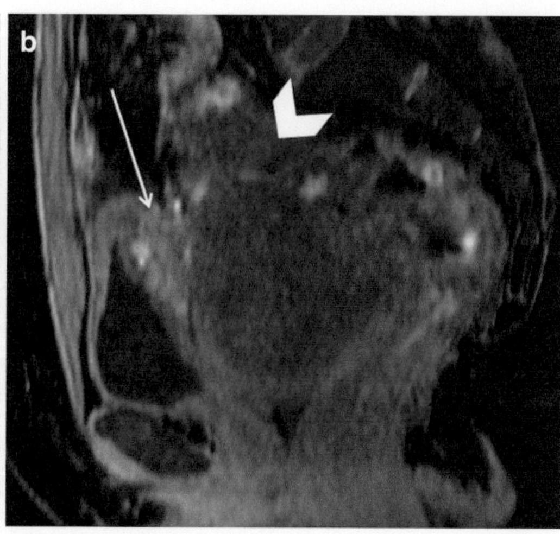

Fig. 7.3 A 28-year-old woman with deep pelvic endometriosis with involvement of anterior and posterior compartments. MRI showed in sagittal T2-weighted (**a**) lesion involved bladder (arrow) sigmoid and rectosigmoid junction (arrowhead) with hyperintense cavities and hemorrhagic foci on bladder (arrow) in sagittal T1-weighted (**b**)

To help surgeons, the radiological report should specify for bowel endometriosis involvement:

- unique, multifocal, and/or multicentric and the location(s) of lesion(s),
- distance to the anal margin for rectosigmoid and rectal involvement,
- lesion's size with height, thickness, and circumference in degree.

Presence of vaginal involvement associated with rectal or rectosigmoid involvement should be clarified because of the higher risk of fistula after surgery (Fig. 7.5).

When the intestinal tract involvement is evolved, it can lead to abnormalities of the **pouch of Douglas**, abnormality of the **rectovaginal septum** and **frozen pelvis**. With this abnormality, a block of tissue is created that simulates carcinoma and is not amenable to complete surgical resection.

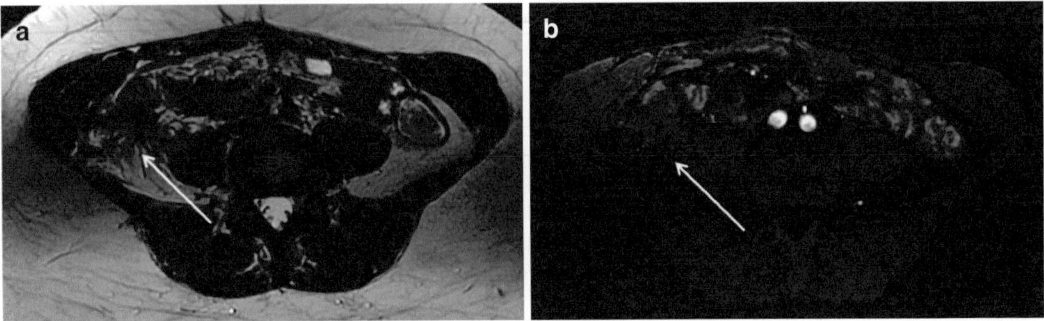

Fig. 7.4 A 39-year-old woman with deep pelvic endometriosis associated with bowel endometriosis. MRI showed in axial T2-weighted (**a**) lesion involved cecum (arrow) with spotted nodule on low signal T2-weigthed. Axial T1-weighted (**b**) showed hemorrhagic foci (arrow) on spikes

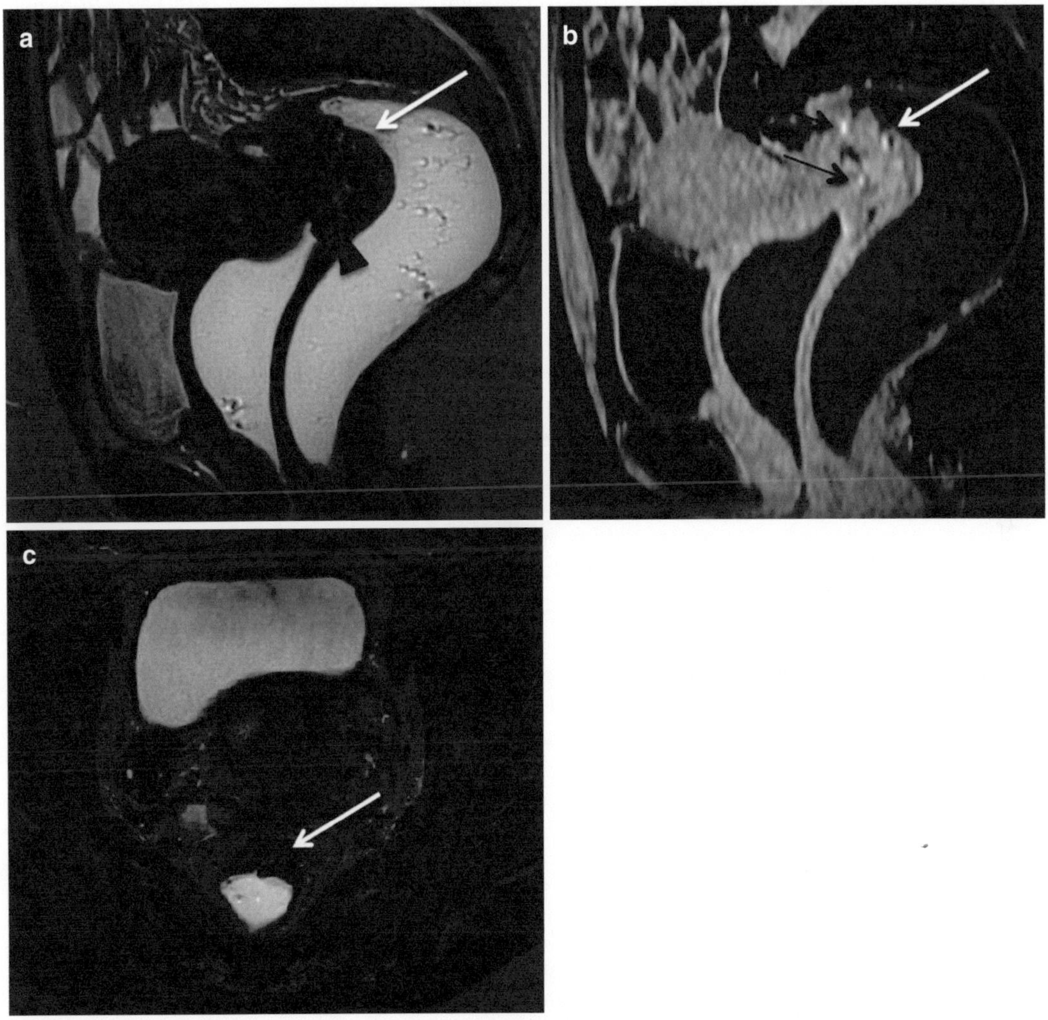

Fig. 7.5 A 30-year-old woman with deep pelvic endometriosis associated with bowel endometriosis. MRI showed in sagittal T2-weighted (**a**) lesion involved posterior vaginal wall (arrowheads), rectovaginal septum, rectum, and rectosigmoid junction (white arrow) with hemorrhagic foci (black arrows) in sagittal T1-weighted (**b**). Axial T2-weigthed (**c**) showed thick lesion with involvement at least 90° circumference

7.3.2 MR Enterography

7.3.2.1 MRI Protocol

MR enterography, which uses anterograde opacification, is a radiation-free imaging technique that is widely used to explore small-bowel and ileocecal diseases.

MR enterography was performed on Rousset et al. study [29] with:

- Patient in the prone position, he had fasted for at least 6 h and ingested a 5% mannitol solution (1000–1500 mL) over a 45–60-min period before the MR examination.
- 3.0-T MR imaging unit (Ingenia; Philips Medical Systems, Best, the Netherlands) equipped with a multichannel phased-array coil.
- First, it is necessary to performed balanced fast field-echo MR sequences to assess small-bowel and cecum distention. If there was inadequate distention, the patient returned to the waiting room to drink more of the oral contrast material solution.
- Then, MR protocol was: respiratory-triggered T2-weighted sequences and breath-hold three-dimensional dual-echo Dixon sequences before and after intravenous administration of gadobenate dimeglumine (0.2 mL of gadolinium per kilogram of body weight).
- Images were acquired at the upper and lower abdomen to cover the entire abdominopelvic region.
- To reduce peristaltic movement artifacts, patients received two intravenous 1 mg doses (1 mg/mL) of glucagon. One dose was administered before the start of MR imaging, and the second dose was administered prior to injection of the gadolinium-containing contrast material.
- The entire MR examination lasted 18 min.

7.3.2.2 MRI Signs

The degree of distention in each colonic segment can be assessed by using a simplified four-point scale previously applied by Taylor et al. [30].

MRE endometriosis diagnosis was based on criteria previously published by Rousset et al. [11, 29]: a bowel deep infiltrating endometriosis (DIE) diagnosis is based on morphologic appearance and contrast material-enhanced sequences, which enables to rule out peristaltic artifacts or fecal content.

A bowel DIE lesion is indicated on T2-weighted studies by an iso- or hypointense (relative to myometrium) nodular or mass-like bowel wall thickening and an associated obliteration of the normal hypointense signal of the wall [12, 31]. On three-dimensional dual-echo Dixon images, the lesion is indicated by the presence of a tissue nodule or mass extending on the bowel wall showing contrast enhancement after gadolinium chelate injection [12, 32]. The lesions may present internal cystic areas on T2-weighted images, with or without hemorrhagic components on precontrast three-dimensional dual-echo Dixon images. The number and the maximum length of the lesions have to be reported (Fig. 7.6).

Other intestinal tract locations (appendicular, cecal, small bowel) are determined by the presence of a solid nodule that penetrated the intestinal wall from outside to the inner surface and bulged toward mucosa (Fig. 7.7).

7.4 Other Examinations

MRI has limited value in assessing multifocality and multicentricity of bowel endometriosis especially when the ileocecal junction is involved. Hence, additional imaging techniques have been recommended, which depend on the surgeon's experience and the nature of the surgery, such as transvaginal sonography, rectal endoscopic ultrasonography, barium enema, computed tomography-based virtual colonoscopy, and computing tomography (CT) enema.

7.4.1 Transvaginal Sonography (TVS)

The distribution of deep endometriosis nodules should be evaluated in the whole pelvic cavity including the anterior, posterior, and subperitoneal lateral compartments:

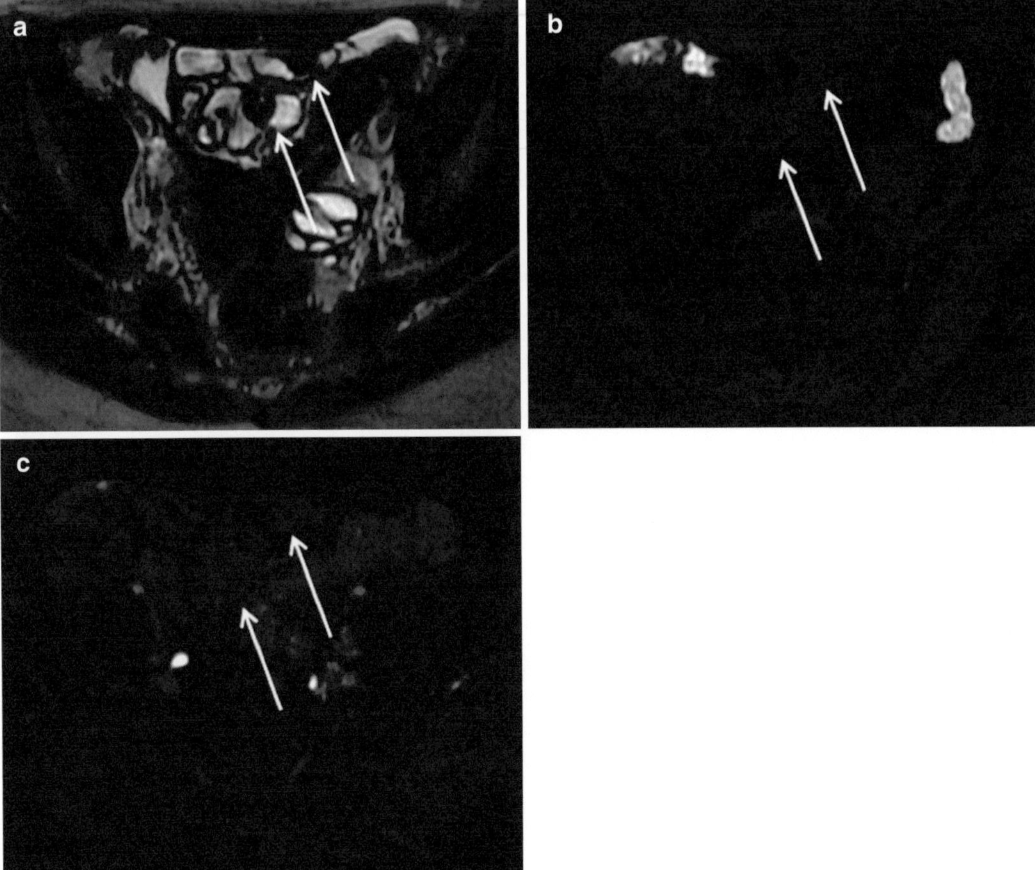

Fig. 7.6 A 33-year-old woman with deep pelvic endometriosis associated with bowel endometriosis. MR enterography showed in axial T2-weighted (**a**) nodule in bowel on low T2 signal intensity (arrows), on iso T1 signal intensity (arrows) axial T1-weighted (**b**) and enhancement after injection of gadolinium in axial T1-weighted after gadolinium injection. (**c**) Rectosigmoid involvement is indicated by a flattened or crenelated aspect of the mucosa or by an extended tissue mass on the bowel wall with slight intravenous contrast enhancement

- Deep endometriosis lesions are most frequently located in the posterior compartment, involving the torus, uterosacral ligaments, vagina, rectovaginal septum, pouch of Douglas, and rectosigmoid colon [5, 6].
- Less frequently, anterior deep endometriosis locations are present involving the vesicouterine pouch, bladder, and round ligaments.
- Rarely described by TVS, lateral compartment involvement includes the parametrium, ureter, visceral fascia, and lateral pelvic wall.

The bowel is considered involved when an irregular hypoechoic mass with or without hypoechoic or hyperechoic foci is found to have penetrated the intestinal wall; in this case the normal hypoechoic aspect of the bowel muscularis propria is replaced by an abnormal tissue mass [33].

While obliteration of the pouch of Douglas does not correspond specifically to deep endometriosis, it is frequently associated with severe deep endometriosis, and especially with rectosigmoid colon endometriosis. In this setting, the TVS "sliding sign" technique to detect pouch of Douglas obliteration in women with suspected endometriosis is highly relevant [34].

Bowel deep endometriosis can take the form of an isolated lesion or can be multifocal (multiple lesions affecting the same intestinal segment) and/or multicentric (multiple lesions affecting different intestinal segments) [35]. The pooled sensitivity and specificity of TVS for rectosigmoid endometriosis are reported as 90% and

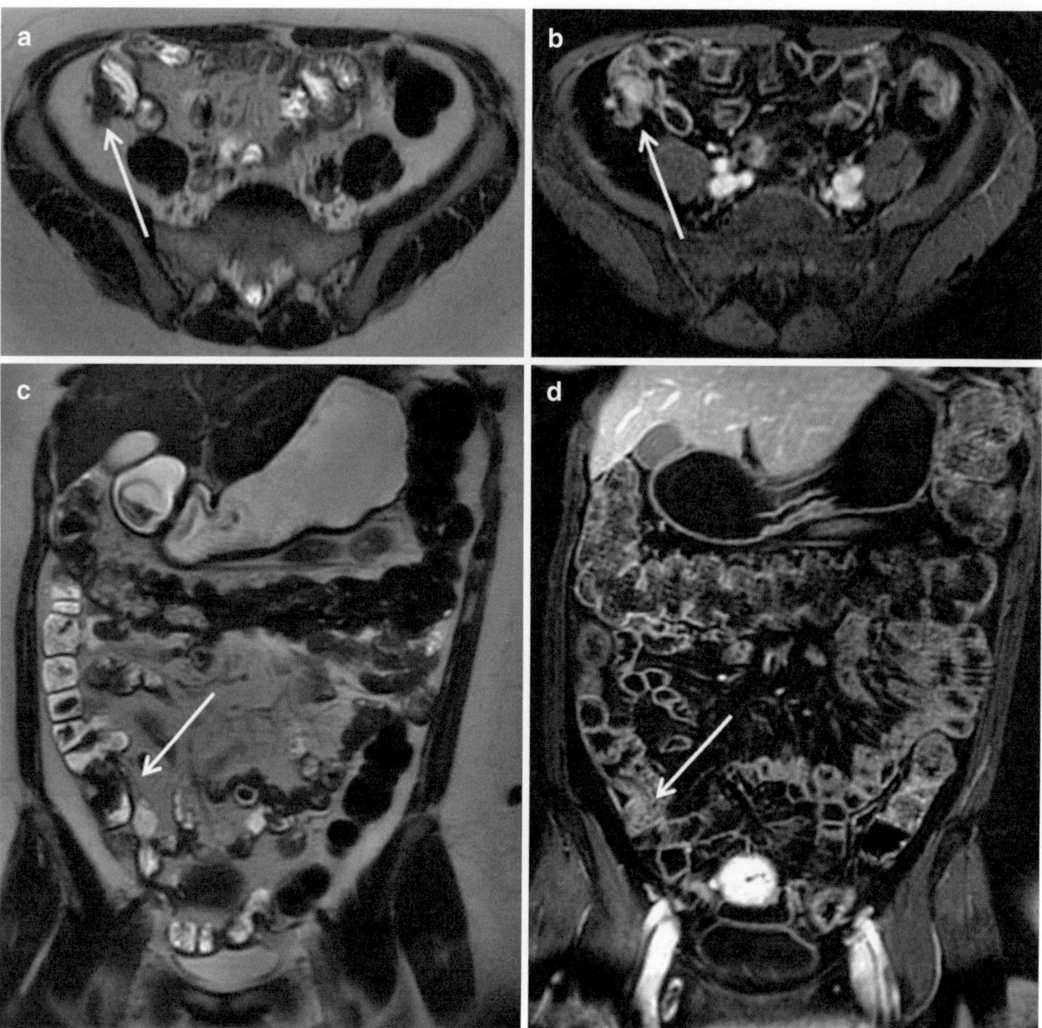

Fig. 7.7 A 43-year-old woman with deep pelvic endometriosis associated with bowel endometriosis. MR enterography showed in axial T2-weighted (**a**) and coronal T2-weighted (**c**) thickened of ileocecum junction on low T2 signal intensity (arrow) with enhancement after injection of gadolinium in axial T1-weighted after gadolinium injection (**b**, **d**)

96%, respectively, with similar results being provided by rectal endoscopic sonography [36].

7.4.2 Fusion Imaging

Fusion imaging [37], also known as real-time virtual sonography, is a new technique that uses magnetic navigation and computer software for the synchronized display of real-time ultrasound and multiplanar reconstructed MR images.

TVS suffers from high interobserver variability in the diagnosis of pelvic endometriosis, and its performance is highly dependent on the sonographer's experience [38]. In contrast, MRI provides visualization of the whole pelvis, with a larger field of view and excellent tissue contrast resolution [12]. Previous studies have reported that TVS and MRI are both highly accurate for the detection of rectal endometriosis [9, 12, 39], with better accuracy for TVS because of its better delineation of the intestinal layers. This is consis-

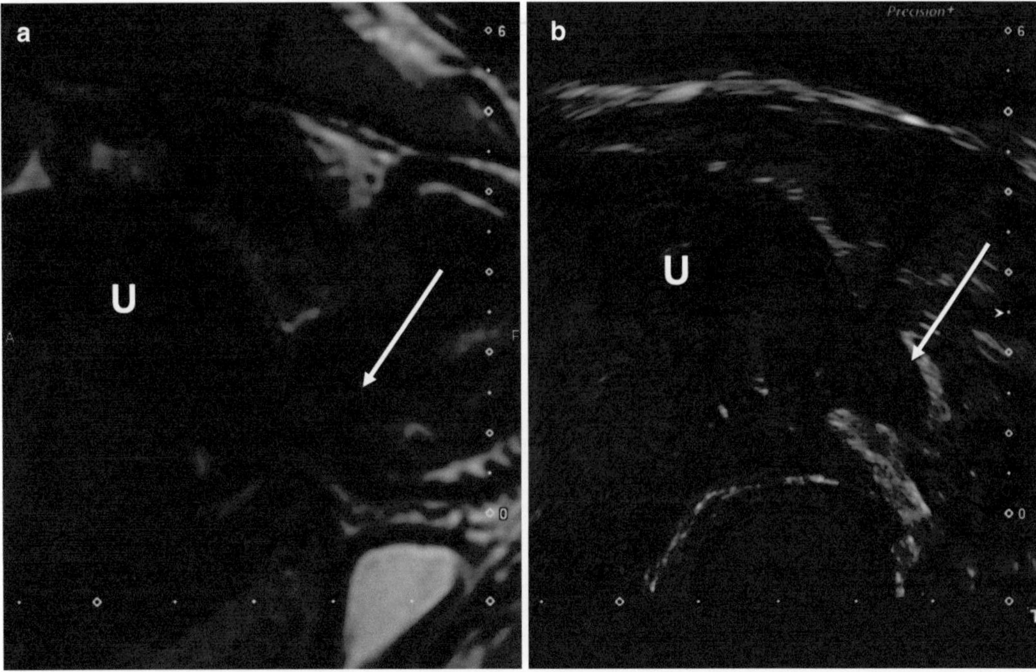

Fig. 7.8 A 31-year-old woman with deep pelvic endometriosis associated with bowel endometriosis. MRI showed in axial T2-weighted (**a**) lesion involved rectosigmoid junction (arrow) and TVUS (**b**) the same lesion with hypoechogenic thin of rectosigmoid junction wall. *U* uterus

tent with Millischer et al. [37] findings (identified in 100% of cases on TVS vs. 82% on MRI), emphasizing the difficulty in identifying pathology of the rectum with MRI, especially when there is fecal impaction. Again, by combining the two modalities, fusion imaging improved on the performance of MRI (Fig. 7.8).

7.4.3 Rectal Endoscopic Sonography

Rectal endoscopic sonography is a complementary technique that often is used to assess the depth of infiltration into the different bowel wall layers [40, 41].

Although transrectal sonography has been reported to have a sensitivity of 80% and a specificity of 97% for the diagnosis of uterosacral ligament involvement [42], no large studies of a comparison of sonography and MR imaging have been published. Endoscopic transrectal sonography has been reported to be useful for the

diagnosis of rectal wall endometriosis, with a sensitivity and specificity of 100% [41, 43, 44].

Bazot et al. [45], however, demonstrated that transvaginal sonography was as performant as endoscopic transrectal sonography for the diagnosis and evaluation of extension of rectal endometriosis. In contrast to MR imaging, which offers an overview of the potential locations of pelvic endometriosis, the main limitation of the sonographic techniques is that they focus on a limited anatomic area of the pelvic cavity and subperitoneal space; none is individually capable of evaluation of overall pelvic extension.

7.4.4 Computed Tomography (CT) Enema

Imaging techniques using an enema strategy have demonstrated overall high performance to detect multicentric digestive lesions [46]. Multidetector CT enema has been advocated due to its excellent sensitivity (98%) and specificity (100%) [47] but this technique requires colonic distension which is painful and uncomfortable and exposes young patients to the potentially harmful effects of ionized radiation.

Belghiti et al. [35] reported a lower accuracy of CT scan enema for the diagnosis of multifocal and multicentric endometriotic lesions in a recent study comparing CT enema to 1.5 T MRI.

CT-based virtual colonography has recently been demonstrated to have high accuracy to explore multicentric lesions when associated with MRI, but the technique requires further studies to be adopted in bowel endometriosis [48].

As demonstrated for most deep endometriosis locations, and particularly in the rectosigmoid colon, TVS and MRI exhibited at least similar sensitivities and specificities to laparoscopy supporting their use as a replacement option. Moreover, the concept of diagnostic laparoscopy should also be discussed taking into account surgical risks.

In conclusion, rectal and rectosigmoid junction lesions can be thoroughly explored with pelvic magnetic resonance imaging. TVS and MRI are both highly accurate for the detection of rectal endometriosis with better accuracy for TVS, so fusion imaging can help. Recently, a new MR classification was published [49] to rate the degree of severity of the deep pelvic endometriotic disease with a high degree of correlation with the risk of post operative disease. The presence of bowel endometriosis needs the referral to expert centers in endometriosis surgery and the use of this type of MR imaging classification is a way to optimize patient management.

MR enterography is widely used to explore small-bowel and ileocecal diseases.

References

1. Clement PB. Endometriosis, lesions of the secondary müllerian system, and pelvic mesothelial proliferations. In: Kurman RJ, editor. Blaustein's pathology of the female genital tract. New York, NY: Springer; 1987. p. 516–59.
2. Olive DL, Schwartz LB. Endometriosis. N Engl J Med. 1993;328:1759–69.
3. Giudice LC, Kao LC. Endometriosis. Lancet. 2004;364:1789–99.
4. Cornillie FJ, Oosterlynck D, Lauweryns JM, Koninckx PR. Deeply infiltrating pelvic endometriosis: histology and clinical significance. Fertil Steril. 1990;53:978–83.
5. Chapron C, Fauconnier A, Vieira M, Barakat H, Dousset B, Pansini V, Vacher-Lavenu MC, Dubuisson JB. Anatomical distribution of deeply infiltrating endometriosis: surgical implications and proposition for a classification. Hum Reprod. 2003;18:157–61.
6. Chapron C, Chopin N, Borghese B, Foulot H, Dousset B, Vacher-Lavenu MC, Vieira M, Hasan W, Bricou A. Deeply infiltrating endometriosis: pathogenetic implications of the anatomical distribution. Hum Reprod. 2006;21:1839–45.
7. Chamié LP, Blasbalg R, Pereira RMA, Warmbrand G, Serafini PC. Findings of pelvic endometriosis at transvaginal US, MR imaging, and laparoscopy. Radiographics. 2011;31:E77–100.
8. Chapron C, Fauconnier A, Dubuisson J-B, Barakat H, Vieira M, Bréart G. Deep infiltrating endometriosis: relation between severity of dysmenorrhoea and extent of disease. Hum Reprod. 2003;18:760–6.
9. Piketty M, Chopin N, Dousset B, Millischer-Bellaische A-E, Roseau G, Leconte M, Borghese B, Chapron C. Preoperative work-up for patients with deeply infiltrating endometriosis: transvaginal ultrasonography must definitely be the first-line imaging examination. Hum Reprod. 2009;24:602–7.
10. Redwine DB. Ovarian endometriosis: a marker for more extensive pelvic and intestinal disease. Fertil Steril. 1999;72:310–5.
11. Nyangoh Timoh K, Stewart Z, Benjoar M, Beldjord S, Ballester M, Bazot M, Thomassin-Naggara I, Darai E. Magnetic resonance enterography to assess multifocal and multicentric bowel endometriosis. J Minim Invasive Gynecol. 2018;25:697–705.
12. Bazot M, Darai E, Hourani R, Thomassin I, Cortez A, Uzan S, Buy J-N. Deep pelvic endometriosis: MR imaging for diagnosis and prediction of extension of disease. Radiology. 2004;232:379–89.
13. Thomassin-Naggara I, Bendifallah S, Rousset P, Bazot M, Ballester M, Darai E. [Diagnostic performance of MR imaging, coloscan and MRI/CT enterography for the diagnosis of pelvic endometriosis: CNGOF-HAS Endometriosis Guidelines]. Gynecol Obstet Fertil Senol. 2018;46:177–84.
14. Fauconnier A, Borghese B, Huchon C, et al. [Epidemiology and diagnosis strategy: CNGOF-HAS Endometriosis Guidelines]. Gynecol Obstet Fertil Senol. 2018;46:223–30.
15. Philip C-A, Dubernard G. [Performances and place of sonography in the diagnostic of endometriosis: CNGOF-HAS Endometriosis Guidelines]. Gynecol Obstet Fertil Senol. 2018;46:185–99.
16. Burla L, Scheiner D, Samartzis EP, Seidel S, Eberhard M, Fink D, Boss A, Imesch P. The ENZIAN score as a preoperative MRI-based classification instrument for deep infiltrating endometriosis. Arch Gynecol

Obstet. 2019;300:109. https://doi.org/10.1007/s00404-019-05157-1.

17. Garry R, Clayton R, Hawe J. The effect of endometriosis and its radical laparoscopic excision on quality of life indicators. BJOG. 2000;107:44–54.

18. Dousset B, Leconte M, Borghese B, Millischer A-E, Roseau G, Arkwright S, Chapron C. Complete surgery for low rectal endometriosis: long-term results of a 100-case prospective study. Ann Surg. 2010;251:887–95.

19. Roman H, Ness J, Suciu N, Bridoux V, Gourcerol G, Leroi AM, Tuech JJ, Ducrotté P, Savoye-Collet C, Savoye G. Are digestive symptoms in women presenting with pelvic endometriosis specific to lesion localizations? A preliminary prospective study. Hum Reprod. 2012;27:3440–9.

20. Belghiti J, Ballester M, Zilberman S, Thomin A, Zacharopoulou C, Bazot M, Thomassin-Naggara I, Daraï E. Role of protective defunctioning stoma in colorectal resection for endometriosis. J Minim Invasive Gynecol. 2014;21:472–9.

21. Daraï E, Zilberman S, Touboul C, Chereau E, Rouzier R, Ballester M. Urological morbidity of colorectal resection for endometriosis. Minerva Med. 2012;103:63–72.

22. Koninckx PR, Ussia A, Adamyan L, Wattiez A, Donnez J. Deep endometriosis: definition, diagnosis, and treatment. Fertil Steril. 2012;98:564–71.

23. Abrão MS, Petraglia F, Falcone T, Keckstein J, Osuga Y, Chapron C. Deep endometriosis infiltrating the recto-sigmoid: critical factors to consider before management. Hum Reprod Update. 2015;21:329–39.

24. Millochau J-C, Stochino-Loi E, Darwish B, Abo C, Coget J, Chati R, Tuech J-J, Roman H. Multiple nodule removal by disc excision and segmental resection in multifocal colorectal endometriosis. J Minim Invasive Gynecol. 2018;25:139–46.

25. Fanfani F, Fagotti A, Gagliardi ML, Ruffo G, Ceccaroni M, Scambia G, Minelli L. Discoid or segmental rectosigmoid resection for deep infiltrating endometriosis: a case-control study. Fertil Steril. 2010;94:444–9.

26. Roman H, Bubenheim M, Huet E, Bridoux V, Zacharopoulou C, Daraï E, Collinet P, Tuech J-J. Conservative surgery versus colorectal resection in deep endometriosis infiltrating the rectum: a randomized trial. Hum Reprod. 2018;33:47–57.

27. Bazot M, Bharwani N, Huchon C, et al. European society of urogenital radiology (ESUR) guidelines: MR imaging of pelvic endometriosis. Eur Radiol. 2017;27:2765–75.

28. Hottat N, Larrousse C, Anaf V, Noël J-C, Matos C, Absil J, Metens T. Endometriosis: contribution of 3.0-T pelvic MR imaging in preoperative assessment--initial results. Radiology. 2009;253:126–34.

29. Rousset P, Peyron N, Charlot M, Chateau F, Golfier F, Raudrant D, Cotte E, Isaac S, Réty F, Valette P-J. Bowel endometriosis: preoperative diagnostic accuracy of 3.0-T MR enterography--initial results. Radiology. 2014;273:117–24.

30. Taylor SA, Halligan S, Goh V, Morley S, Bassett P, Atkin W, Bartram CI. Optimizing colonic distention for multi-detector row CT colonography: effect of hyoscine butylbromide and rectal balloon catheter. Radiology. 2003;229:99–108.

31. Busard MPH, van der Houwen LEE, Bleeker MCG, Pieters van den Bos IC, Cuesta MA, van Kuijk C, Mijatovic V, Hompes PGA, van Waesberghe JHTM. Deep infiltrating endometriosis of the bowel: MR imaging as a method to predict muscular invasion. Abdom Imaging. 2012;37:549–57.

32. Scardapane A, Bettocchi S, Lorusso F, Stabile Ianora AA, Vimercati A, Ceci O, Lasciarrea M, Angelelli G. Diagnosis of colorectal endometriosis: contribution of contrast enhanced MR-colonography. Eur Radiol. 2011;21:1553–63.

33. Bazot M, Thomassin I, Hourani R, Cortez A, Darai E. Diagnostic accuracy of transvaginal sonography for deep pelvic endometriosis. Ultrasound Obstet Gynecol. 2004;24:180–5.

34. Reid S, Lu C, Casikar I, Mein B, Magotti R, Ludlow J, Benzie R, Condous G. The prediction of pouch of Douglas obliteration using offline analysis of the transvaginal ultrasound "sliding sign" technique: inter- and intra-observer reproducibility. Hum Reprod. 2013;28:1237–46.

35. Belghiti J, Thomassin-Naggara I, Zacharopoulou C, Zilberman S, Jarboui L, Bazot M, Ballester M, Daraï E. Contribution of computed tomography enema and magnetic resonance imaging to diagnose multifocal and multicentric bowel lesions in patients with colorectal endometriosis. J Minim Invasive Gynecol. 2015;22:776–84.

36. Nisenblat V, Prentice L, Bossuyt PMM, Farquhar C, Hull ML, Johnson N. Combination of the non-invasive tests for the diagnosis of endometriosis. Cochrane Database Syst Rev. 2016;7:CD012281.

37. Millischer A-E, Salomon LJ, Santulli P, Borghese B, Dousset B, Chapron C. Fusion imaging for evaluation of deep infiltrating endometriosis: feasibility and preliminary results. Ultrasound Obstet Gynecol. 2015;46:109–17.

38. Bazot M, Daraï E, Biau DJ, Ballester M, Dessolle L. Learning curve of transvaginal ultrasound for the diagnosis of endometriomas assessed by the cumulative summation test (LC-CUSUM). Fertil Steril. 2011;95:301–3.

39. Kinkel K, Chapron C, Balleyguier C, Fritel X, Dubuisson JB, Moreau JF. Magnetic resonance imaging characteristics of deep endometriosis. Hum Reprod. 1999;14:1080–6.

40. Bazot M, Bornier C, Dubernard G, Roseau G, Cortez A, Daraï E. Accuracy of magnetic resonance imaging and rectal endoscopic sonography for the prediction of location of deep pelvic endometriosis. Hum Reprod. 2007;22:1457–63.

41. Chapron C, Dumontier I, Dousset B, Fritel X, Tardif D, Roseau G, Chaussade S, Couturier D, Dubuisson JB. Results and role of rectal endoscopic ultrasonography for patients with deep pelvic endometriosis. Hum Reprod. 1998;13:2266–70.

42. Fedele L, Bianchi S, Portuese A, Borruto F, Dorta M. Transrectal ultrasonography in the assessment of rectovaginal endometriosis. Obstet Gynecol. 1998;91:444–8.

43. Dumontier I, Roseau G, Vincent B, Chapron C, Dousset B, Chaussade S, Moreau JF, Dubuisson JB, Couturier D. [Comparison of endoscopic ultrasound and magnetic resonance imaging in severe pelvic endometriosis]. Gastroenterol Clin Biol. 2000;24:1197–204.

44. Roseau G, Dumontier I, Palazzo L, Chapron C, Dousset B, Chaussade S, Dubuisson JB, Couturier D. Rectosigmoid endometriosis: endoscopic ultrasound features and clinical implications. Endoscopy. 2000;32:525–30.

45. Bazot M, Detchev R, Cortez A, Amouyal P, Uzan S, Daraï E. Transvaginal sonography and rectal endoscopic sonography for the assessment of pelvic endometriosis: a preliminary comparison. Hum Reprod. 2003;18:1686–92.

46. Biscaldi E, Ferrero S, Fulcheri E, Ragni N, Remorgida V, Rollandi GA. Multislice CT enteroclysis in the diagnosis of bowel endometriosis. Eur Radiol. 2007;17:211–9.

47. Ferrero S, Biscaldi E, Morotti M, Venturini PL, Remorgida V, Rollandi GA, Valenzano Menada M. Multidetector computerized tomography enteroclysis vs. rectal water contrast transvaginal ultrasonography in determining the presence and extent of bowel endometriosis. Ultrasound Obstet Gynecol. 2011;37:603–13.

48. Roman H, Carilho J, Da Costa C, De Vecchi C, Suaud O, Monroc M, Hochain P, Vassilieff M, Savoye-Collet C, Saint-Ghislain M. Computed tomography-based virtual colonoscopy in the assessment of bowel endometriosis: the surgeon's point of view. Gynecol Obstet Fertil. 2016;44:3–10.

49. Thomassin-Naggara I, Lamrabet S, Crestani A, Bekhouche A, Abdel-Wahab C, Kermarrec E, Touboul C, Darai E. Magnetic resonance imaging classification of deep pelvic endometriosis: description and impact on surgical management. Hum Reprod. 2020;35(7):1589–1600.

Multidetector Computerized Tomography Enema

8

Ennio Biscaldi, Fabio Barra, Gaby Moawad, Umberto Leone Roberti Maggiore, and Simone Ferrero

8.1 Multidetector Computerized Tomography Enema

Multidetector computerized tomography enema (MDCT-e) is a computerized tomography technique relying on the distention of the colon using water. Several studies have shown its excellent accuracy for the detection of colon cancer [1–4]. Based on these experiences, approximately 10 years ago, MDCT-e was applied to the investigation of intestinal endometriosis.

E. Biscaldi (✉)
Department of Radiology, Galliera Hospital, Genoa, Italy

F. Barra · S. Ferrero
Academic Unit of Obstetrics and Gynecology, IRCCS Ospedale Policlinico San Martino, Genova, Italy

Department of Neurosciences, Rehabilitation, Ophthalmology, Genetics, Maternal and Child Health (DiNOGMI), University of Genova, Genova, Italy

G. Moawad
The George Washington University School of Medicine and Health Sciences, Washington, DC, USA

U. Leone Roberti Maggiore
Fondazione IRCCS Istituto Nazionale dei Tumori, Milan, Italy

8.2 Multidetector Computerized Tomography Enema Technique

Bowel cleansing is required before MDCT-e to improve diagnostic accuracy. A low-residue diet is usually administered on 1 [5] to 3 days [6–10] before the exam. Furthermore, on the day prior to the exam, the patients usually receive osmotic laxatives such as polyethylene glycol [5–9, 11]. A small amount of liquid with limited CT density may remain in the bowel lumen at the time of the exam maintaining in suspension the bowel content.

Colonic distention is usually performed with the patient in the left lateral decubitus on the CT table [5, 8–10]. A dedicated catheter is introduced in the anal canal (Fig. 8.1) and 2000–2500 ml of warm (37 °C) water is injected into the bowel [5, 7] (Fig. 8.2a, b). Some radiologists ask to the patient to drink 1.5 l of water 30–50 min before the exam with the aim to distend the small bowel [5]. However, the simultaneous distention of both the small and large bowel is not systematically applied because it may to be painful for the patient.

Intestinal hypotonization is usually performed during colonic distention by intramuscular injection of hyoscine-N-butylbromide [5–9, 11]. The hypotonization aims to minimize bowel peristalsis and to decrease the risk of examining the abdomen colonic spams, improving patient

© Springer Nature Switzerland AG 2020
S. Ferrero, M. Ceccaroni (eds.), *Clinical Management of Bowel Endometriosis*,
https://doi.org/10.1007/978-3-030-50446-5_8

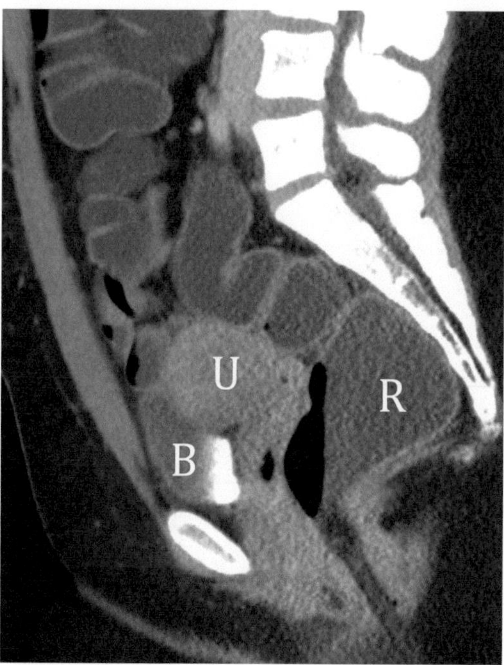

Fig. 8.1 Multidetector computerized tomography enema, sagittal reconstruction. A rectal catheter is introduced in the anal canal until the first part of the rectum (R). *U* uterus, *B* bladder

comfort, and facilitating the distention of the colon and the terminal ileum permitting imaging of a larger intestinal surface.

Intravenous iodinated contrast medium (CM) is used during MDCT-e. Patients receive an intravenous injection of iodinated CM (iodine concentration of 350 mg I/ml) [5]. The same iodine load adjusted for patient's body weight (1.5 mg/kg) is administered [5, 10]. The rate of intravenous injection of CM is standardized (2.5–3 ml/s) [8]. Ideally the flow rate should be standardized considering the dose of Iodine per kg of patient weight and the administration may be theoretically considered in mg of Iodine per second. A bolus-tracking software designed to quantitatively and qualitatively monitor organ contrast enhancement is used by some radiologists to maximize the quality of MDCT-e images [7, 8, 10]. Forty to 50 ml of saline solution at a rate of 2.5–3 ml/s are injected after CM administration [5]. The injection of the iodinated CM is useful to better examine the intestinal wall and to enhance the visualization of the endometriotic nodules and the assessment of its characteristics. In par-

ticular, the enhancement allows the radiologist in evaluating the depth of penetration of the nodule in the intestinal wall. Furthermore, CM improves the evaluation of the abdominal organs. No scan should be performed before CM injection [5, 8]. The acquisition without CM may be used to detect opaque findings (such as urinary stones) or when doubtful images should be evaluated (such as surgical clips of medical devices in patients who underwent previous surgery). Some radiologists inject the CM accordingly to the "double split" bolus technique [9]. A pre-bolus of iodinated CM (20% of the total dose calculated using the patient's body weight) is injected simultaneously to colonic distention and intestinal hypotonization (7–8 min before the volumetric acquisition) at a rate of 1 ml/s. At the end of this step, 150 ml of saline solution is infused to accelerate the urinary CM excretion and to increase the concentration of CM in the renal cavities and ureters. The remaining dose is injected and a volumetric acquisition is performed in the portal phase (40 s after the arterial peak). No published study investigating the use of MDCT-e in the diagnosis of bowel endometriosis reported adverse reaction to iodinated CM [6, 7].

The exams are ideally performed using a 64-row scanner [5, 6], although some authors have used a 16-row scanner [7–11]. The following parameters are usually chosen: 64 × 0.5/0.625 mm collimation, rotation time 0.5–0.7 s, tube voltage 120 kV, effective mA 340, effective slice thickness 5 mm, reconstruction increment 1.25 mm [5, 6]. The scanning is ideally performed in the supine position during retrograde colonic distention [5, 9]. The supine position is better tolerated by the patient compared with the prone position. A single scan is performed in craniocaudal direction from the dome of the diaphragm to the pubic symphysis during a single breath hold [10].

The volumetric acquisition is performed in portal phase (40 s after the arterial peak) after the injection of the intravenous CM.

The criterion to diagnose bowel endometriosis requires the presence of solid nodules with positive enhancement, contiguous or infiltrating the thickened colonic wall. Infiltration of the muscularis propria is diagnosed when the fat plane

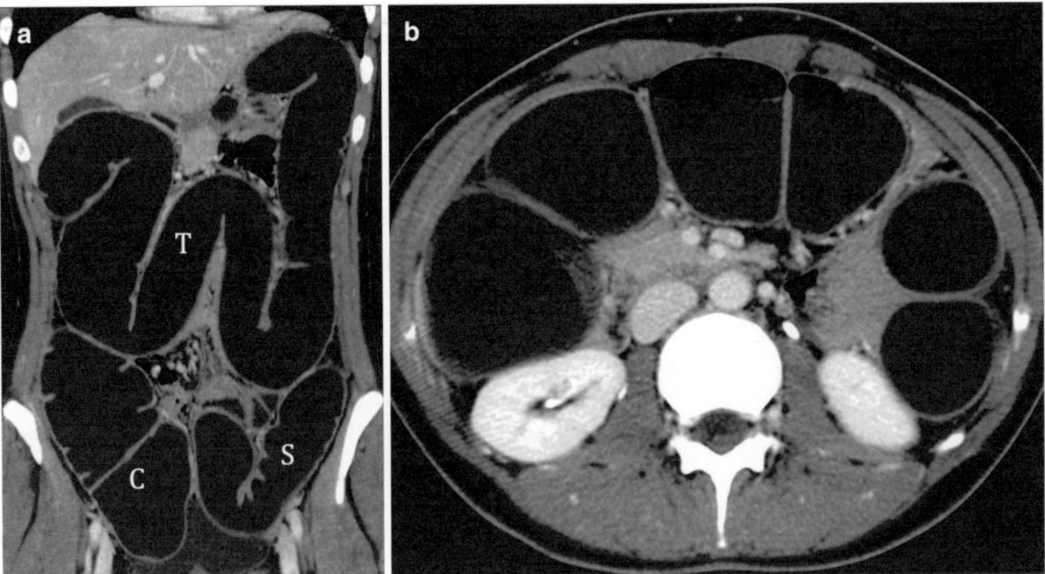

Fig. 8.2 Multidetector computerized tomography enema. (a) The coronal reconstruction shows as a good distension that allows to evaluate whole the colonic wall, also in a case of long colic extension. *C* cacum, *S* sigmoid, *T* transverse colon. (b) The corresponding axial image across the mid abdomen. Colonic loops are retrogradely dilated

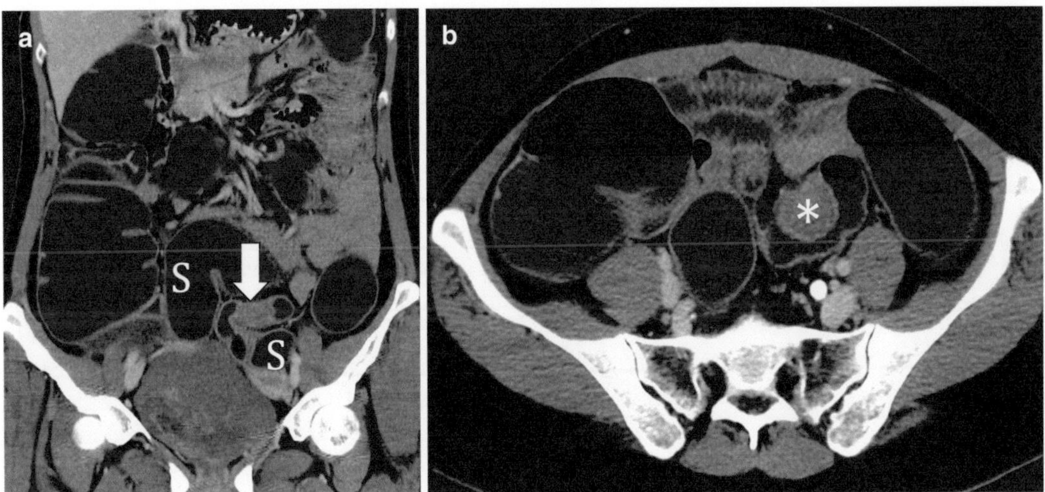

Fig. 8.3 Multidetector computerized tomography enema. (a) Coronal reconstruction. The sigmoid colon (S) is stenosed where the endometriotic lesion infiltrates the colonic wall (arrow). (b) Axial scan. The rectal nodule (asterisk) bulges into the lumen

between the nodule and the bowel disappears and the nodule penetrates the intestinal wall from outside, abuts the inner surface and bulges toward the mucosa (Fig. 8.3a, b). A pathological multi-layered aspect of the wall may sometimes be detectable (Fig. 8.4a, b). The submucosa may appear as a hypodense layer located between the muscularis and the mucosa [7]. Endometriosis infiltrating only the intestinal serosa (peritoneal endometriosis) is characterized by the presence of a nodule with an irregular profile adjacent to the bowel loop (persisting despite pharmacologic hypotonization and forced distension with water); in these cases, a hypodense layer (which separates the serosa from the lesion) is observed (Fig. 8.5) [7].

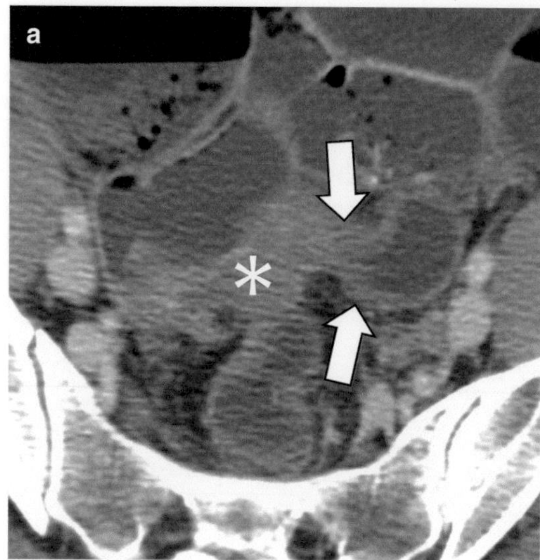

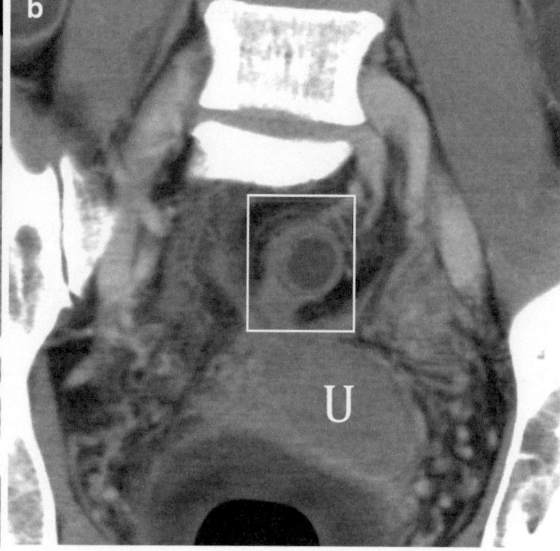

Fig. 8.4 Multidetector computerized tomography enema. The paracoronal reconstruction (**a**) shows the layered pattern (arrows) of the sigmoid wall, immediately before the infiltrating endometriotic nodule (asterisk). This aspect of the colonic wall is well demonstrated in the coronal reconstruction, the involved sigmoid loop is shown in the white box (**b**). *U* uterus

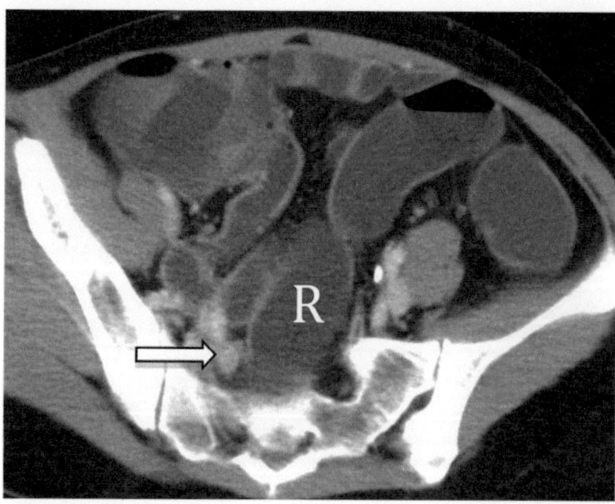

Fig. 8.5 Multidetector computerized tomography enema, axial plane. The arrow shows a small endometriotic nodule, which is not penetrating the intestinal wall. A subtle fat plane between the nodule (arrow) and the rectum (R) is present

A strength of MDCT-e is that it can reliably differentiate bowel endometriosis from other intestinal pathologies [10]. For example, the contrast enhancement of bowel adenocarcinoma is intense; the lesion originates from the mucosa and infiltrates the whole thickness of the bowel wall. Another rare condition that should be considered in the differential diagnosis is intestinal lymphoma which originates in the submucosa and progresses toward the serosa or the mucosa. Using MDCT-e, the growth of the lymphoma progressively divides bowel wall layers separating the mucosa from the serosa; thus, the appearance of these lesions is different from endometriosis. Patients with bowel endometriosis may sometimes complain of symptoms similar to those of patients with inflammatory bowel diseases [12]. Ulcerative colitis has a variable CT pattern; colonic involvement is more extensive than in endometriosis and it can be easily differentiated. Ulcerative colitis is characterized by a thickened and sometimes layered aspect of the colonic wall and the mucosa is frequently hyperdense (Fig. 8.6). No pericolic lesion is detectable in case of inflammatory disease. Crohn's disease is characterized by a multilayered pattern; in the majority of cases it involves small bowel and intense hyperemia of the mucosa can be observed.

Axial and multiplanar reconstructed (MPR) images are evaluated [8] (Fig. 8.7a–c). Curved multiplanar reconstructions are used to better define the location and longitudinal extension of bowel lesions. Maximum intensity-projection (MIP) reconstructions are used to visualize the ureters [5].

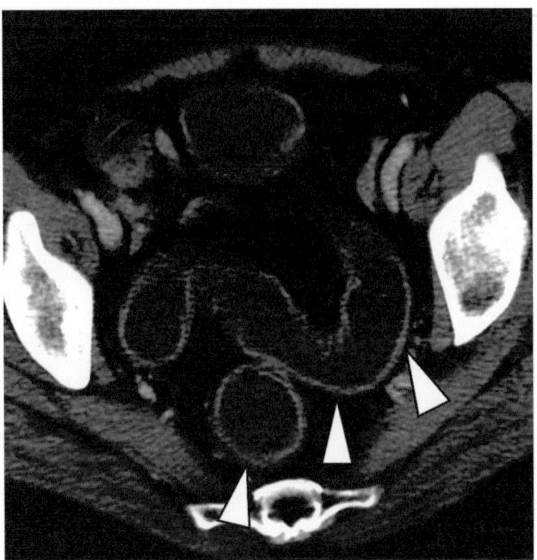

Fig. 8.6 Multidetector computerized tomography enema. A case of ulcerative colitis in a 45-year-old woman. The disease involves extensively the colonic wall: the sigmoid colon shows a pathologic wall (head arrows), homogeneously thickened

The average radiation dose delivered to each patient ranges between 12 and 15.8 mSv for patients receiving scanning in two phases (venous and excretory) [5–8, 10] and 9.2 mSv for those undergoing MDCT-e with slit-bolus technique [5].

The published studies show that the colonic distention is well tolerated, and no patient has needed to interrupt the exam because of pain. The introduction of the rectal enema tube may be painful in patients with hemorrhoids or anal fissures [10]. Some studies investigated the pain caused by MDCT-e using a 10 cm visual analogue scale (VAS) [6]. The mean intensity of pain experienced by the patients during MDCT-e ranges between 5.2 and 5.8 cm [6, 7].

Image reconstructions are generated on a workstation. In addition to axial images, coronal and sagittal reformatted multiplanar reconstructions (MPRs) and maximum-intensity-projection (MIP) and average-intensity-projection images are generated. Enhanced thick-slab MIP images including both kidneys and ureters are elaborated when the exam aims to investigate ureteral involvement [9]. The time required to perform MDCT-e is approximately 30 min [6].

8.3 Multidetector Computerized Tomography Enema in the Diagnosis of Bowel Endometriosis

In 2007, a single-center prospective study proposed the use of MDCT-e for the diagnosis of bowel endometriosis [8]. Ninety-eight patients were included in the study and 76 patients had bowel endometriosis; 116 bowel endometriotic nodules were identified in these patients at surgery. MDCT-e had sensitivity of 98.7%, specificity of 100%, positive predictive value (PPV) of 100%, and negative predictive value (NPV) of 95.7% in identifying women with bowel endometriosis. MDCT-e identified 94.8% (110/116) of the bowel endometriotic nodules observed at surgery. In particular, MDCT-e identified all nodules located on the sigmoid colon, cecum, and ileum; 47 of 53 (88.7%) rectal nodules were diagnosed. Out of 25 nodules infiltrating the intestinal submucosa at histology, the depth of infiltration was correctly identified by MDCT-e in 19 nodules (70.0%), while in six cases it was underestimated. MDCT-e correctly estimated the size of intestinal endometriotic nodules.

Subsequently, a prospective study including 103 women with clinical suspicion of bowel endometriosis investigated the accuracy of MDCT-e with a split-bolus technique in detecting ureteral compression caused by endometriosis [9]. Sixty-seven women (65.0%) had bowel endometriotic nodules at surgery. The sensitivity of MDCT-e in identifying bowel nodules was 93.3%, the specificity was 96.6%, the PPV was 95.5%, the NPV was 94.9%, the accuracy was 95.1%, the positive likelihood ratio (LR+) was 27.07, and negative likelihood ratio (LR−) was 0.07. Ureteral compression was observed at MDCT-e urography in 36 ureters (17.4%); surgery confirmed the presence of ureteral compression in 34 ureters (16.4%). The sensitivity of MDCT-e urography in identifying ureteral compression was 97.1%, the specificity was 98.8%, the PPV was 94.4%, the NPV was 99.4%, the accuracy was 99.0%, the LR+ was 83.54, and LR− was 0.03 (Figs. 8.8a–c, 8.9a, b, and 8.10a–c).

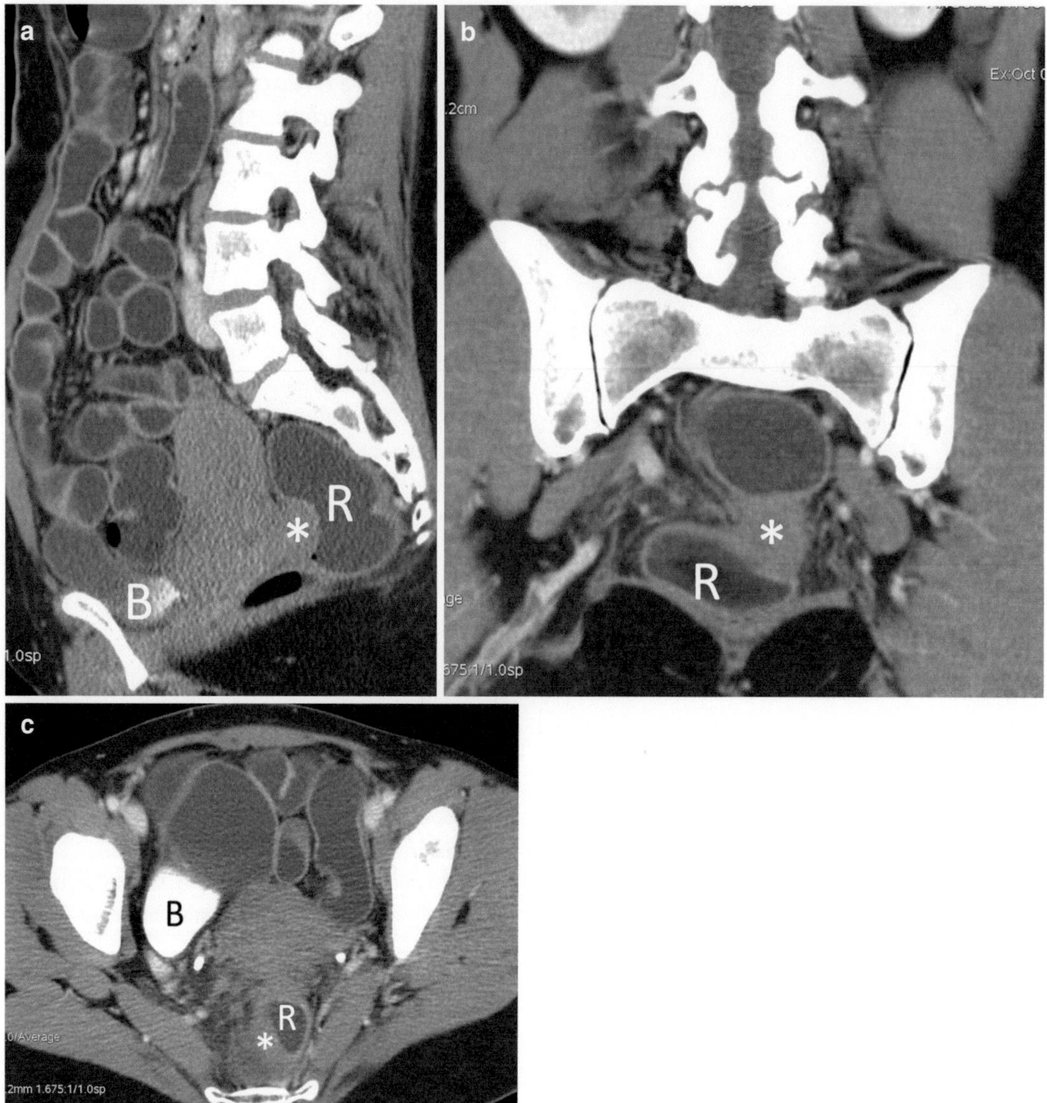

Fig. 8.7 Multidetector computerized tomography enema showing a rectal nodule infiltrating the muscularis propria in sagittal (**a**), coronal reconstruction (**b**) and in axial plane (**c**). The asterisk indicates the nodule. *B* bladder, *R* rectum

An Italian retrospective single-center study investigated the accuracy of MDCT-e in the diagnosis of bowel and ureteral endometriosis [5]. The study included 94 women (64 underwent laparoscopy and 20 women had intestinal endometriosis). The radiologist classified colonic distention as good in 92% of cases and moderate in 8% of cases; in no colonic distention was judged to be unsatisfactory. MDCT-e had sensitivity of 100%, specificity of 97.6%, diagnostic accuracy of 98.4%, PPV of 95.6%, and NPV of 100% for diagnosing bowel endometriosis. Twenty-three intestinal nodules were excised at surgery. The two radiologists involved in the study tried to distinguish lesions involving only the subserosa from those infiltrating at least the intestinal muscularis. Regarding intestinal wall involvement, the sensitivity was 95% and the specificity was

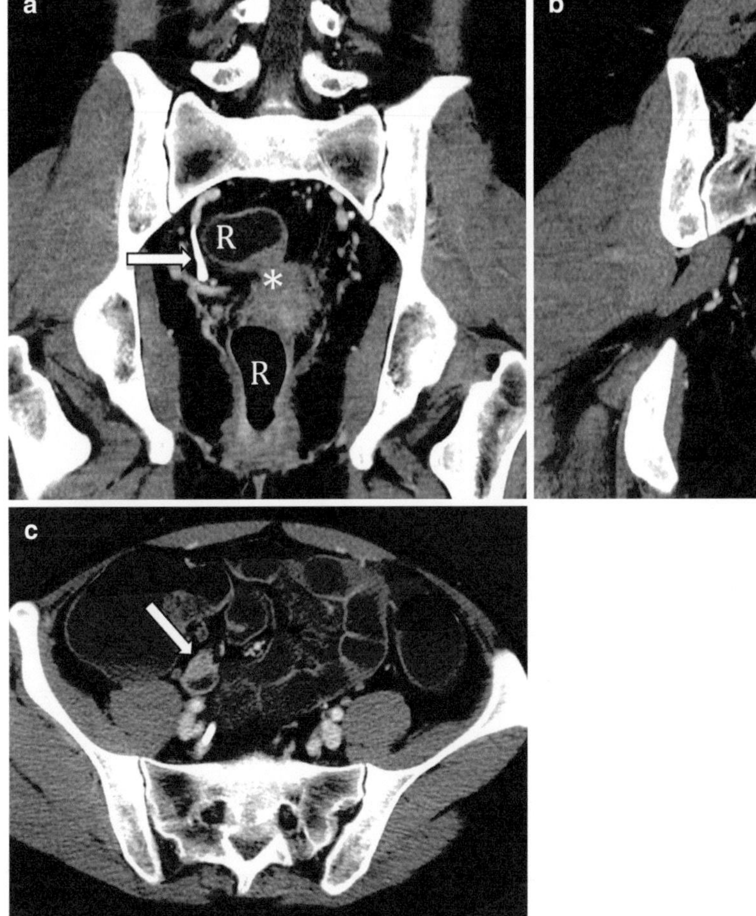

Fig. 8.8 Multidetector computerized tomography enema with "split-bolus technique". (**a**) Coronal reconstruction. The pelvis is infiltrated by endometriosis (asterisk). It involves extensively the rectum (R). The arrow indicates on the right ureter opacified by the split bolus. (**b**) Coronal plane posterior to **a**; the asterisk indicates the endometriotic nodule. (**c**) In the same patient, a cranial axial plane shows a tiny endometriotic nodule adherent to an ileal loop

50%. In addition, in this study MDCT-e had sensitivity of 72.2%, specificity of 100%, diagnostic accuracy of 88.8%, PPV of 100%, and NPV of 87.5% for detecting ureteral endometriosis. The exam also was able to diagnose endometriomas, lesions of the pouch of Douglas, nodules of the rectovaginal septum, lesions of the uterosacral ligaments and bladder lesions. A strength of this study was that it showed an excellent interobserver agreement in the identification of the presence of intestinal endometriosis.

8.4 Comparison Between Multidetector Computerized Tomography Enema and Other Imaging Techniques Used in the Diagnosis of Bowel Endometriosis

Several studies compared the performance of MDCT-e and other imaging techniques commonly used in the diagnosis of bowel endometriosis.

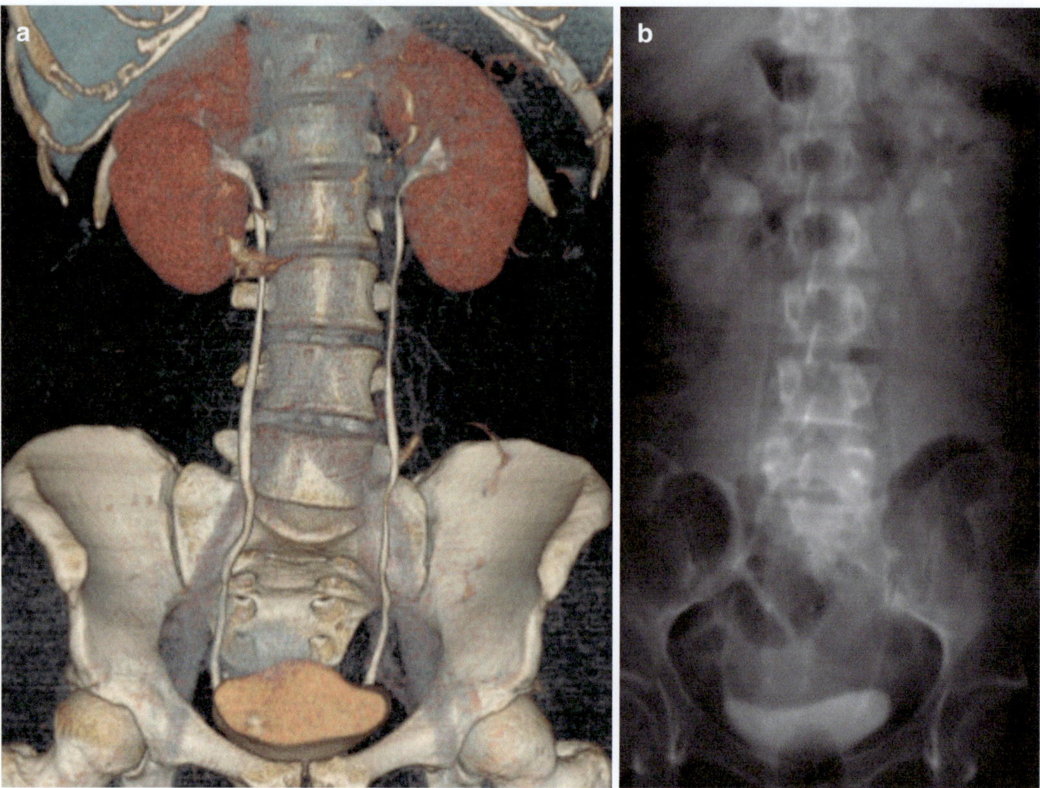

Fig. 8.9 Multidetector computerized tomography enema with "split-bolus technique". (**a**) The 3D image shows the complete opacification of the excretory renal cavities, of the ureters and of the bladder. The "split-bolus technique" allows to acquire a single volume during the excretory phase of the pre-bolus of iodinated contrast medium. (**b**) In the same exam, it is possible to create a virtual "urography," applying a protocol of computerized reconstruction, obtaining an image similar to conventional radiology

8.4.1 Multidetector Computerized Tomography Enema Versus Transvaginal Ultrasonography

An Italian single-center prospective study compared the accuracy of MDCT-e and rectal water contrast transvaginal ultrasonography (RWC-TVS) in the diagnosis of bowel endometriosis. RWC-TVS is a transvaginal ultrasonography that is performed after the distention of the rectosigmoid with 100–350 ml of saline solution that is injected in the bowel using a catheter connected to a syringe [13–15]. Ninety-six patients were included in the study, 51 had surgical diagnosis of bowel endometriosis [7]. TVS did not identify two ileal nodules and one cecal nodule that were detected by MDCT-e. The two techniques had similar accuracy in the diagnosis of bowel endometriosis and in the diagnosis of rectosigmoid endometriosis. MDCT-e had sensitivity of 96.1%, specificity of 100%, PPV of 100%, NPV of 95.7%, LR− of 0.04, and accuracy of 97.9% in diagnosing bowel endometriosis (including nodules located above the sigmoid). The performance of MDCT-e in diagnosing rectosigmoid endometriosis was: sensitivity 95.8%, specificity 100%, PPV 100%, NPV 96.0%, LR− 0.04, and accuracy 97.9%. MDCT-e and RWC-TVS had similar performance in estimating the depth of infiltration of endometriosis in the intestinal wall. Both MDCT-e and RWC-TVS underestimated the size of the endometriotic nodules; however, the underestimation was greater for RWC-TVS than for MDCT-e. In addition, in both imaging techniques the underestimation was greater for nodules with diameter ≥30 mm. There was no

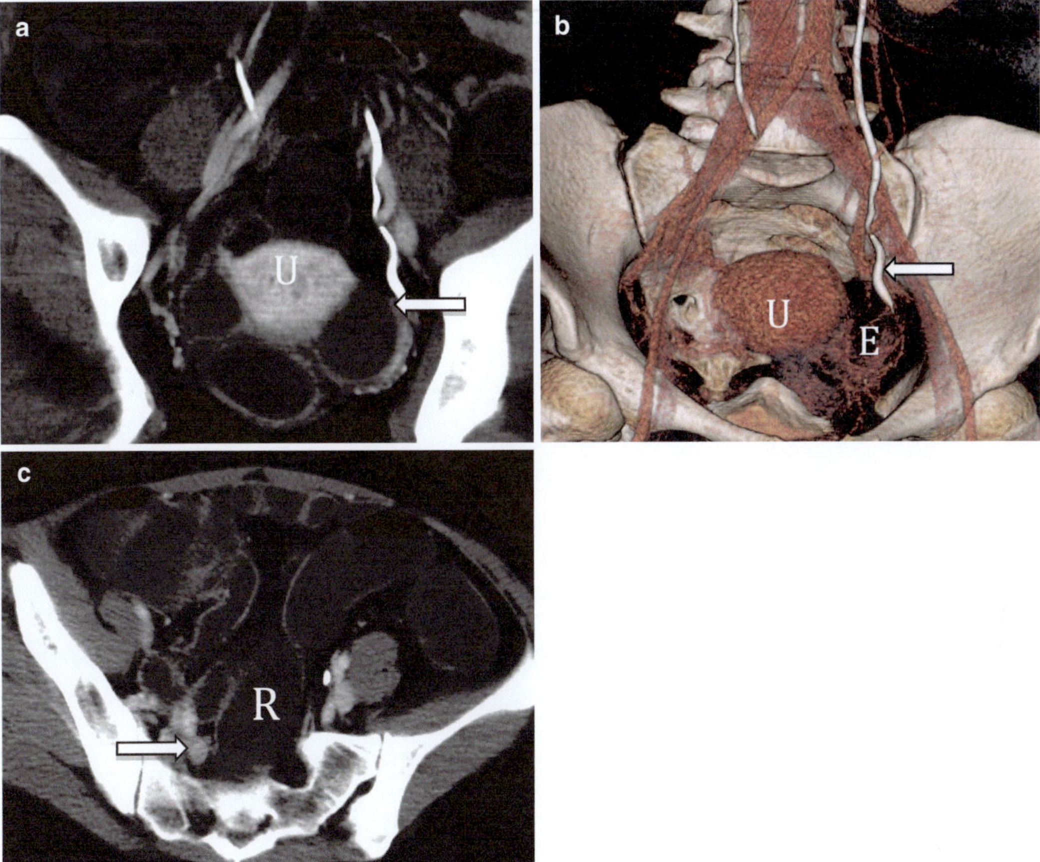

Fig. 8.10 Multidetector computerized tomography enema with "split-bolus technique". (**a**) Coronal reconstruction showing two endometriomas at the sides of the uterus (U). The arrow indicates the left ureter which is compressed by the unilateral endometrioma. The ureter is enhanced by the contrast medium. (**b**) The 3D image shows the same finding demonstrated in Fig. 8.16a. (**c**) Axial image of the same patient. The arrow shows a small endometriotic nodule, which is not penetrating the intestinal wall. A subtle fat plane between the nodule (arrow) and the rectum (R) is present

significant difference in the proportion of patients in whom MDCT-e and RWC-TVS correctly identified the number of rectosigmoid nodules. MDCT-e identified seven out of nine nodules infiltrating only the intestinal serosa.

8.4.2 Multidetector Computerized Tomography Enema Versus Magnetic Resonance Enema

A single-center prospective study compared the accuracy of MDCT-e and magnetic resonance enema (MR-e) in assessing the presence and characteristics of rectosigmoid endometriosis [6]. Following an initial presentation of the preliminary results of this study in the abstract form [16], the final study included 260 women (176 had rectosigmoid endometriotic nodules). The nodules were located on the sigmoid in 54.5% of the patients, on the rectosigmoid junction in 15.9% and on the rectum in 29.6%. The accuracy, sensitivity, specificity, PPV, NPV, LR+, and LR− of MDCT-e in the diagnosis of rectosigmoid endometriosis were 98.5%, 98.3%, 98.8%, 99.4%, 96.5%, 81.59, 0.02. This study demonstrated that MDCT-e and MRI-e had similar accuracy in the diagnosis of rectosigmoid

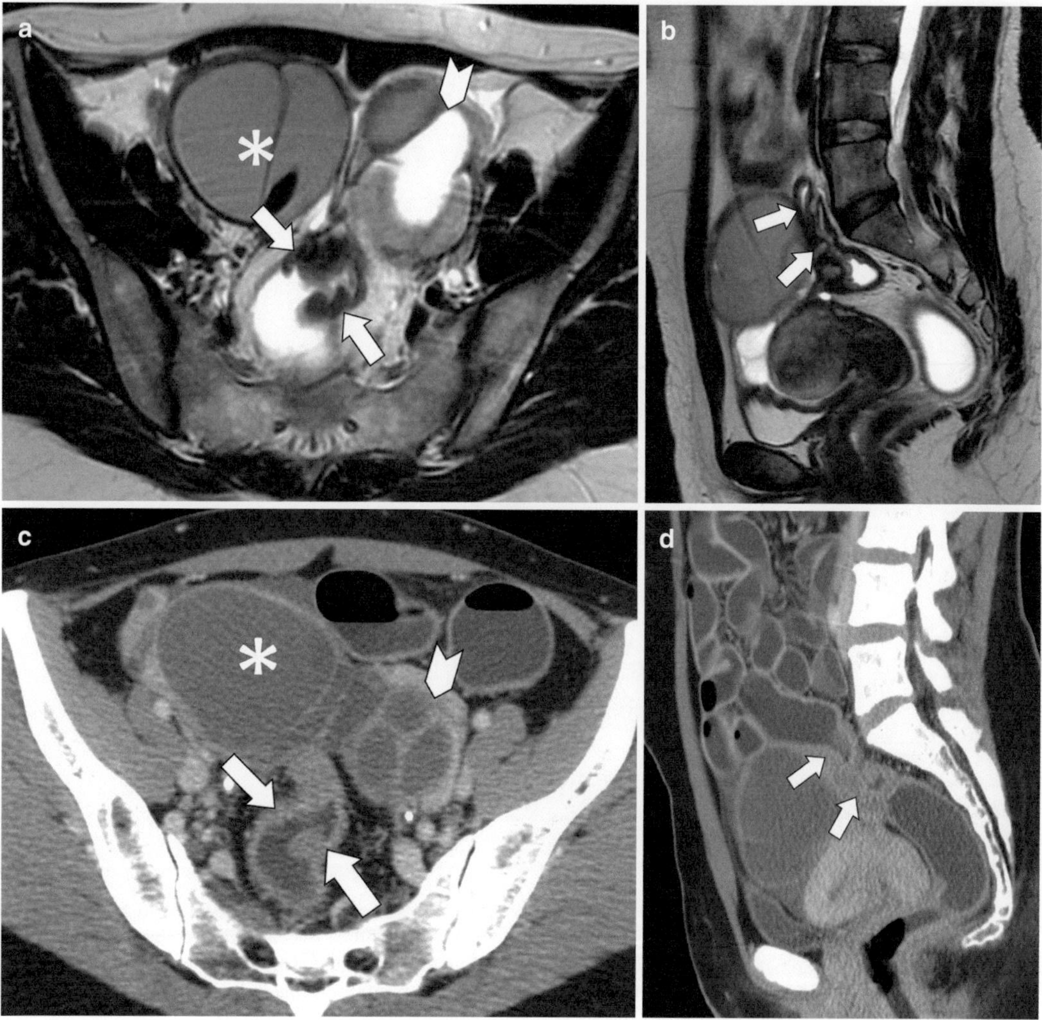

Fig. 8.11 Multidetector computerized tomography enema and magnetic resonance enema. Magnetic resonance enema FrFSE T2W sequence in axial plane (**a**) and in sagittal plane (**b**). The arrows show the stenosis of the rectum caused by the endometriotic nodule. A right ovarian endometrioma (asterisk) can be observed. On the left side, there is an ovarian cyst with mixed liquid (white T2 signal) and endometriotic content (hypointense signal) (arrow head). Multidetector computerized tomography enema of the same patient in the axial plane (**c**) and in sagittal reconstruction (**d**). The MDCT-e image overestimates the rectosigmoid stenosis if compared with the corresponding MR-e image

endometriosis (Figs. 8.11a–d, 8.12a–d, and 8.13a–c). MDCT-e identified three nodules located on the cecum that were not diagnosed by MRI-e. Both imaging techniques underestimated the size of the intestinal endometriotic nodules, and the underestimation was greater for nodules with diameter ≥30 mm.

8.4.3 Multidetector Computerized Tomography Enteroclysis

No large study investigated the use of MDCT enteroclysis in the diagnosis of ileal endometriosis. However, Zouari-Zaoui et al. described two patients with ileal endometriosis diagnosed

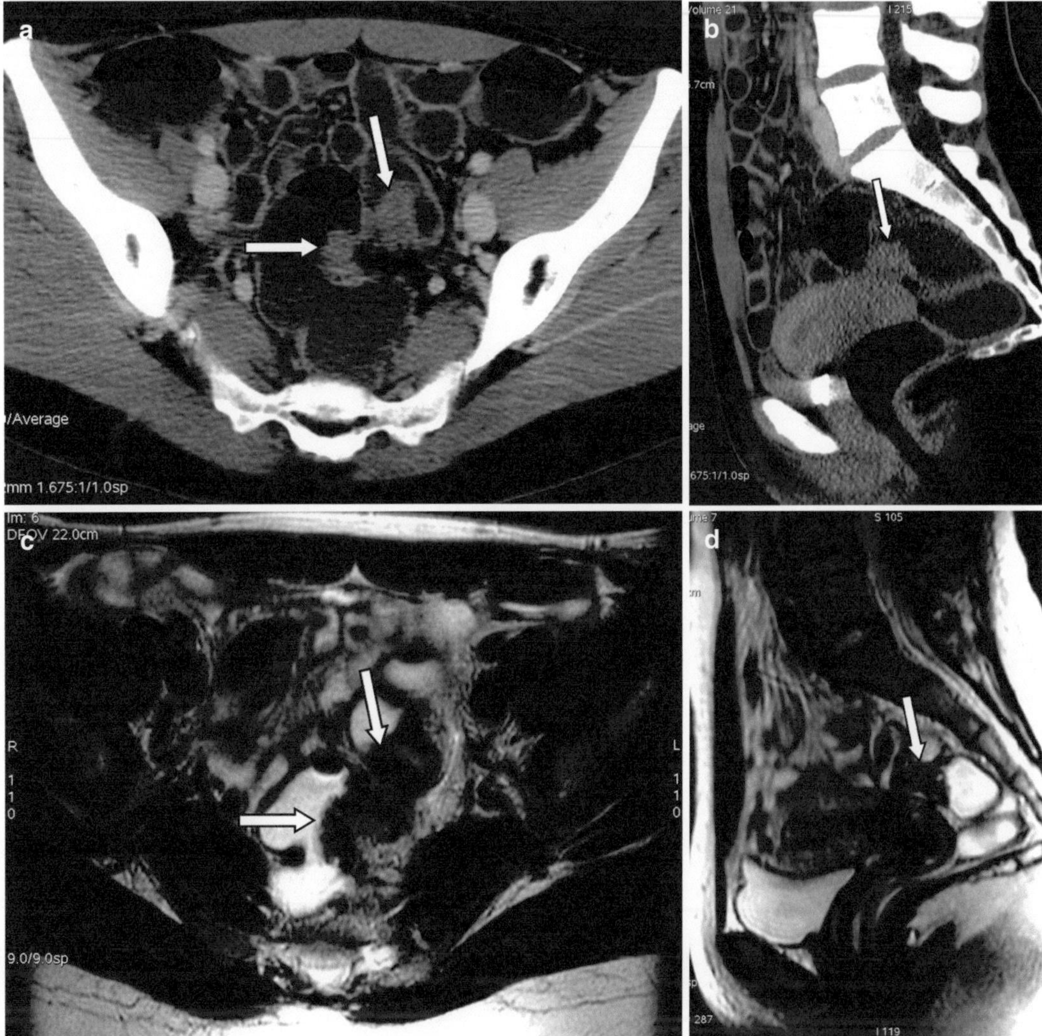

Fig. 8.12 Multidetector computerized tomography enema and magnetic resonance enema. (**a**) Multidetector computerized tomography enema, axial reconstruction. The arrows indicate two endometriotic rectosigmoid nodules. (**b**) Multidetector computerized tomography enema, the sagittal reconstruction shows the rectal nodule. (**c**) Magnetic resonance enema, T2W scan. The axial scan shows the nodules demonstrated in **a**. (**d**) Magnetic resonance enema, T2W scan. The sagittal scan shoes the nodule demonstrated in **b**

by MDCT enteroclysis [17]. In one patient the exam demonstrated dilated small bowel up to an area of stenosis due to circumferential parietal thickening in the distal ileum and, in the other patient, an ileal parietal solid nodule was observed. MDCT enteroclysis was performed positioning an 8-F nasojejunal tube into the duodenojejunal junction by using fluoroscopic guidance. Room temperature water (less than 2000 ml) was infused with a pressure-controlled pump at a rate of 150–200 ml/min. Intestinal hypotonization and intravenous injection of nonionic iodinated CM was performed before image acquisition [18].

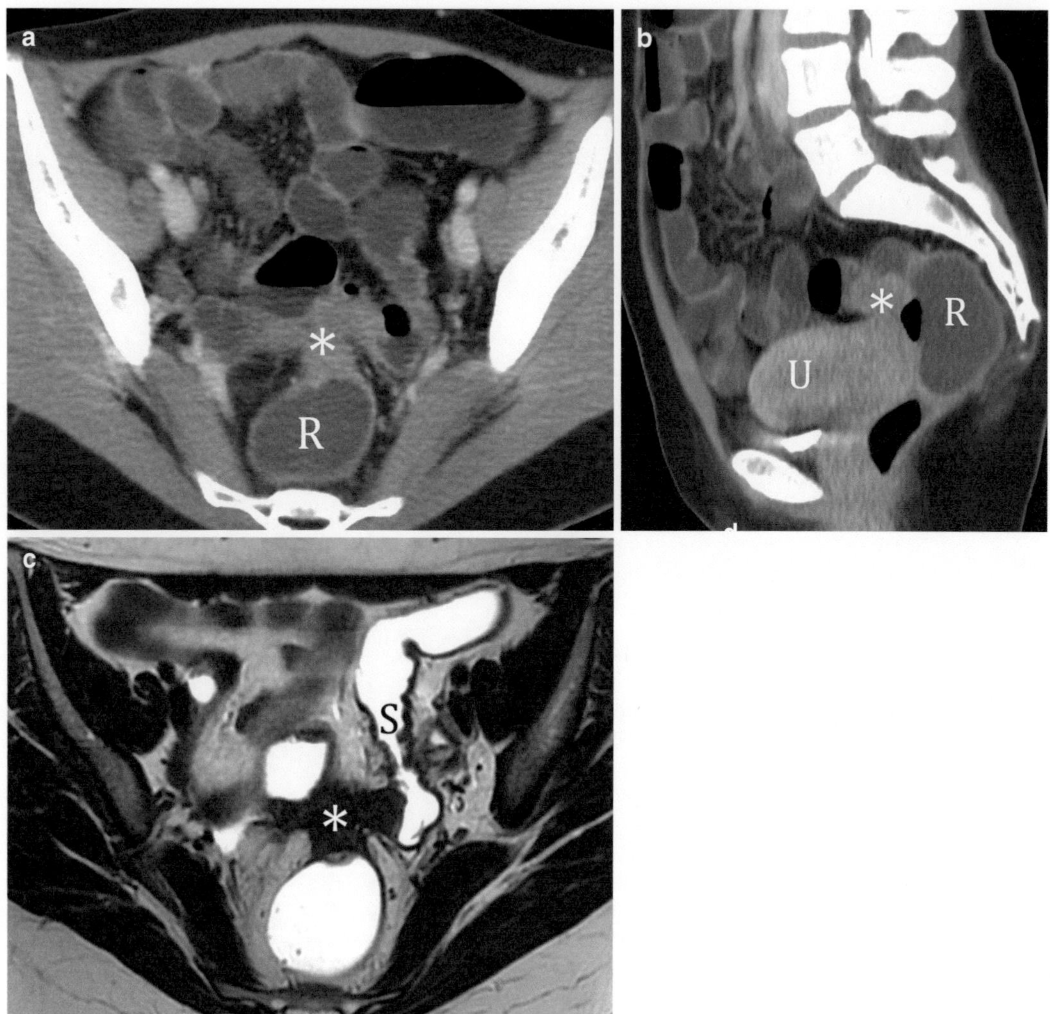

Fig. 8.13 Multidetector computerized tomography enema and magnetic resonance enema. (**a**) Multidetector computerized tomography enema, the asterisk shows an endometriotic nodule that infiltrates the rectum (R) and the sigmoid colon. (**b**) Multidetector computerized tomography enema, sagittal reconstruction shows the sigmoid colon (S) which is infiltrated. *R* rectum, *U* uterus. (**c**) Magnetic resonance enema, SE T2W image in axial plane shows the nodule (asterisk) demonstrated in Fig. 8.7a. *S* sigmoid colon

8.5 Conclusion

MDCT-e allows a "panexploring" study of the entire colon from the rectum to the cecum and the last ileal loops (Figs. 8.14a–c and 8.15a–d). This is one of the major advantages of MDCT-e. The noninvasive diagnosis of multiple endometriotic nodules located in different bowel segment (multicentric disease) allows the surgeon to provide the patient an adequate preoperative informed consent. In fact, these patients may require multiple segmental bowel resections or disc excisions.

The studies presented in this chapter show that MDCT-e is accurate and reproducible in diagnosing intestinal endometriosis. The forced distension of the lumen highlights the decreased distensibility of the bowel wall due to endometriotic infiltration [8]. The images have high spatial resolution and their evaluation in axial, sagittal, and coronal planes allows higher diagnostic con-

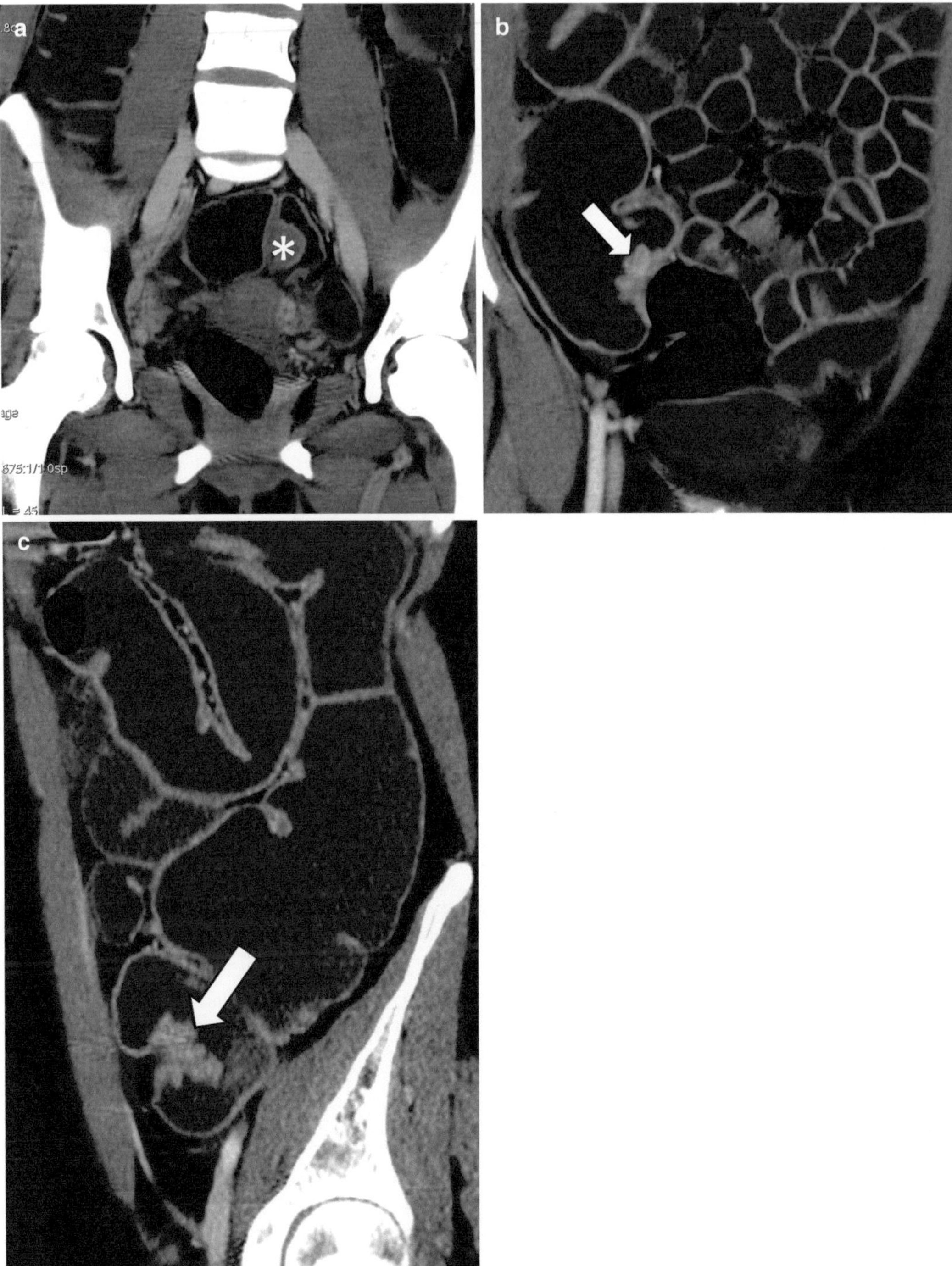

Fig. 8.14 Multidetector computerized tomography enema. A rectal endometriotic nodule is observed in the coronal reconstruction (asterisk, **a**). The intestinal disten- tion allows to identify in the same patient a cecal endometriotic nodule in paracoronal reconstruction (**b**) and in sagittal reconstruction (**c**)

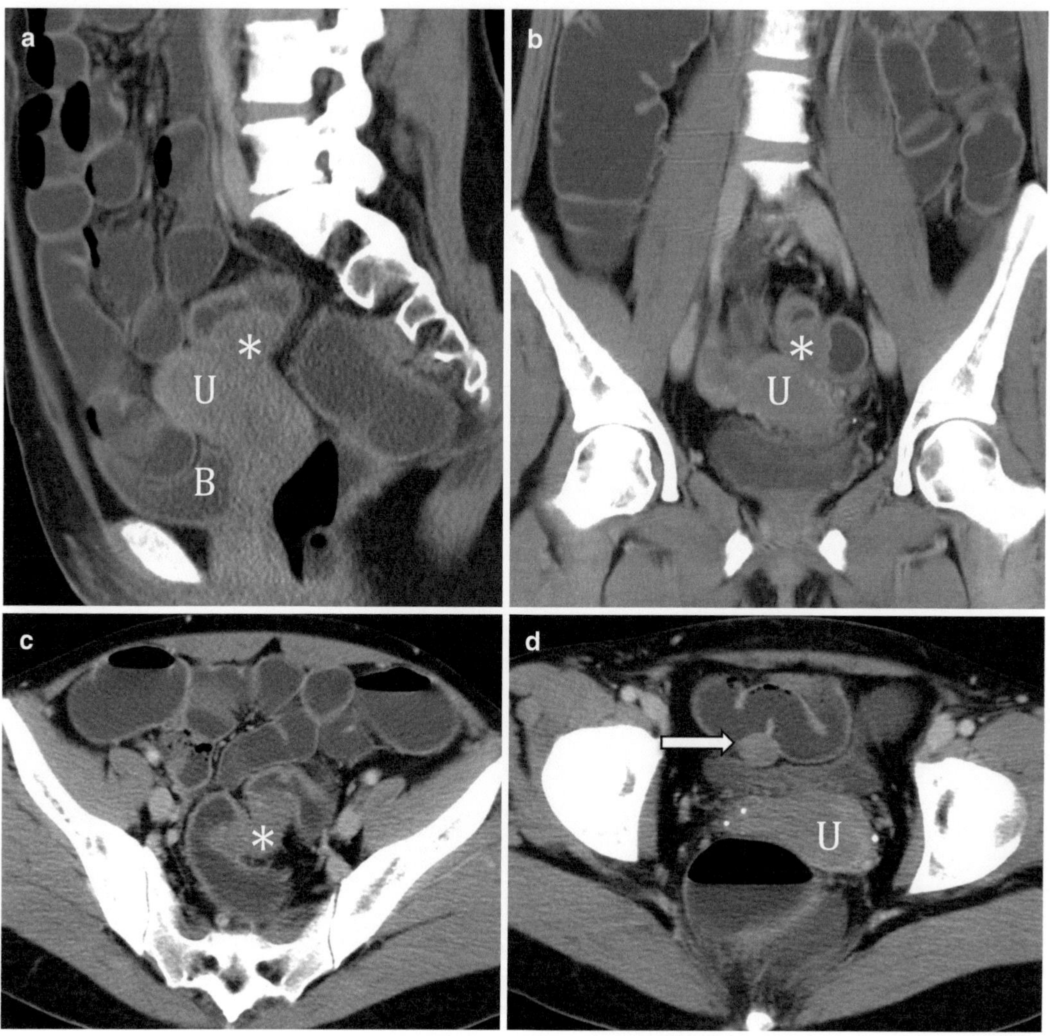

Fig. 8.15 Multidetector computerized tomography enema. Endometriotic nodule (asterisk) infiltrating the sigmoid colon in sagittal (**a**), coronal (**b**), and axial (**c**) reconstruction. Another axial scan (**d**) demonstrates that the nodule infiltrates the distal loops of the ileum. *U* uterus, *B* bladder

fidence. In addition, coronal images obtained by multiplanar reconstruction are more easily understandable both for radiological diagnosis and for clinical discussion with surgeons and clinicians [10]. A recent Cochrane review concluded that, compared with other imaging techniques, MDCT-e displayed the highest diagnostic performance for rectosigmoid and other bowel endometriosis and met the criteria for both SpPin triage test (ruling in the diagnosis with a positive result) and SnNout triage tests (ruling out the diagnosis with a negative result), but studies were too few to provide meaningful results [19].

MDCT-e not only identifies precisely the presence of intestinal endometriotic nodules, but it also estimates the characteristics of these lesions. MDCT-e accurately estimates the size of endometriotic nodules [5]. Curved MPR images permit to measure the distance of the endometriotic nodule from the anal verge. MDCT-e carried out using the split-bolus technique allows to detect endometriotic lesions involving the ureters [5, 9]. MDCT-e allows to estimate the depth of infiltration of endometriosis in the intestinal wall (Fig. 8.16a–c) [5]. However, a better assessment of the depth of intestinal wall involvement is

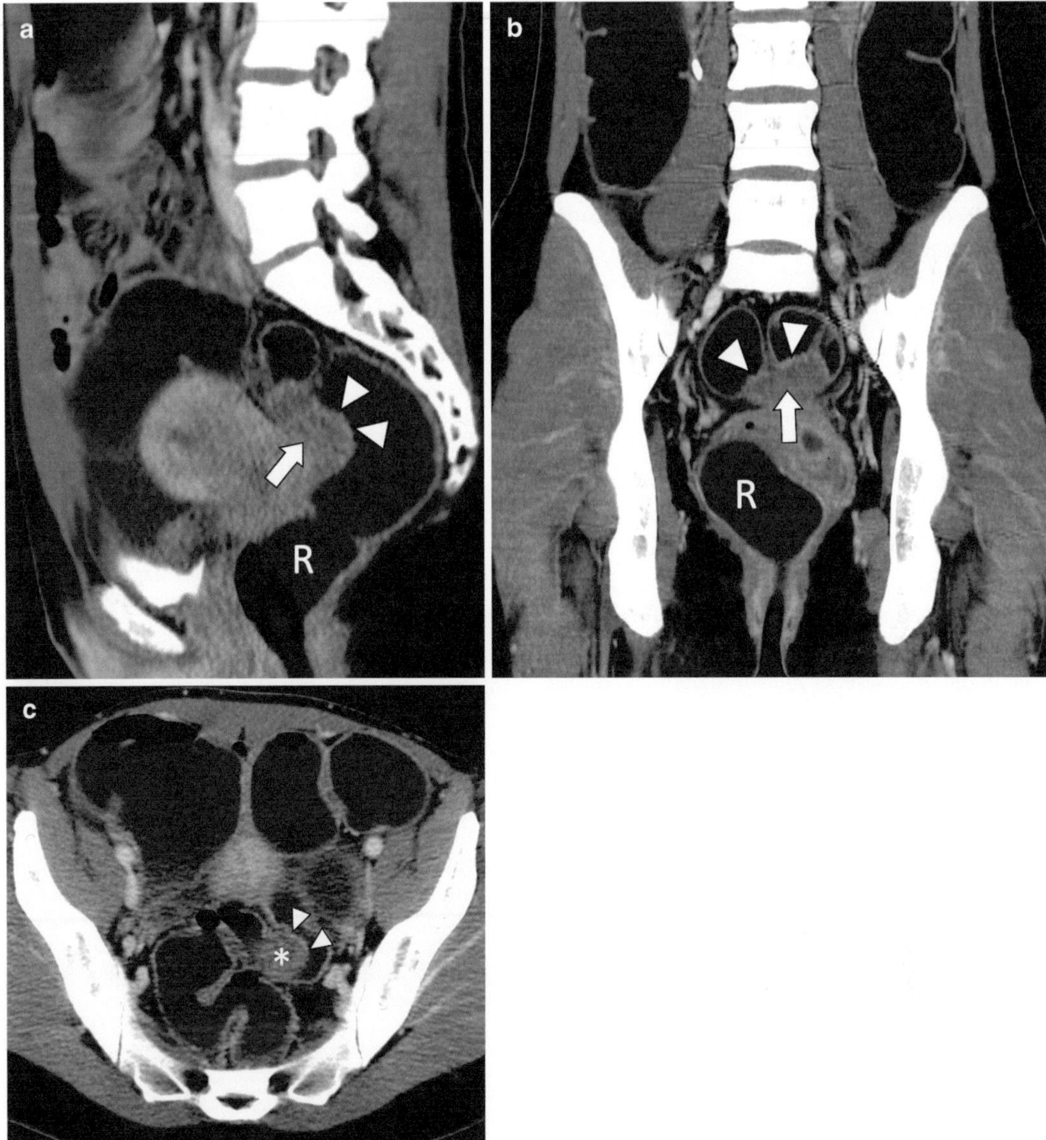

Fig. 8.16 Multidetector computerized tomography enema. (**a**) Sagittal reconstruction shows the endometriotic nodule (arrow) infiltrating the low sigmoid colon and the high rectum. (**b**) Coronal reconstruction shows the nodule (arrow) demonstrated in **a**. (**c**) The axial reconstruction shows the nodule demonstrated in **a** and **b**. In all the images the arrowheads show the mucosa which is not infiltrated

probably obtained by other imaging techniques such as transvaginal ultrasonography [20–22]. Obviously, MDCT-e can diagnose ovarian endometrioma (Fig. 8.10a–c). However, because of its low intrinsic resolution, MDCT-e is less precise than other imaging techniques (such as TVS and MRI) in assessing the presence of deep endometriotic nodules (such as those on the uterosacral ligaments and on the rectovaginal septum).

The main limitation of MDCT-e in the assessment of bowel endometriosis is the radiation dose delivered to the patients. A significant reduction in the radiation dose can be obtained by dedicated algorithmic reconstruction normally implemented in modern CT scanners (such as the adaptive statistical iterative reconstruction, ASiR-v algorithm; GE Healthcare, Milwaukee, WI, USA). Obviously, another limitation of

MDCT-e is the intravenous administration of iodinated CM, which can potentially cause various degrees of adverse reactions [23].

The experience of the radiologist performing MDCT-e is crucial in diagnosing bowel endometriosis. However, one study documented an excellent interobserver agreement in the identification of intestinal endometriosis [5].

In conclusion, MDCT-e has the ideal advantage of evaluating the whole colon, the cecum and the last ileal loops. The studies described in this chapter show that MDTC-e has similar performance to MR-e [6] and to RWC-TVS [7] in diagnosing rectosigmoid endometriosis. Based on the similar diagnostic performance and the disadvantages of MDCT-e (exposure to radiation and use of iodinated CM), this technique is currently not routinely used as the first-line investigation of patients with suspicion of intestinal endometriosis. However, MDCT-e may have a role in the diagnosis of intestinal nodules located above the sigmoid and in assessing the degree of stenosis of the intestinal lumen in patients with bowel endometriosis.

References

1. Pilleul F, Bansac-Lamblin A, Monneuse O, Dumortier J, Milot L, Valette PJ. Water enema computed tomography: diagnostic tool in suspicion of colorectal tumor. Gastroenterol Clin Biol. 2006;30(2):231–4.
2. Ridereau-Zins C, Aube C, Luet D, Vielle B, Pilleul F, Dumortier J, et al. Assessment of water enema computed tomography: an effective imaging technique for the diagnosis of colon cancer: colon cancer: computed tomography using a water enema. Abdom Imaging. 2010;35(4):407–13.
3. Soyer P, Sirol M, Dray X, Place V, Pautrat K, Hamzi L, et al. Detection of colorectal tumors with water enema-multidetector row computed tomography. Abdom Imaging. 2012;37(6):1092–100.
4. Soyer P, Hamzi L, Sirol M, Duchat F, Dray X, Hristova L, et al. Colon cancer: comprehensive evaluation with 64-section CT colonography using water enema as intraluminal contrast agent-a pictorial review. Clin Imaging. 2012;36(2):113–25.
5. Iosca S, Lumia D, Bracchi E, Duka E, De Bon M, Lekaj M, et al. Multislice computed tomography with colon water distension (MSCT-c) in the study of intestinal and ureteral endometriosis. Clin Imaging. 2013;37(6):1061–8.
6. Biscaldi E, Ferrero S, Leone Roberti Maggiore U, Remorgida V, Venturini PL, Rollandi GA. Multidetector computerized tomography enema versus magnetic resonance enema in the diagnosis of rectosigmoid endometriosis. Eur J Radiol. 2014;83(2):261–7.
7. Ferrero S, Biscaldi E, Morotti M, Venturini PL, Remorgida V, Rollandi GA, et al. Multidetector computerized tomography enteroclysis vs. rectal water contrast transvaginal ultrasonography in determining the presence and extent of bowel endometriosis. Ultrasound Obstet Gynecol. 2011;37(5):603–13.
8. Biscaldi E, Ferrero S, Fulcheri E, Ragni N, Remorgida V, Rollandi GA. Multislice CT enteroclysis in the diagnosis of bowel endometriosis. Eur Radiol. 2007;17(1):211–9.
9. Biscaldi E, Ferrero S, Remorgida V, Rollandi GA. MDCT enteroclysis urography with split-bolus technique provides information on ureteral involvement in patients with suspected bowel endometriosis. AJR Am J Roentgenol. 2011;196(5):W635–40.
10. Biscaldi E, Ferrero S, Remorgida V, Rollandi GA. Bowel endometriosis: CT-enteroclysis. Abdom Imaging. 2007;32(4):441–50.
11. Telegrafo M, Lorusso V, Rubini G, Rella L, Pezzolla A, Stabile Ianora AA, et al. [Sigmoid endometriosis: a diagnostic dilemma on multidetector CT]. Recenti Prog Med. 2013;104(7–8):438–41.
12. Guadagno A, Grillo F, Vellone VG, Ferrero S, Fasoli A, Fiocca R, et al. Intestinal endometriosis: mimicker of inflammatory bowel disease? Digestion. 2015;92(1):14–21.
13. Valenzano Menada M, Remorgida V, Abbamonte LH, Nicoletti A, Ragni N, Ferrero S. Does transvaginal ultrasonography combined with water-contrast in the rectum aid in the diagnosis of rectovaginal endometriosis infiltrating the bowel? Hum Reprod. 2008;23(5):1069–75.
14. Menada MV, Remorgida V, Abbamonte LH, Fulcheri E, Ragni N, Ferrero S. Transvaginal ultrasonography combined with water-contrast in the rectum in the diagnosis of rectovaginal endometriosis infiltrating the bowel. Fertil Steril. 2008;89(3):699–700.
15. Morotti M, Ferrero S, Bogliolo S, Venturini PL, Remorgida V, Valenzano Menada M. Transvaginal ultrasonography with water-contrast in the rectum in the diagnosis of bowel endometriosis. Minerva Ginecol. 2010;62(3):179–85.
16. Ferrero S, Leone Roberti Maggiore U, Venturini PL, Rollandi GA, Biscaldi E. Multidetector computerized tomography enteroclysis versus magnetic resonance enteroclysis in the diagnosis of colorectal endometriosis. Fertil Steril. 2013;100(3 Suppl):S103.
17. Zouari-Zaoui L, Soyer P, Merlin A, Boudiaf M, Nemeth J, Rymer R. Multidetector row helical computed tomography enteroclysis findings in ileal endometriosis. Clin Imaging. 2008;32(5):396–9.
18. Boudiaf M, Jaff A, Soyer P, Bouhnik Y, Hamzi L, Rymer R. Small-bowel diseases: prospective evaluation of multi-detector row helical CT entero-

clysis in 107 consecutive patients. Radiology. 2004;233(2):338–44.

19. Nisenblat V, Bossuyt PM, Farquhar C, Johnson N, Hull ML. Imaging modalities for the non-invasive diagnosis of endometriosis. Cochrane Database Syst Rev. 2016;(2):CD009591.

20. Ferrero S, Barra F, Stabilini C, Vellone VG, Leone Roberti Maggiore U, Scala C. Does bowel preparation improve the performance of rectal water contrast transvaginal ultrasonography in diagnosing rectosigmoid endometriosis? J Ultrasound Med. 2018;38(4):1017–25.

21. Ferrero S, Scala C, Stabilini C, Vellone VG, Barra F, Leone Roberti Maggiore U. Transvaginal ultraso-nography with or without bowel preparation in the diagnosis of rectosigmoid endometriosis: prospective study. Ultrasound Obstet Gynecol. 2018;53(3):402–9.

22. Guerriero S, Condous G, Van den Bosch T, Valentin L, Leone FP, Van Schoubroeck D, et al. Systematic approach to sonographic evaluation of the pelvis in women with suspected endometriosis, including terms, definitions and measurements: a consensus opinion from the International Deep Endometriosis Analysis (IDEA) group. Ultrasound Obstet Gynecol. 2016;48:318.

23. Singh J, Daftary A. Iodinated contrast media and their adverse reactions. J Nucl Med Technol. 2008;36(2):69–74; quiz 6–7.

Computed Tomography Colonoscopy

9

Fabio Barra, Ennio Biscaldi, and Simone Ferrero

9.1 Introduction

Computed tomography colonoscopy (CTC) also named virtual colonoscopy was originally developed by Vining et al. in 1994 with the aim to diagnose polyps and early colorectal cancers [1]. Over 20 years from its introduction, CTC is nowadays widely used for colorectal cancer screening [2]. The performance of CTC in diagnosing colorectal cancer is superior to that of barium enema. In fact, several studies showed that CTC with bowel preparation has sensitivity from 73% to 98% and specificity from 89% to 91% in detecting adenomas ≥ 6 mm; these diagnostic values are comparable with those obtained using optical colonoscopy [3]. In addition, CTC is less invasive than colonoscopy, it is easy to perform, and its technique is quite standardized [2]. The reduced bowel preparation and the colonic distention obtained using carbon dioxide (CO_2) increase the compliance of the patients. In addition, the improvements in image reconstruction algorithms decrease radiation exposure. Therefore, the European Society of Gastrointestinal and Abdominal Radiology (ESGAR) and the European Society of Gastrointestinal Endoscopy (ESGE) recommend CTC as the radiological examination of choice in the context of colorectal cancer [4]. Over the last 10 years, CTC has been used to diagnose bowel endometriosis.

9.2 Computed Tomography Colonoscopy Technique

Bowel cleansing is important in CTC; in fact, residual stools in the bowel lumen may either mimic intestinal pathologies or hide a lesion [2]. However, although complete bowel cleansing is useful for the interpretation of CTC, it is not mandatory for the successful performance of CTC which can be performed with the aid of fecal tagging. Several methods for bowel cleansing have been used in patients with suspicion of intestinal endometriosis. A low-fiber diet in the 1–3 days before the exam is used by some radiologist [5, 6] with the aim to decrease fecal volume and improve tagging. In contrast, other radiologists do not require a diet before the exam

Electronic Supplementary Material The online version of this chapter (https://doi.org/10.1007/978-3-030-50446-5_9) contains supplementary material, which is available to authorized users.

F. Barra (✉) · S. Ferrero
Academic Unit of Obstetrics and Gynecology, IRCCS Ospedale Policlinico San Martino, Genova, Italy

Department of Neurosciences, Rehabilitation, Ophthalmology, Genetics, Maternal and Child Health (DiNOGMI), University of Genova, Genova, Italy

E. Biscaldi
Department of Radiology, Galliera Hospital, Genoa, Italy

© Springer Nature Switzerland AG 2020
S. Ferrero, M. Ceccaroni (eds.), *Clinical Management of Bowel Endometriosis*,
https://doi.org/10.1007/978-3-030-50446-5_9

[7]. In order to facilitate bowel cleansing, some authors ask the patient to use a liquid diet in the 24 h before the exam [8]. Fasting from solid food is usually required in the 6 h before the CTC exam [6]. Bowel purgation is usually performed in the 24 h or less before the exam. Polyethylene glycol (PEG) [5, 6], sodium phosphate [9], magnesium citrate [8] and bisacodyl [9] are widely used laxatives for bowel preparation. Sodium phosphate and magnesium citrate are preferred for CTC because they typically leave little fluid in the colon after the preparation [10]. Laxatives are usually administered in the evening before the exam [8, 11]. When virtual colonoscopy is used to evaluate intestinal endometriosis, it must be underlined that the diagnostic goal is not the detection of small polyps or the evaluation of subtle mucosal lesions. Intestinal cleansing improves a correct intestinal distension, but it is not so relevant for precise diagnosis compared to when the CTC is used for colorectal cancer screening.

Fecal and fluid tagging is performed by the oral administration of iodine-based solution [9] or barium-based solution [8, 11] or their combinations. There is no consensus on the most effective method of fecal tagging: type of agent, dose, administration protocol [10]. The contrast agent is administered orally at each meal, typically the day before CTC. The contrast material mixes with the ingested food starting from the stomach and it becomes an integral part of the stool. Part of the tagged feces are evacuated after bowel preparation, while the rest remains in the colon. Absorption of iodine and barium by the intestinal mucosa is negligible. Therefore, fecal tagging facilitates the visualization of bowel pathologies and decrease the number of false-positive exams. In fact, after fecal tagging, residual bowel content appears hyperdense or white and, thus, it can be distinguished from the homogeneous soft tissue density of intestinal lesions [12]. Electronic stool subtraction software allows the colon to be cleansed of tagged residues and this procedure facilitates virtual navigation. Iodinated contrasts usually allow more homogeneous tagging; the risk of allergic reactions is extremely rare. The tagging is not essential to perform the diagnosis of intestinal endometriosis. Minimal fecal residues do not usually impair the correct detection of endometriotic nodules. Nevertheless, the tagging allows detection and subtraction of fecal remnants.

Some radiologists advise to insert a large obstetrical tampon high into the vagina immediately before the exam [8, 13]. This tampon stretches the rectovaginal septum and creates a gas interface with the distended gas filled rectum.

Colon distention is very important in CTC because a suboptimally distended colon limits the detection of the lesions [10]. It is obtained by inflating the colon with air [5, 14] or CO_2 [6–9, 11, 13, 15–17] using a small-caliber, flexible tube inserted into the distal rectum. Some authors use a 12F or 24F Foley catheter for colonic distention [6]; notably, the catheter bulb is not inflated or it is minimally distended in order to prevent distortion of the rectovaginal septum [8]. CO_2 distention decreases postprocedural discomfort compared with air distention due to the fast absorption of CO_2 through the intestinal mucosa [18]. Most radiologists use automatic insufflation with CO_2 [8] which optimizes the distention and minimize the discomfort of the patient, but it increases the cost of the exam. The distention is started with the patient in the left lateral decubitus at a pressure of 15–20 mmHg. After 1–1.5 l has been introduced, the patient is turned supine and the pressure is increased to 15–20 mmHg (without exceeding 25 mmHg) [7, 13, 15, 17]. Intestinal distention is usually well tolerated without relevant adverse effects [19].

Several authors use spasmolytic agents (such as hyoscine butylbromide) to facilitate the distention by relieving colonic spams [5–7, 15, 20]; this may decrease the discomfort of the patients. The use of spasmolytic agents is not unequivocally established by guidelines [4]; this is the reason why the use of intestinal hypotonization is not mandatory but suggested, to improve the compliance of the patients.

A multidetector computed tomography scanner ($\geq$16 rows) is required to obtain high quality images. A slice collimation $\leq$3 mm with a reconstruction interval $\leq$1.5 mm provides optimal images [7, 15].

Both supine and prone scans are usually obtained [9, 15]; this combination allows higher diagnostic performance compared with either position alone [21, 22] and it ensure that all segments are adequately visualized. The prone scan is particularly important, because this position improves the distention of the rectosigmoid colon and it promotes the best evaluation of the recto-uterine space, minimizing the extrinsic compression by the uterus.

The radiation dose can be decreased, without impairing the diagnostic performance, to as low as 80 mA with a total effective dose of 2.4 mSv in women [23], which is less than half the radiation dose of a barium enema [10]. Published studies in patients with endometriosis used a mean dose per patient ranging of about 12 mSv [5]. In order to decrease the X-ray dose administered to the patient, the field of view may be limited to the pelvic bowel (rectosigmoid, distal descending colon, proximal ascending colon, and cecum) which is more frequently affected by endometriosis. The entire abdomen is scanned only in particular cases (such as doubtful localizations of endometriosis outside the pelvis, patient with suspicion of hydronephrosis) [8].

Intravenous contrast medium (CM) may be useful for differentiating intestinal pathologies from fecal residues [24, 25] and for improving the detection of pathologies in poorly prepared colons [26]. However, it is not routinely used in CTC [10]. The use of CM in the diagnosis of bowel endometriosis is debated with some radiologists who use it [7, 17] and others who do not use it [8, 16]. The ideal evaluation of the depth of penetration of the endometriotic nodules in the intestinal wall is allowed by the use of the iodinated CM. CTC shows the profile of the nodule which penetrates the intestinal wall but the distinction between nodule and colonic wall is maximally improved by the injections of the CM. However, the integrated use of bidimensional images (axial scans) and pseudoendoscopic images allow a good detection of the endometriotic nodule event without the use of iodinated CM (Video 9.1). From another point of view, intravenous CM must be added when CTC aims to investigate the urinary tract. In this case,

a dose of 1.5 ml/kg of iodinated product is injected at an iodine delivery rate between 1.2 and 1.4 mg I/s through the antecubital vein with an automatic power injector, followed by approximately 250 ml of saline solution which accelerate the urinary CM excretion. Patients are firstly scanned in the supine position during the portal phase, 80–90 s after the intravenous administration of CM. A second scan is performed in the prone position during the urographic phase [5, 6].

Image post-processing is performed using workstations suitable for 3D data management and reconstruction. The evaluation of CTC is based on both 2D and 3D images. 2D evaluations consist in the review of the colon from the rectum to the cecum by scrolling through serial transverse images in a stack mode. It requires tracing of the colonic outline on each image to find small contour abnormalities. 3D review typically refers to an optical colonoscopy-like endoluminal flythrough of a 3D reconstructed colon. This type of review consists of four different fly-throughs: antegrade and retrograde in both the supine and prone positions.

In case of examination performed without CM injection, intestinal endometriotic nodules appear as nodules protruding on the profile of the distended colon. The nodule is normally detected as a lesion infiltrating the intestinal wall and bulging toward the lumen (Fig. 9.1a, b). Differently, in case of use of iodinated CM, the nodule is detectable not only due to its morphology, as before described (Fig. 9.2). Although the morphological aspect with or without CM is the same, iodine injection enhances the visualization of the nodule as well as of the intestinal wall, improving the detection of the lesion. Moreover, it facilitates the assessment of the depth of infiltration of the nodule in the intestinal wall. In this situation, it is easier to distinguish if the nodule is contiguous or penetrating the intestinal wall, causing an extrinsic mass effect [5]. Bowel endometriosis is suspected in the presence of shortening, tethering or flattening of the bowel wall and/or retraction of the mucosa [16], in both presence or absence of the CM.

The time required to perform CTC examinations is variable due to the different compliance

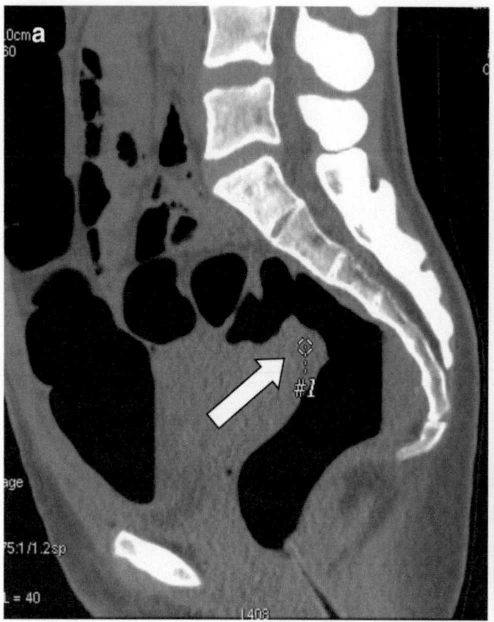

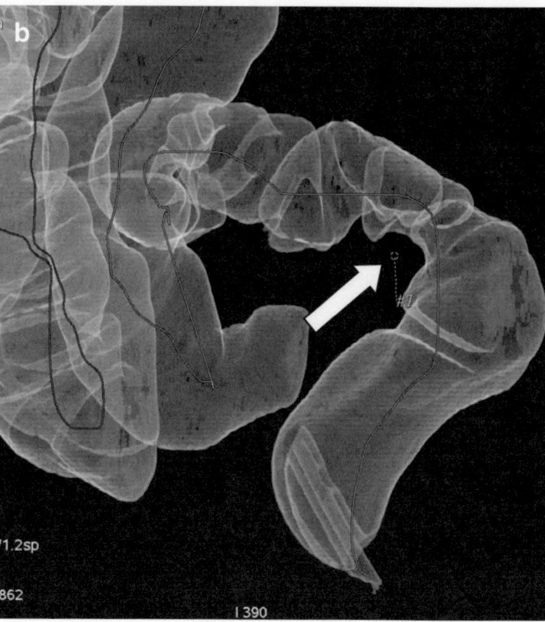

Fig. 9.1 Computerize tomography colonoscopy reconstruction. (**a**) Computerize tomography colonoscopy sagittal reconstruction. A marker shows the endometriotic nodule. (**b**) The "double contrast like" image gives to the surgeon a "tridimensional" idea of the spatial position of the nodule

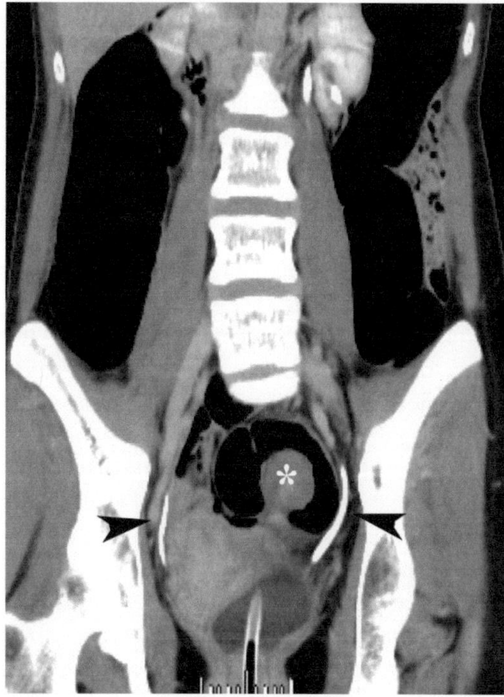

Fig. 9.2 Computerize tomography colonoscopy with contrast medium injection: coronal reconstruction. The ureters can be detected (arrowheads). The sigmoid colon is dilated and the endometriotic nodule bulges into the lumen. The nodule is positively enhanced by contrast injection

levels of the patient, in case of colonic distension. The quality of the distension influences the effectiveness of the examination: that is the reason why it is difficult to report a standardized time to complete a CTC examination. Following the literature, it usually ranges between 15 and 24 min [19], but it is important to consider the variability among different patients, especially if a population of young women is considered.

9.3 Computed Tomography Colonoscopy in the Diagnosis of Bowel Endometriosis

The use of CTC in the diagnosis of bowel endometriosis was originally reported in 2002 in a 29-year-old woman admitted to the hospital because of pain, constipation, and cyclical rectal bleeding. The exam demonstrated a severe stenosis of the sigmoid caused by a submucosal mass. The diagnosis of endometriosis was subsequently based on optical colonoscopy and biopsy [27].

The use of CTC in the diagnosis of intestinal endometriosis was systematically described by van der Wat and Kaplan in 2007 [8]. The authors demonstrated the following forms of endometriosis. "Extrinsic bowel wall involvement" was defined as an impression of the bowel wall caused by extrinsic endometriotic lesions (such as endometriomas) that were not necessarily infiltrating the intestinal muscularis. In these cases, the mucosa is usually smooth with no serrations or puckering. "Bowel strictures" were defined as a circumferential involvement of the intestinal wall; these strictures are observed on both supine and prone scans confirming that they are not caused by underdistention or by spasm. CTC allows to differentiate intestinal endometriosis from colorectal cancer that usually appears as an intrinsic exophytic mass. "Invasive colorectal endometriosis" was defined as transmural invasion with mucosal involvement that can be observed at multiplanar and fly-through reconstructions. "Rectovaginal septum involvement" was defined as a nodularity and asymmetrical thickening of the septum that is clearly visible on multiplanar reconstructions. In case of ureteral stenosis causing ureteral distention and/or hydronephrosis, urinary tract involvement can be diagnosed without intravenous CM. However, in general the urinary tract can be adequately assessed administering IV contrast. Finally, CTC was also used to assess the quality of the anastomosis after segmental colorectal resection.

Subsequently Koutoukos et al. used CTC in patients with suspected intestinal endometriosis and obstructive symptoms [11]. CTC could diagnose bowel endometriosis in all the patients and it also allowed to diagnose extracolonic disease in some patients. However, the authors did not declare the number of patients who underwent CTC and they did not provide information on the characteristics of the intestinal nodules.

A French study described the use of CTC in 27 patients who underwent laparoscopic excision of deep endometriosis [17]. CTC precisely estimated the length of the intestinal stenosis (mean, 54 mm in patients treated by segmental colorectal resection and 50 mm in the other patients). In addition, it estimated the diameter of the intestinal lumen at the level of the stenosis (10 mm in patients treated by segmental

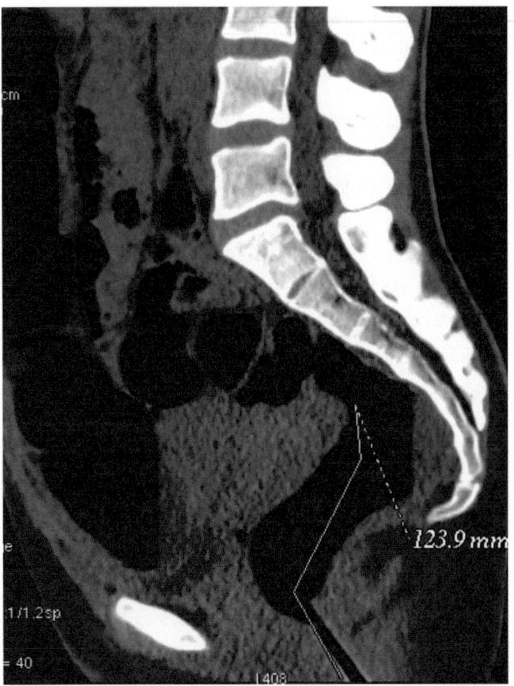

Fig. 9.3 Computerize tomography colonoscopy. Sagittal reconstruction. An electronic estimation of the distance between the endometriotic nodule and the anal verge is performed. The measure is performed on the volume of images and along a curvilinear trace

colorectal resection and 14 mm in the other patients). In addition, the authors showed that CTC was precise in estimating the distance between the intestinal stenosis and the anal verge (Fig. 9.3).

A single-center prospective pilot study published only in the abstract form investigated the accuracy of CTC in the diagnosis of rectosigmoid endometriosis [14]. Out of 53 patients included in the study 42 underwent laparoscopy and were included in the analysis (24 patients had rectosigmoid endometriosis at surgery). The sensitivity, specificity, positive predictive value (PPV), negative predictive value (NPV), positive likelihood ratio (LR+), and negative likelihood ratio (LR−) of CTC in diagnosing bowel endometriosis were 95.8%, 88.9%, 92.0%, 94.1%, 8.62 and 0.05, respectively.

Recently, an Italian retrospective study investigated the diagnostic performance of CTC with intravenous CM and urographic phase in 73 women with strong clinical suspicion of deep endometriosis [6]. CTC had sensitivity of 82.3%, specificity of 66.7%, PPV of 92.7% and NPV of 42.1% in diagnosing rectosigmoid endometriosis. However, the sensitivity of CTC was higher in detecting nodules located on the rectosigmoid junction (57.7%) and on the sigmoid colon (63.6%) and lower rectal lesions (18.8%). When considering the diagnosis of deep endometriosis of the urinary tract, CTC had sensitivity of 45.9%, specificity of 78.4%, PPV of 68.0%, and NPV of 59.1%.

9.4 Comparison Between Computed Tomography Colonoscopy and Other Imaging Techniques for the Diagnosis of Bowel Endometriosis

Some studies compared the diagnostic performance of CTC and other imaging techniques commonly used in the diagnosis of intestinal endometriosis.

9.4.1 Computed Tomography Colonoscopy Versus Magnetic Resonance Imaging

Magnetic resonance imaging (MRI) is commonly used not only to diagnose rectosigmoid endometriosis but also other forms of deep pelvic endometriosis and ovarian endometriomas [28].

A Korean retrospective study compared the diagnostic performance of CTC and MRI in diagnosing rectosigmoid endometriosis [9]. The study included 50 patients (37 with rectosigmoid endometriosis at surgery). CTC had significantly higher diagnostic accuracy for rectosigmoid endometriosis than that of MRI. With CTC, the luminal alteration of the rectosigmoid was detected with sensitivity of 96.0%, specificity of 48.0%, PPV of 64.9%, and NPV of 92.3%. In this study both CTC and MRI were sensitive in the detection of rectosigmoid endometriosis, but they lacked specificity.

A French retrospective study based on a prospectively collected database investigated the role of CTC in the preoperative assessment of bowel endometriosis [7]. One hundred and twenty-seven patients underwent CTC, MRI and endorectal ultrasonography (ERUS). CTC had sensitivity of 97.2%, specificity of 84.2%, PPV of 97.2%, and NPV of 84.2% in diagnosing rectal endometriosis. The sensitivity was 92.6%, the specificity 87.7%, the PPV 84.8%, and the NPV 94.1% in diagnosing sigmoid nodules. Finally, when considering intestinal lesions located above the sigmoid colon, the sensitivity was 91.7%, the specificity 86.6%, the PPV 85.9%, and the NPV 92.1%. In addition, the sensibility and specificity of CTC were over 90% in identifying bowel stenosis. CTC performed better than ERUS in the diagnosis of stenosis and of sigmoid nodules. Furthermore, the information provided by CTC on height and length of colorectal nodules (Fig. 9.4) were close to those measured intraoperatively. When compared to intraoperative data, the estimation of the height and length of colorectal involvement was significantly different using ERUS, while that of the length of bowel

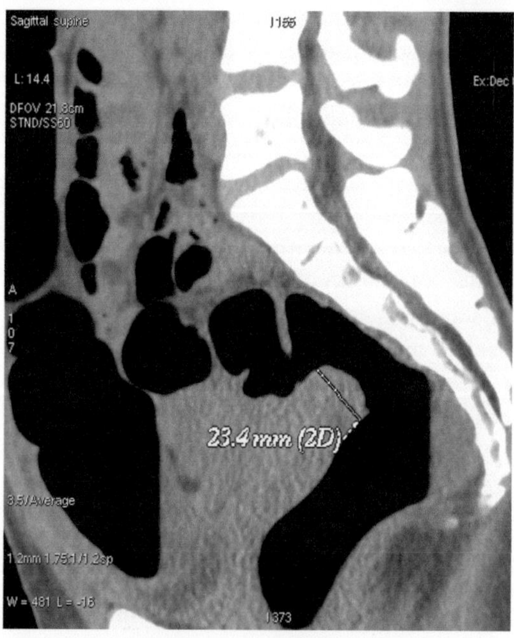

Fig. 9.4 Computerize tomography colonoscopy reconstruction. A system of electronic caliper allows to evaluate the main diameter of the endometriotic nodule

infiltration was significantly different using MRI (Fig. 9.5a, b). Therefore, the authors concluded that the data provided by CTC are very useful in choosing the surgical technique (intestinal shaving, disk excision or segmental resection). A potential limitation of this study was that the surgeons were not blinded to the findings of CTC; therefore, knowledge of preoperative data could

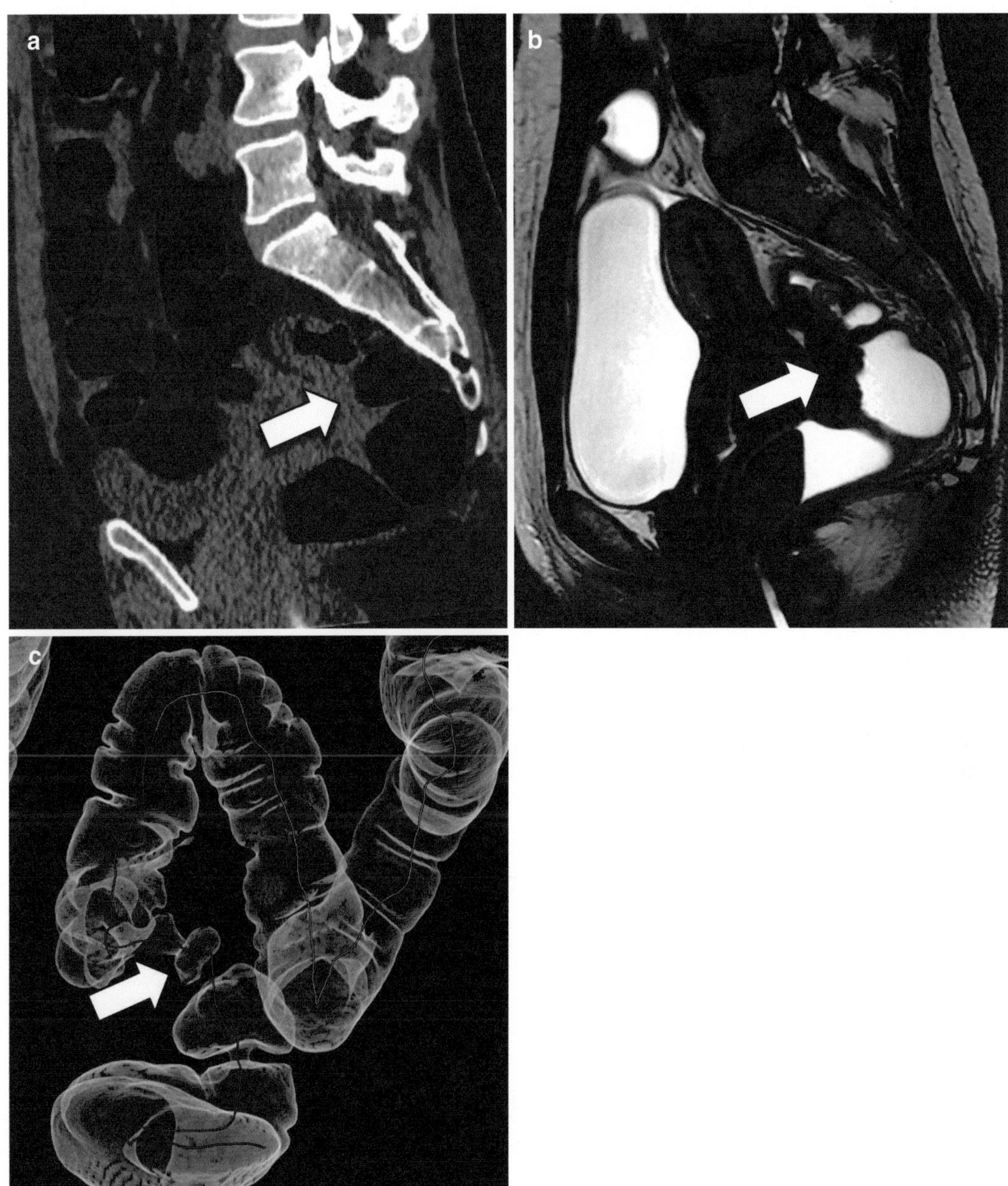

Fig. 9.5 Computed tomography colonoscopy and magnetic resonance enema. (**a**) CTC sagittal reconstruction: the endometriosis infiltrates the anterior wall of the rectum. (**b**) Magnetic resonance sagittal FSE T2W acquisition confirms the infiltration of the intestinal muscularis. The mucosa is continuous and the endometriotic nodule does not overcome it. (**c**) "Double contrast like" reconstruction shows the stenosis of the intestinal lumen caused by infiltration of the intestinal muscularis

interfere with intraoperative estimation of stenosis, length, and height of the intestinal nodules (Fig. 9.6a–c).

A retrospective analysis of a prospectively collected database (71 patients with rectosigmoid endometriosis) investigated whether combining CTC with MRI (with vaginal and rectal opacification) improves the preoperative assessment of patient with suspicion of colorectal endometriosis compared with MRI alone [15]. When colorectal endometriosis was diagnosed by clinical examination and/or MRI, patients underwent CTC in order to assess the stenosis of the intestinal lumen, the distance between the bowel nodule and the anal verge, the length of colorectal wall infiltration and to establish the presence of multicentric disease (associated lesions of the colon or small bowel). The average height of rec-

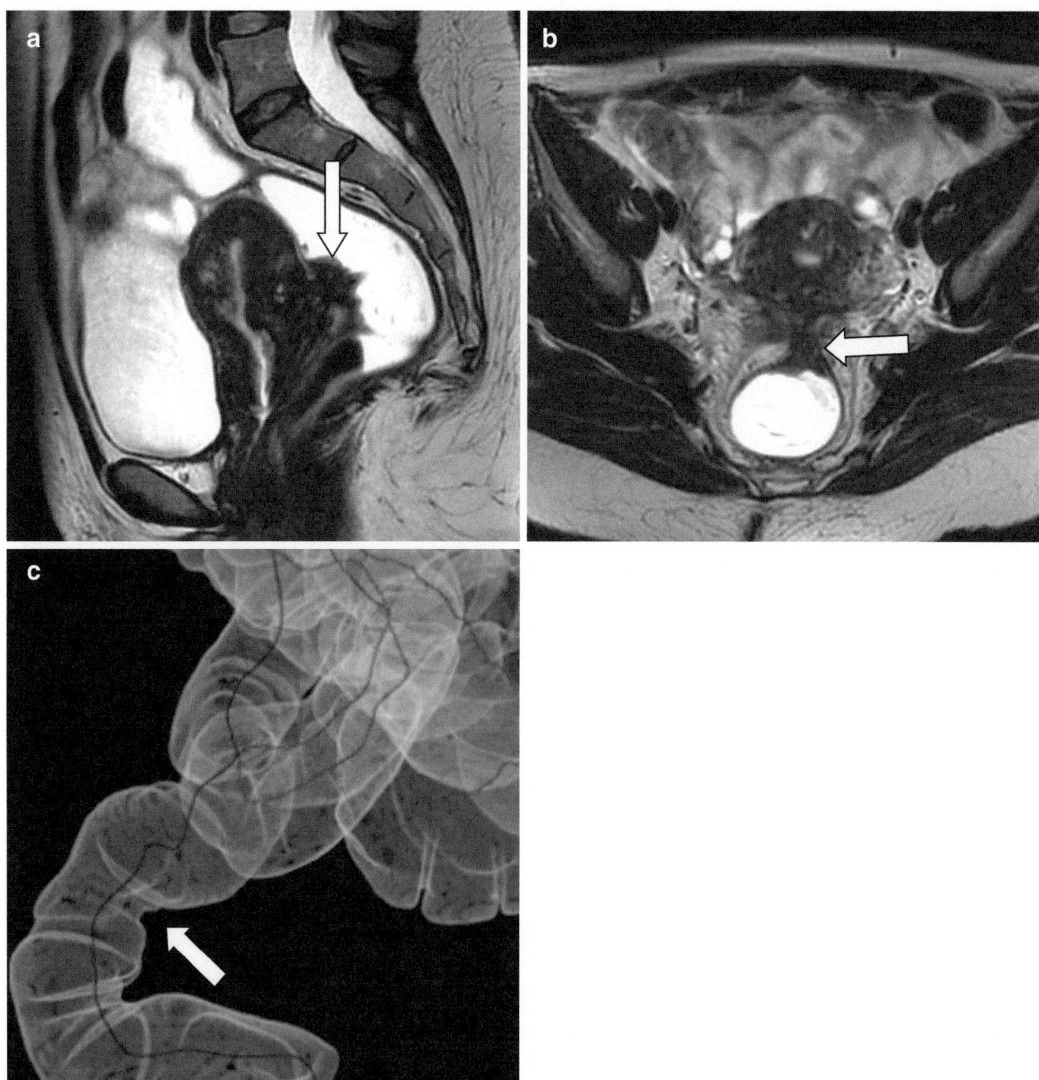

Fig. 9.6 Computed tomography colonoscopy and magnetic resonance enema. (**a**) Magnetic resonance enema FSE T2W sequence, sagittal plane, the endometriotic rectal nodule (arrow) infiltrates the low rectum wall. (**b**) Coronal plana of the nodule shown in (**a**). (**c**) Computerize tomography colonoscopy "double contrast like" image; it is possible to observe the extrinsic compression (arrow) of the presence of the nodule on the anterior rectal wall

tal nodules provided by CTC and the average length of sigmoid nodules provided by MRI were significantly different from those measured intraoperatively. The concordance between intraoperative and preoperative findings provided by MRI combined with CTC regarding the presence of rectal nodules was high. CTC was effective for establishing the degree of stenosis for rectal nodules. For sigmoid nodules intraoperative assessment and CTC showed moderate concordance. Given that sigmoid nodules cause stenosis to a greater degree than rectal nodules, CTC was found to have greater accuracy in the diagnosis of the former than MRI. Combining MRI and CTC increased the accuracy of the diagnosis of both rectal and sigmoid nodules.

9.4.2 Computed Tomography Colonoscopy Versus Transvaginal Ultrasonography

Transvaginal ultrasonography (TVS) is the first-line investigation for the diagnosis of deep endometriosis, including rectosigmoid nodules [29]. Three prospective studies with small sample size compared the performance of CTC and transvaginal ultrasonography (TVS) in diagnosing bowel endometriosis.

A single-center Italian prospective study included 92 patients with clinical suspicion of deep endometriosis, but CTC was performed only in 37 patients (21 of them with bowel endometriosis) [16]. CTC had higher accuracy in detecting bowel endometriosis than TVS. The sensitivity of CTC was 68%, the specificity 67%, the PPV 81%, and the NPV 50%. TVS had sensitivity of 41%, specificity of 93%, PPV of 91%, and NPV of 58%. The authors of this study underlined that the low diagnostic performance of CTC and TVS were related to inexperience of the operators in diagnosing endometriosis. Furthermore, a relevant limitation of this study was the small sample size.

A prospective cross-sectional pilot study including 47 patients compared the diagnostic accuracy of TVS and CTC in diagnosing deep infiltrating endometriosis [5]. TVS had sensitivity of 97.5%, specificity of 33.3%, PPV of 90.9%,

NPV of 66.6%, LR+ of 1.46, and LR− of 0.07 in diagnosing intestinal endometriosis. CTC had sensitivity of 78.0%, specificity of 50.0%, PPV of 90.6%, NPV of 20.0%, LR+ of 1.41, and LR− of 0.59 in diagnosing intestinal endometriosis. TVS had higher accuracy in diagnosing rectal and sigmoid endometriosis. In contrast, a similar accuracy for the two imaging methods was observed for the diagnosis of overall intestinal endometriosis. CTC had higher accuracy than TVS in diagnosing ureteral endometriosis.

A prospective study including 70 patients compared the performance of CTC and rectal water contrast transvaginal ultrasonography (RWC-TVS) in assessing the presence and characteristics of rectosigmoid endometriosis [19] (Fig. 9.7). RWC-TVS is a TVS combined with retrograde water distention of the rectosigmoid (200–300 ml) that has been shown to be accurate for the diagnosis of rectosigmoid endometriosis in several prospective studies [30–33]. Forty patients had surgical diagnosis of rectosigmoid endometriosis. CTC and RWC-TVS had similar accuracy in diagnosing rectosigmoid endometriosis. In particular, CTC had accuracy of 90.0%, sensitivity of 92.5%, specificity of 86.7%, PPV of 90.2%, NPV of 89.7%, LR+ of 6.94, and LR− of 0.09. CTC was significantly more precise than RWC-TVS in estimating the distance between the lower margin of the rectosigmoid nodule and the anal verge. However, CTC was less accurate than RWC-TVS in diagnosing multifocal disease (presence of one or more lesions that affected the rectosigmoid that was associated with the colorectal primary lesion). CTC was significantly less tolerated than RWC-TVS with main intensity of pain measured on a 10 cm visual analogue scale of 39 mm for CTC and 28 mm for RWC-TVS.

9.4.3 Computed Tomography Colonoscopy Versus Magnetic Resonance Imaging Versus Transvaginal Ultrasonography

A recent abstract reported the results of a prospective comparative study who enrolled 43 women with rectosigmoid endometriosis under-

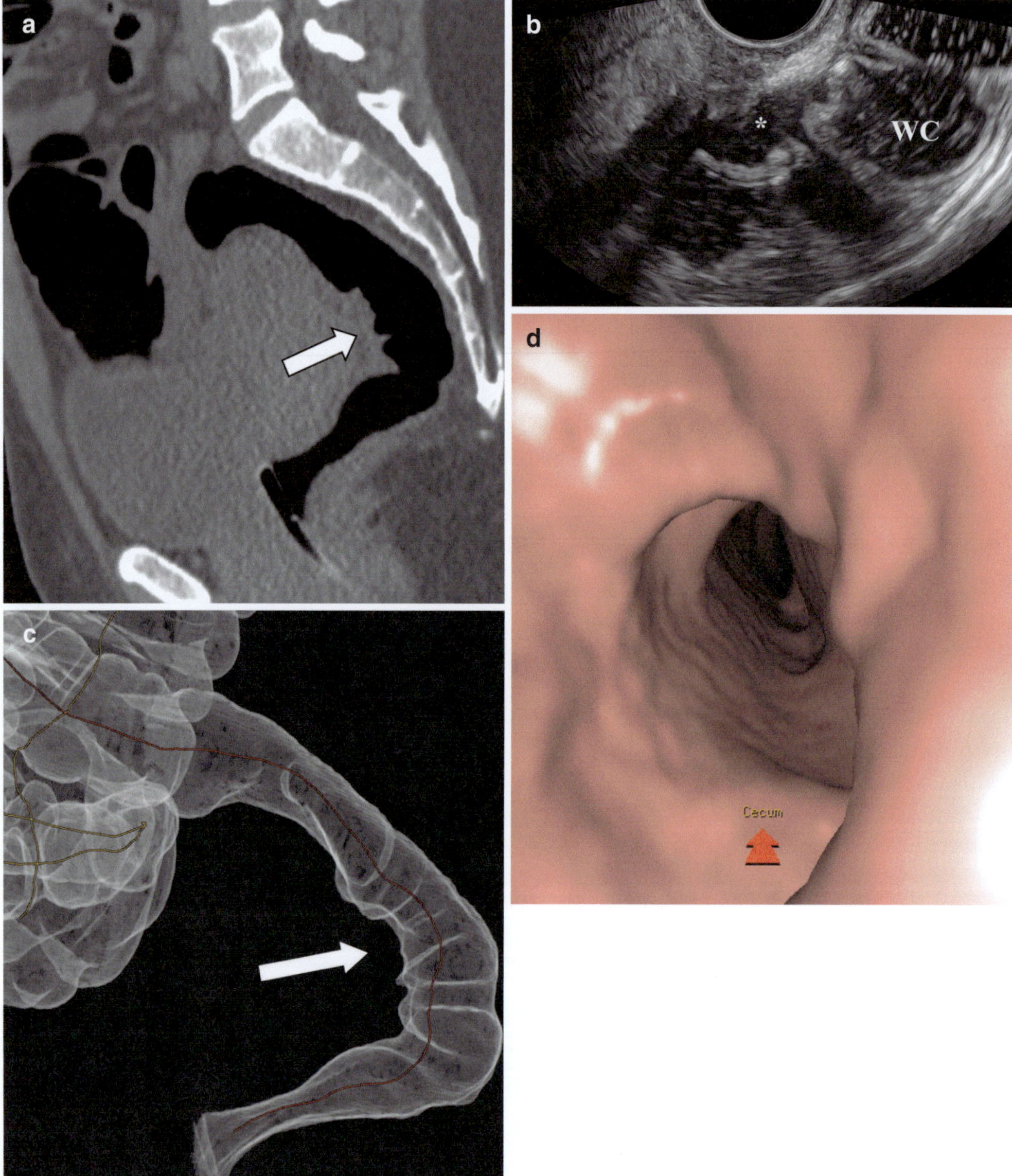

Fig. 9.7 Computed tomography colonoscopy and rectal water contrast transvaginal ultrasonography. (**a**) Computerize tomography colonoscopy: sagittal reconstruction. In this figure the rectal infiltration is detectable: the endoluminal profile is irregular and the lumen is substenosed by the nodular infiltration (arrow). (**b**) Rectal water contrast transvaginal ultrasonography image: a rectal nodule infiltrating the muscularis mucosa of the rectum is observed (asterisk). The intestinal lumen is distended by the water contrast (WC) image, sagittal scan: the rectal distension confirms the endometriotic nodule (arrow) and the "crenulation" of the mucosal layer on the luminal surface suggests the infiltration of the mucosa; (**c**) Computerize tomography colonoscopy: the "double contrast like" image detects the rectal compression caused by the anterior nodule (arrow). (**d**) Computerize tomography colonoscopy: the flying through reconstruction shows the substenosed lumen in the middle of the endometriotic infiltrated tract

going segmental bowel resection. This study aimed to estimate the accuracy of different imaging methods for evaluating the degree of bowel stenosis in women affected by rectosigmoid endometriosis. TVS, RWC-TVS, CTC, and MRI with rectal enema were preoperatively performed. The examinations were done by physicians blinded to the results of the other imaging methods; the specimens obtained from surgery underwent pathological examination. Overall, the mean (±SD) degree of the bowel lumen stenosis was 64.1% (±15.6%). The Kruskal–Wallis one-way analysis of variance on ranks demonstrated that the imaging methods had different accuracy in estimating the bowel stenosis degree ($P < 0.001$). The Tukey test showed that CTC was more accurate than other methods in estimating the bowel stenosis degree ($P < 0.05$); MRI with rectal enema was more accurate than TVS ($P < 0.05$). The authors concluded that the highest precision of CTC may have been due to the fact that bowel distention is uniform below and above the endometriotic nodules [34].

9.5 Conclusion

The studies presented in this chapter show that CTC has good performance in the diagnosis of intestinal endometriosis.

CTC has several advantages compared with other techniques used for the diagnosis of bowel endometriosis. A major advantage of CTC is that it provides an overview of the whole colon and, in particular, of the intestinal nodules located above the sigmoid colon (such as those on the transverse colon and the cecum). These nodules cannot be diagnosed by TVS because they are beyond the field of view of the transvaginal probe. In addition, they can also be difficult to be diagnosed by MRI. However, considering that in 39% of cases bowel lesions are multifocal [35], a complete assessment of the colon is essential to detect all endometriotic lesions before surgery. Multiple endometriotic nodules on the digestive tract may require multiple segmental bowel resections or disc excisions. The patient must be informed of this possibility before surgery. Another advantage of CTC is that it is a quick outpatient exam; it has high spatial resolution (for example when compared with MRI) and it allows scanning the abdomen within seconds. Furthermore, it is safe and minimally painful for the patients; no analgesia or sedation is required [19]. The patient can return to work and social activities immediately after the exam because the exam is minimally painful at most. A further advantage of CTC is that it allows to estimate digestive tract stenosis. Colonic distension with CO_2 and combination of prone and supine positions provide better estimation of digestive tract narrowness than that of any other imaging techniques. Although MRI performance can be enhanced by opacification with ultrasound of the rectum and/or the vagina [36–39], improvement only concerns diagnosis of rectal and sigmoid nodules. CTC precisely assess the distance between the intestinal endometriotic nodule and the anal verge [17, 19]. Finally, compared with optical colonoscopy, CTC allows to study patients with severe stenosis of the intestinal lumen that would block the progression of the endoscope.

A disadvantage of CT is radiation exposure. This limit is particularly relevant when the exam is performed in young women of reproductive age. However, the CTC protocol has been standardized to decrease radiation exposure. In fact, the average radiation dose administered to the patient is around 9 mSv that is lower than that usually used for a barium enema.

CTC allows to scan the entire abdomen, therefore additional extracolonic organ information can be obtained. However, CTC should not be considered as an alternative to TVS or MRI, because these imaging techniques provide a better assessment of deep pelvic endometriosis, ovarian endometriomas and uterine adenomyosis [7]. In contrast, CTC provides better information on the characteristic of intestinal nodules.

References

1. Vining DJ, Gelfand DW, Bechtold RE, Scharding ES, Grishaw EK, Shifrin RY. Technical feasibility of colon imaging with helical CT and virtual reality. AJR Am J Roentgenol. 1994;162:104.
2. Laghi A. Computed tomography colonography in 2014: an update on technique and indications. World J Gastroenterol. 2014;20(45):16858–67.

3. Lin JS, Piper MA, Perdue LA, Rutter CM, Webber EM, O'Connor E, et al. Screening for colorectal cancer: updated evidence report and systematic review for the US Preventive Services Task Force. JAMA. 2016;315(23):2576–94.

4. Spada C, Stoker J, Alarcon O, Barbaro F, Bellini D, Bretthauer M, et al. Clinical indications for computed tomographic colonography: European Society of Gastrointestinal Endoscopy (ESGE) and European Society of Gastrointestinal and Abdominal Radiology (ESGAR) guideline. Endoscopy. 2014;46(10):897–915.

5. Zannoni L, Del Forno S, Coppola F, Papadopoulos D, Valerio D, Golfieri R, et al. Comparison of transvaginal sonography and computed tomography-colonography with contrast media and urographic phase for diagnosing deep infiltrating endometriosis of the posterior compartment of the pelvis: a pilot study. Jpn J Radiol. 2017;35(9):546–54.

6. Coppola F, Paradisi R, Zanardi S, Papadopoulos D, Gramenzi A, Valerio D, et al. Computed tomography-colonography with intravenous contrast medium and urographic phase for the evaluation of pelvic deep infiltrating endometriosis of intestinal and urinary tract. J Comput Assist Tomogr. 2019;43(3):513–8.

7. Roman H, Carilho J, Da Costa C, De Vecchi C, Suaud O, Monroc M, et al. Computed tomography-based virtual colonoscopy in the assessment of bowel endometriosis: the surgeon's point of view. Gynecol Obstet Fertil. 2016;44(1):3–10.

8. van der Wat J, Kaplan MD. Modified virtual colonoscopy: a noninvasive technique for the diagnosis of rectovaginal septum and deep infiltrating pelvic endometriosis. J Minim Invasive Gynecol. 2007;14(5):638–43.

9. Jeong SY, Chung DJ, Myung Yeo D, Lim YT, Hahn ST, Lee JM. The usefulness of computed tomographic colonography for evaluation of deep infiltrating endometriosis: comparison with magnetic resonance imaging. J Comput Assist Tomogr. 2013;37(5):809–14.

10. Park SH, Yee J, Kim SH, Kim YH. Fundamental elements for successful performance of CT colonography (virtual colonoscopy). Korean J Radiol. 2007;8(4):264–75.

11. Koutoukos I, Langebrekke A, Young V, Qvigstad E. Imaging of endometriosis with computerized tomography colonography. Fertil Steril. 2011;95(1):259–60.

12. Mahgerefteh S, Fraifeld S, Blachar A, Sosna J. CT colonography with decreased purgation: balancing preparation, performance, and patient acceptance. AJR Am J Roentgenol. 2009;193(6):1531–9.

13. van der Wat J, Kaplan MD. Modified virtual colonoscopy in the diagnosis and quantification of bowel and disseminated endometriosis. Surg Technol Int. 2015;26:19–24.

14. Racca A, Biscaldi E, Remorgida V, Leone Roberti Maggiore U, Vellone VG, Venturini PL, et al. Computed tomographic colonography in the diagnosis of recto-sigmoid endometriosis: a pilot study. J Minim Invasive Gynecol. 2015;22(6S):S28–S9.

15. Mehedintu C, Brinduse LA, Bratila E, Monroc M, Lemercier E, Suaud O, et al. Does computed tomography-based virtual colonoscopy improve the accuracy of preoperative assessment based on magnetic resonance imaging in women managed for colorectal endometriosis? J Minim Invasive Gynecol. 2018;25(6):1009–17.

16. Baggio S, Zecchin A, Pomini P, Zanconato G, Genna M, Motton M, et al. The role of computed tomography colonography in detecting bowel involvement in women with deep infiltrating endometriosis: comparison with clinical history, serum Ca125, and transvaginal sonography. J Comput Assist Tomogr. 2016;40(6):886–91.

17. Vassilieff M, Suaud O, Collet-Savoye C, Da Costa C, Marouteau-Pasquier N, Belhiba H, et al. [Computed tomography-based virtual colonoscopy: an examination useful for the choice of the surgical management of colorectal endometriosis]. Gynecol Obstet Fertil. 2011;39(6):339–45.

18. Shinners TJ, Pickhardt PJ, Taylor AJ, Jones DA, Olsen CH. Patient-controlled room air insufflation versus automated carbon dioxide delivery for CT colonography. AJR Am J Roentgenol. 2006;186(6):1491–6.

19. Ferrero S, Biscaldi E, Vellone VG, Venturini PL, Leone Roberti Maggiore U. Computed tomographic colonography vs rectal water-contrast transvaginal sonography in diagnosis of rectosigmoid endometriosis: a pilot study. Ultrasound Obstet Gynecol. 2017;49(4):515–23.

20. Taylor SA, Halligan S, Goh V, Morley S, Bassett P, Atkin W, et al. Optimizing colonic distention for multi-detector row CT colonography: effect of hyoscine butylbromide and rectal balloon catheter. Radiology. 2003;229(1):99–108.

21. Yee J, Kumar NN, Hung RK, Akerkar GA, Kumar PR, Wall SD. Comparison of supine and prone scanning separately and in combination at CT colonography. Radiology. 2003;226(3):653–61.

22. Chen SC, Lu DS, Hecht JR, Kadell BM. CT colonography: value of scanning in both the supine and prone positions. AJR Am J Roentgenol. 1999;172(3):595–9.

23. Iannaccone R, Laghi A, Catalano C, Brink JA, Mangiapane F, Trenna S, et al. Detection of colorectal lesions: lower-dose multi-detector row helical CT colonography compared with conventional colonoscopy. Radiology. 2003;229(3):775–81.

24. Neri E, Vagli P, Picchietti S, Vannozzi F, Linsalata S, Bardine A, et al. CT colonography: contrast enhancement of benign and malignant colorectal lesions versus fecal residuals. Abdom Imaging. 2005;30(6):694–7.

25. Oto A, Gelebek V, Oguz BS, Sivri B, Deger A, Akhan O, et al. CT attenuation of colorectal polypoid lesions: evaluation of contrast enhancement in CT colonography. Eur Radiol. 2003;13(7):1657–63.

26. Morrin MM, Farrell RJ, Kruskal JB, Reynolds K, McGee JB, Raptopoulos V. Utility of intravenously administered contrast material at CT colonography. Radiology. 2000;217(3):765–71.

27. Tzambouras N, Katsanos KH, Tsili A, Papadimitriou K, Efremidis S, Tsianos EV. CT colonoscopy for

obstructive sigmoid endometriosis: a new technique for an old problem. Eur J Intern Med. 2002;13(4):274–5.

28. Nisenblat V, Bossuyt PM, Farquhar C, Johnson N, Hull ML. Imaging modalities for the non-invasive diagnosis of endometriosis. Cochrane Database Syst Rev. 2016;(2):CD009591.

29. Guerriero S, Condous G, Van den Bosch T, Valentin L, Leone FP, Van Schoubroeck D, et al. Systematic approach to sonographic evaluation of the pelvis in women with suspected endometriosis, including terms, definitions and measurements: a consensus opinion from the International Deep Endometriosis Analysis (IDEA) group. Ultrasound Obstet Gynecol. 2016;48:318.

30. Menada MV, Remorgida V, Abbamonte LH, Fulcheri E, Ragni N, Ferrero S. Transvaginal ultrasonography combined with water-contrast in the rectum in the diagnosis of rectovaginal endometriosis infiltrating the bowel. Fertil Steril. 2008;89(3):699–700.

31. Valenzano Menada M, Remorgida V, Abbamonte LH, Nicoletti A, Ragni N, Ferrero S. Does transvaginal ultrasonography combined with water-contrast in the rectum aid in the diagnosis of rectovaginal endometriosis infiltrating the bowel? Hum Reprod. 2008;23(5):1069–75.

32. Ferrero S, Biscaldi E, Morotti M, Venturini PL, Remorgida V, Rollandi GA, et al. Multidetector computerized tomography enteroclysis vs. rectal water contrast transvaginal ultrasonography in determining the presence and extent of bowel endometriosis. Ultrasound Obstet Gynecol. 2011;37(5):603–13.

33. Leone Roberti Maggiore U, Biscaldi E, Vellone VG, Venturini PL, Ferrero S. Magnetic resonance enema vs rectal water-contrast transvaginal sonography in diagnosis of rectosigmoid endometriosis. Ultrasound Obstet Gynecol. 2017;49(4):524–32.

34. Barra F, Carolina S, Vellone VG, Stabilini C, Ferrero S. A prospective comparative study for the evaluation of bowel stenosis degree in women with rectosigmoid endometriosis. Category – Gynaecological imaging. BJOG. 2019;126(S2):1470–0328.

35. Chapron C, Fauconnier A, Vieira M, Barakat H, Dousset B, Pansini V, et al. Anatomical distribution of deeply infiltrating endometriosis: surgical implications and proposition for a classification. Hum Reprod. 2003;18(1):157–61.

36. Loubeyre P, Petignat P, Jacob S, Egger JF, Dubuisson JB, Wenger JM. Anatomic distribution of posterior deeply infiltrating endometriosis on MRI after vaginal and rectal gel opacification. AJR Am J Roentgenol. 2009;192(6):1625–31.

37. Loubeyre P, Copercini M, Frossard JL, Wenger JM, Petignat P. Pictorial review: rectosigmoid endometriosis on MRI with gel opacification after rectosigmoid colon cleansing. Clin Imaging. 2012;36(4): 295–300.

38. Biscaldi E, Ferrero S, Leone Roberti Maggiore U, Remorgida V, Venturini PL, Rollandi GA. Multidetector computerized tomography enema versus magnetic resonance enema in the diagnosis of rectosigmoid endometriosis. Eur J Radiol. 2014;83(2):261–7.

39. Kikuchi I, Kuwatsuru R, Yamazaki K, Kumakiri J, Aoki Y, Takeda S. Evaluation of the usefulness of the MRI jelly method for diagnosing complete cul-de-sac obliteration. Biomed Res Int. 2014;2014: 437962.

Part III

Treatment

Ted Lee and Noah Rindos

10.1 Preoperative Work Up

Bowel involvement is relatively common in women with endometriosis, affecting 3.8–37% of patients [1]. The rectum and rectosigmoid account for 65% of bowel involvement, with the sigmoid colon (17%), appendix (6%) cecum and ileocecal junction (4%), and small bowel (5%) accounting for the remainder [1]. Women that remain symptomatic with medical therapy, especially those with diarrhea, hematochezia, or dyschezia should be evaluated for bowel endometriosis [2]. Identifying patients with bowel endometriosis preoperatively can prevent the need for a second surgery if more extensive disease than was originally expected is encountered.

Selecting the appropriate surgical candidate for a discoid resection begins during the history and physical portion of the initial visit. A carefully history is taken for symptoms such as cyclic

Link to video (https://www.youtube.com/watch?v=Ub1j7um6Tco).

Electronic Supplementary Material The online version of this chapter (https://doi.org/10.1007/978-3-030-50446-5_10) contains supplementary material, which is available to authorized users.

T. Lee (✉) · N. Rindos
Department OB/GYN/RS, Magee-Womens Hospital of UPMC, University of Pittsburgh Medical Center, Pittsburgh, PA, USA
e-mail: leextt@upmc.edu

rectal bleeding or dyschezia, as well as reviewing operative notes if available from earlier surgeries. The physical exam allows for the detection of nodules in the distal most 5 cm of the rectum but is limited in its ability to detect higher nodules. Patients in whom a nodule is suspected must be properly counseled prior to surgery on preoperative risks including need for resection, bowel reanastamosis, and osteomy.

It is important to thoroughly discuss treatment techniques with the patient during this visit as the optimal surgical approach may not be clear until the nodule is visualized. There is not always a consensus among surgeons on the optimal technique for resection of deep infiltrating endometriosis [2, 3]. In addition to a discoid resection, surgical removal of the rectal nodule can be performed using multiple techniques including shaving of the nodule, laparoscopic stapling or full thickness excision and bowel resection with reanastamosis [4].

Laparoscopic shaving is performed by peeling the bowel serosal layer and subserosal endometriotic nodules off of the underlying bowel. It is best utilized for resection of small, more superficial nodules that are on the surface of the bowel and not infiltrating into the lumen. The nodule is separated from adhesions to the uterus or vagina. The lesion is then excised from the bowel, taking care to not enter the mucosa. Any resultant defect at the site of the shaving can be reinforced with a delayed absorbable suture. Proctoscopy can be

© Springer Nature Switzerland AG 2020
S. Ferrero, M. Ceccaroni (eds.), *Clinical Management of Bowel Endometriosis*,
https://doi.org/10.1007/978-3-030-50446-5_10

performed to ensure that the lumen of the bowel has not been entered [4].

Ideally shaving minimizes the amount of unaffected bowel that needs to be removed. It may also prevent entry into the lumen of the bowel. This technique is limited to smaller lesions that are more superficial in distribution. Additionally full thickness nodules cannot be resected using this technique so a careful preoperative work up is essential [4].

Laparoscopic discoid resection of endometriotic nodules can be performed utilizing a circular stapler. The bowel is mobilized free of any adhesions, the nodule is isolated, and overlying fat is removed to provide a fresh plane for the stapler. A suture is passed through the nodule to aid in mobilization and positioning. An appropriately sized stapler is selected and the proximal portion of the anterior bowel wall including the endometriotic nodule is resected. The stapler is reintroduced and the distal portion of the nodule and the original staple line are excised [3, 5].

One series described resection of nodules as large as 4.2 cm using the double circular staple technique. The authors reported urinary retention in only 1 out of 11 patients (9%) using this technique compared with 14 out of 45 who underwent a bowel resection [3].

Segmental resection bowel resection offers the benefit of complete removal endometriotic lesions. Patients with multiple lesions, larger nodules, and full thickness disease, especially where greater than 50% of the circumference of the bowel is involved are most likely to benefit from resection. Major complications in one meta-analysis were reported in as many as 11% of patients and included bowel leaks, fistulas, bowel obstructions, hemorrhage, and infections. Minor complications such as temporary bladder and bowel dysfunction occurred in 14% of women [6].

A comparison between discoid resection and segmental resection with 31 patients in each arm found a shorter operative time with discoid resection and higher rate and duration of postoperative voiding dysfunction [7]. The decision to perform a segmental resection or a discoid resection was determined intraoperatively by the surgeon based on the characteristics of the lesion. This decision was influenced by the size of the lesion, circumferential involvement and presence of multiple lesions; with more extreme disease favoring segmental resection [7].

10.2 Imaging

Endoanal ultrasound can be utilized but we favor MRI with vaginal and rectal contrast gel for evaluation of rectal nodules. In our practice we counsel patients with multiple nodules or a single nodule larger than 5 cm that they are not good candidates for discoid resection but would rather favor a segmental resection.

10.3 Preoperative Collaboration

Patients with likely bowel endometriosis should undergo evaluation with a colorectal surgeon preoperatively in case the nodule is larger than can be managed with a discoid resection alone. It is important to communicate with the colorectal surgeon ahead of time to ensure that the patient undergoes the proper preoperative work up, bowel prep, and surgical clearance. The use of intraoperative antibiotics should be discussed prior to the procedure as well as what portions of the case each surgeon will be responsible for.

10.4 Surgical Technique

Good candidates for an anterior discoid resection are women with a single endometriotic nodule in the rectosigmoid that is less than 3 cm and involves less than half of the circumference of the bowel (Fig. 10.1). In part this is because full thickness lesions are likely to involve 40% or more of the bowel, so the closure may lead to a significant reduction in the diameter of the bowel and cause a stricture [8]. Larger nodules may be approached using this technique, but the surgeon should be aware that the nodule may be larger within the lumen of the bowel than it appears initially at the level of the serosa. The determination

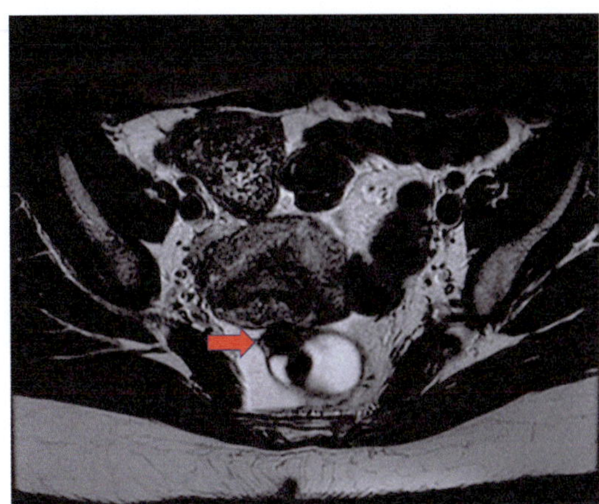

Fig. 10.1 MRI showing a rectosigmoid nodule that was amenable to excision using a discoid resection. Note that the nodule (as illustrated by the red arrow) is small in relation to the lumen of the bowel

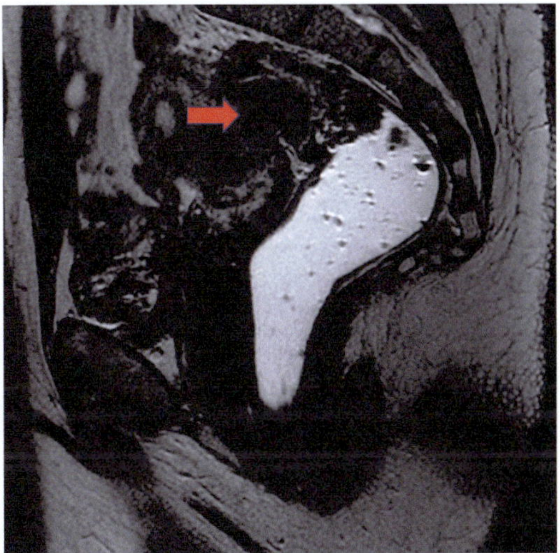

Fig. 10.2 Nodule that was not amenable to discoid resection but rather required a segmental resection. The nodule (as illustrated by the red arrow) occupied most of the diameter of the lumen of the bowel

of the size of the nodule is partially made based on preoperative imaging as well as the intraoperative assessment (Fig. 10.2).

Bowel endometriosis can be divided into two groups—superficial and full thickness disease. Patients with full thickness involvement, the nodule invades into the lumen of the bowel whereas superficial disease does not penetrate fully through the bowel [1]. Endometriosis involving only the serosa is not considered to be true bowel endometriosis, rather the deeper layers of the bowel must be involved. In one study, the muscularis propria was found to contain endometriosis in 95.1% of cases. The submucosa and mucosa were involved in 37.8% and 6.4% of pathologically confirmed endometriosis [1].

Partial thickness nodules can be treated with bowel shaving or a discoid resection. If the lumen is not entered a single layer closure may be employed rather than a two-layer closures. Full thickness nodules warrant complete excision and re-approximation of the bowel layers. A discoid resection, stapler or segmental resection can all be utilized in these situations. The goal is complete resection of all involved tissue with clear margins, although the theoretical benefits of avoiding residual disease are not completely understood [3].

Before tackling any bowel endometriosis, we perform the rest of the excision of endometriosis and hysterectomy if needed. This allows for easier access to the rectal nodules, mobilization of the ureters has already been performed and the uterus is either removed or can be easily deflected out of the way with the uterine manipulator. We will generally perform an oophoropexy to keep the ovaries out of the operative field and then remove the stitch on postoperative day 3 (Fig. 10.3). This both keeps the adnexa away from the surgical field during the discoid resection as well as prevents retroperitonealization of the ovaries after surgery. We use a 2-0 prolene on a Keith needle which is passed through the ante-

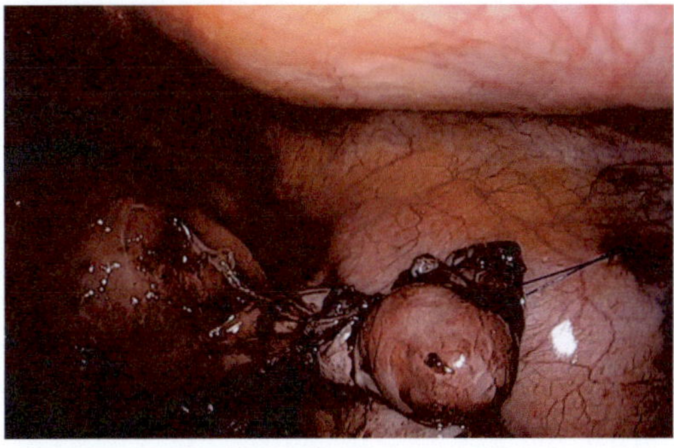

Fig. 10.3 Oophoropexy, suspension of the ovary out of the operative field, may assist with

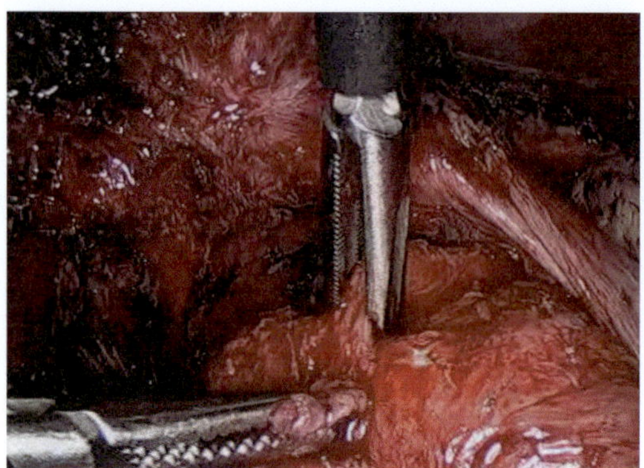

Fig. 10.4 The squeeze technique is performed by using an atraumatic grasper to outline the borders of the rectal nodule. This allows the surgeon to determine if the nodule is amenable to discoid resection or if it is too large and a segmental resection should be performed instead

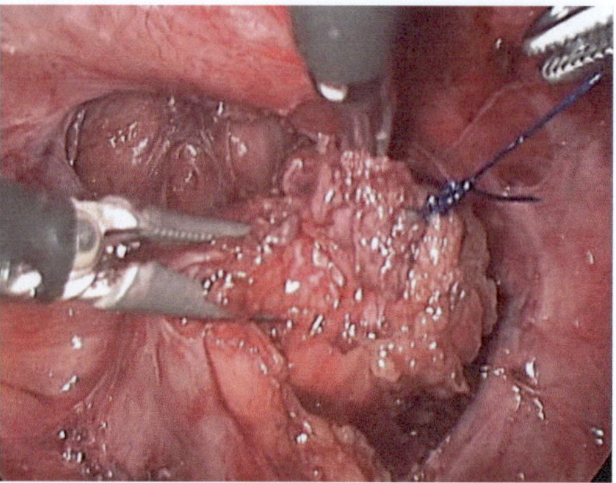

Fig. 10.5 A suture passed through the nodule can be employed to aid with mobilization and intraoperative dissection

rior abdominal wall, through the ovary and back through the abdominal wall. It is temporarily secured to the skin using a sterile button.

Endometriotic nodules of the rectosigmoid are generally associated with advanced disease but the pararectal spaces are generally preserved. By approaching the nodule laterally through these avascular spaces, it is possible to mobilize the bowel off of the uterus and posterior aspects of the vagina. Care must be taken to prevent thermal bowel injury by favoring cold scissors rather than electrosurgical instruments.

Once the uterus and vagina have been mobilized off of the bowel, an atraumatic grasper can be used to define the location and size of the nodule (Fig. 10.4). These graspers can squeeze the nodule and bounce off of the unaffected bowel. This allows the surgeon to evaluate the percentage of the bowel that has nodule involvement. We favor discoid resection in nodules that are 3 cm or less and involving less than half of the circumference of the bowel as that allows an adequately sized lumen after surgery. Intraoperatively, we use a rectal probe to evaluate the diameter of the bowel lumen. If the rectal probe passes easily beyond the nodule, a discoid resection will be able to be performed and leave adequate space for a primary closure. In patients where the rectal probe does not pass easily, a segmental resection should be performed instead.

Once the nodules have been identified and any adhesions mobilized off of it, a suture can be passed through the nodule to assist with manipulation during dissection and allows the surgeon to confidently identify the uninvolved margins of the tissue (Fig. 10.5).

An advanced bipolar device with a cutting blade is then used to dissect the nodule away from the unaffected tissue. We favor the ENSEAL bipolar (Ethicon, Somerville, N.J.) as it bounces off of the hard tissues of the nodule, helping guide the surgeon toward the correct plane and minimizing the size of the defect created.

The dissection is started at the level of the serosa and continued circumferentially around the lesion until the nodule is completely defined (Fig. 10.6). The nodule may initially appear smaller at the level of the serosa and then become larger by the time the lumen is entered.

The bowel incision is created once the nodule has been well circumscribed (Fig. 10.7). The border of the endometriosis can then be followed in a circumferential fashion until the lesion is completely freed from the underlying rectum. Electrosurgery can be judiciously used to obtain hemostasis but should be minimized to avoid unnecessary thermal injury to healthy tissue.

Once the lesion has been completely removed and nearby tissues inspected for any additional disease or inadvertent injury, closure of the colpotomy can be performed. A rectal probe is

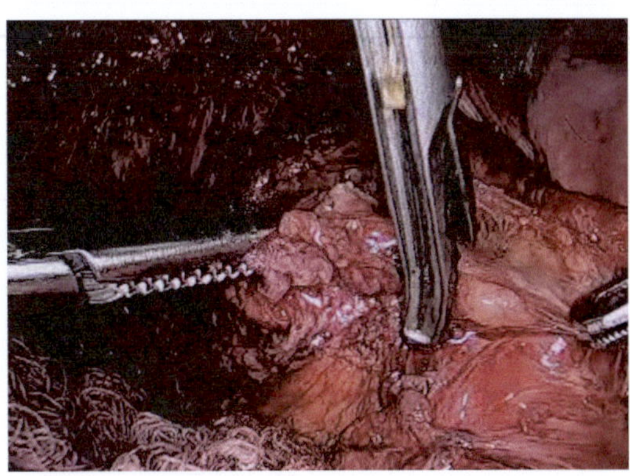

Fig. 10.6 Advanced bipolar is used for dissection of fat off of bowel. We favor this as it minimizes thermal spread while aiding hemostasis

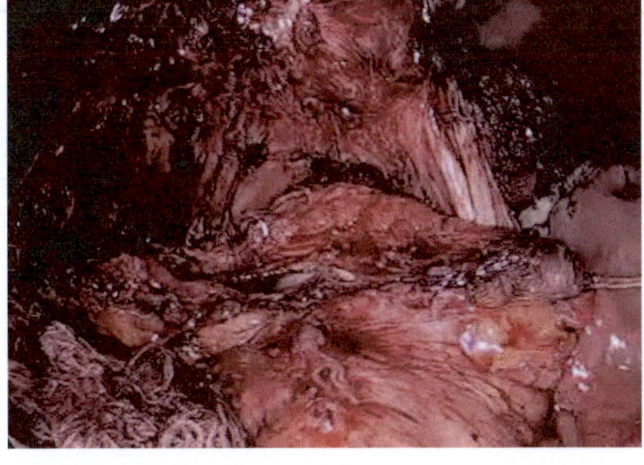

Fig. 10.9 Anchoring the lateral borders of the defect in preparation for closure

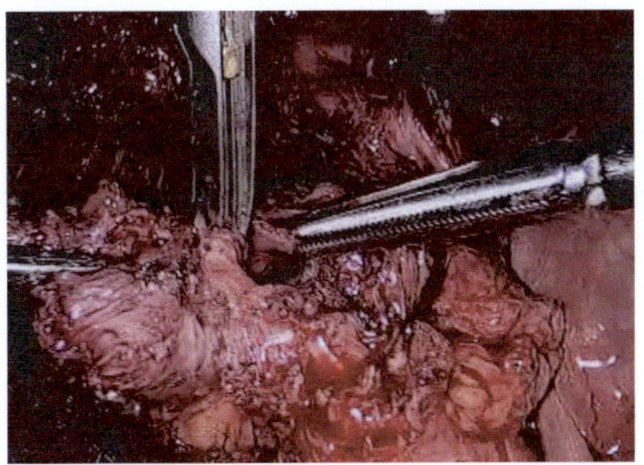

Fig. 10.7 Entry into the lumen of the bowel is performed using sharp dissection

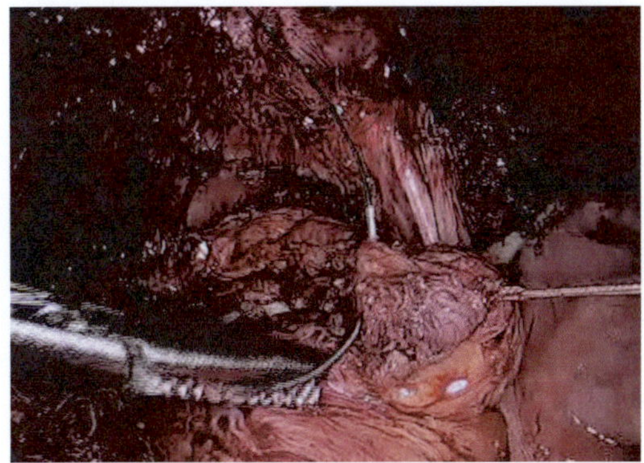

Fig. 10.10 First layer of the closure with unidirectional barbed suture

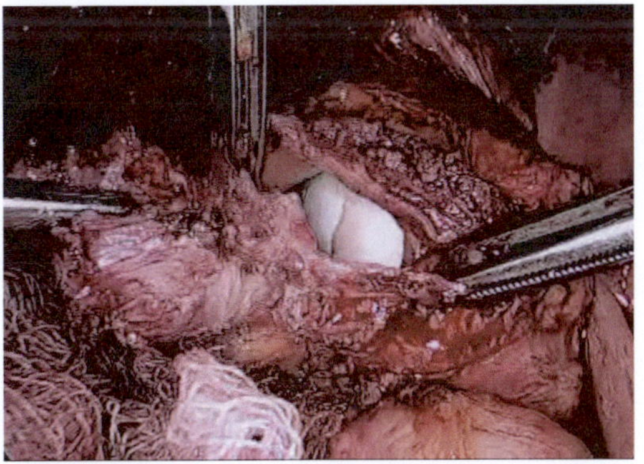

Fig. 10.8 Resection of the bowel nodule is aided by visualization of rectal probe

inserted to the level of the defect and serves as a guide during the repair (Fig. 10.8). The probe helps to ensure that the repair will be without ten-sion and that the lumen is not being inadvertently being reduced. If at this point the nodule was larger than expected, or the lumen will be too small after closure, a reanastamosis by the general surgeons should be considered instead.

In cases where the dissection results in a large defect, both corners may be anchored with a delayed absorbable suture. This aids in the closure by elevating the edges of the defect and ensuring an even re-approximation of the bowel (Fig. 10.9). The colpotomy closure is performed using a unidirectional barbed suture with a two-layer closure. We favor a V-Loc (Medtronic, Minneapolis, M.N.) for ability to provide a tension free repair (Fig. 10.10).

The closure is performed in two layers with a similar approach as closing a vaginal cuff after a hysterectomy (Fig. 10.11). The sutures should be

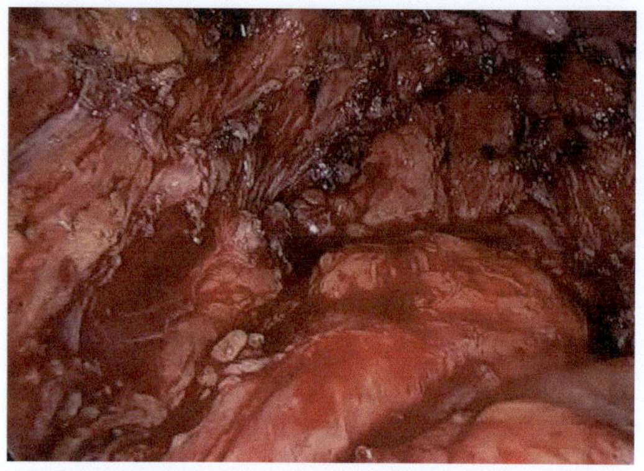

Fig. 10.11 Second layer of the closure

close enough to ensure a tight seal but not so frequently as to strangulate the tissues.

An air leak test is then performed to assess the repair and look for any defects in the closure. This is done by placing a rigid proctoscope into the rectum, filling the pelvis with saline and placing a bowel clamp above the level of the repair. The closure should be below the saline for the test to be effective. If bubbles are not seen then the closure is considered adequate and at low risk for developing a leak. If there are bubbles, the affected area should be re-inspected and the leak repaired.

A video is available that demonstrates Dr. Lee performing a discoid resection employing this technique at https://www.youtube.com/watch?v=Ub1j7um6Tco.

Postoperatively we admit the patient to the hospital and slowly advance their diet until they are tolerating a soft diet and passing flatus. We keep them on a bowel regimen with the goal of daily bowel movements for the first month postoperatively. The major complication following discoid resection that we encounter is a bowel stricture that generally resolves with time and laxative use.

Case

A 36-year-old G1P1 with history of longstanding pelvic pain and cyclic hematochezia presents for evaluation in clinic. A pelvic exam reveals a fixed, retroverted uterus with uterosacral nodularity and tenderness. A rectal exam does not reveal any nodule. What are the appropriate next steps?

Answer

This patient is at high risk for a rectal nodule given her history and exam findings. A pelvic MRI with rectal and vaginal contrast or an endoanal ultrasound can be performed. If imaging reveals a bowel nodule, surgical management may be warranted. Patients with solitary nodules 3 cm or less in size are good candidates for discoid resections. An available colorectal surgeon is important in case she is found to have a larger nodule intraoperatively that requires a segmental resection.

References

1. Meuleman C, Tomassetti C, D'Hoore A, Van Cleynenbreugel B, Penninckx F, Vergote I, et al. Surgical treatment of deeply infiltrating endometriosis with colorectal involvement. Hum Reprod Update. 2011;17(3):311–26.
2. Abrão MS, Petraglia F, Falcone T, Keckstein J, Osuga Y, Chapron C. Deep endometriosis infiltrating the recto-sigmoid: critical factors to consider before management. Hum Reprod Update. 2015;21(3): 329–39.
3. Oliveira MAP, Crispi CP, Oliveira FM, Junior PS, Raymundo TS, Pereira TD. Double circular stapler technique for bowel resection in rectosigmoid endometriosis. J Minim Invasive Gynecol. 2014;21(1):136–41.
4. Laganà AS, Vitale SG, Trovato MA, Palmara VI, Rapisarda AMC, Granese R, et al. Full-thickness excision versus shaving by laparoscopy for intestinal deep infiltrating endometriosis: rationale and potential treatment options. Biomed Res Int. 2016;2016:3617179.
5. Kondo W, Ribeiro R, Zomer MT, Hayashi R. Laparoscopic double discoid resection with a circular stapler for bowel endometriosis. J Minim Invasive Gynecol. 2015;22(6):929–31.
6. De Cicco C, Corona R, Schonman R, Mailova K, Ussia A, Koninckx P. Bowel resection for deep endometriosis: a systematic review. BJOG. 2011;118(3): 285–91.
7. Jayot A, Nyangoh Timoh K, Bendifallah S, Ballester M, Darai E. Comparison of laparoscopic discoid resection and segmental resection for colorectal endometriosis using a propensity score matching analysis. J Minim Invasive Gynecol. 2018;25(3):440–6.
8. Abrão MS, Podgaec S, Dias JA, Averbach M, Silva LFF, Marino de Carvalho F. Endometriosis lesions that compromise the rectum deeper than the inner muscularis layer have more than 40% of the circumference of the rectum affected by the disease. J Minim Invasive Gynecol. 2008;15(3):280–5.

Philippe R. Koninckx, Ussia Anastasia,
Leila Adamian, Shaima Alsuwaidi, Bedaya Amro,
Hanan Gharbi, Muna Tahlak, and Arnaud Wattiez

11.1 Introduction

The surgical treatment of deep bowel endometriosis is a confusing debate [1]. In the literature, variable definitions of deep endometriosis are used [2, 3]. The use of preoperative imaging is variable and varies from an indication for surgery [4], to a prediction of the type and severity of the disease [5, 6], based on the prediction of the depth of invasion into the bowel and of the degree of bowel stenosis. The aim of the surgery varies from emphasising radical excision of all endometriosis like tissue to a more conservative excision leaving at least a rim of fibrosis [3]. The surgical outcome varies from the treatment of pain and infertility, to the prevention of recurrences and the absence of complications. The debate gets even more confused since the surgical difficulty is variable and poorly defined. Variable personal skills and preferences of instruments and energy sources together with the variable local and medicolegal aspect of gynecologists performing bowel surgery further complicate the debate.

With these many variables, many of which are personal preferences, solid data resulting from a multivariate analysis with all variables do not exist and will not exist soon. A prospective study taking into account all variables would require prohibitively large numbers of interventions, with in addition the difficulty to define surgeon factor—the singer or the song [7]. Moreover, techniques of surgery and our understanding of endometriosis vary over time and would make a trial outdated before being finished.

A chapter or article on deep endometriosis bowel surgery will necessarily be colored by personal opinions, preferences, beliefs, and by the history of the authors' past. We therefore will describe briefly the history of deep endometriosis surgery, our concepts of diagnostic methods and

P. R. Koninckx (✉)
Latifa Hospital, Dubai, United Arab Emirates

Gruppo Italo Belga, Villa del Rosario and Gemelli Hospital Università Cattolica, Rome, Italy

Prof em Department of Obstetrics and Gynecology, University Hospital, Catholic University Leuven, Leuven, Belgium

U. Anastasia
Gruppo Italo Belga, Villa del Rosario and Gemelli Hospital Università Cattolica, Rome, Italy

L. Adamian
Department of Operative Gynecology, Federal State Budget Institution V. I. Kulakov Research Centre for Obstetrics, Gynecology and Perinatology, Ministry of Health of the Russian Federation, Moscow, Russia

Department of Reproductive Medicine and Surgery, Moscow State University of Medicine and Dentistry, Moscow, Russia

S. Alsuwaidi · B. Amro · H. Gharbi · M. Tahlak
Latifa Hospital, Dubai, United Arab Emirates

A. Wattiez
Latifa Hospital, Dubai, United Arab Emirates

University of Strassbourg, Strassbourg, France

© Springer Nature Switzerland AG 2020
S. Ferrero, M. Ceccaroni (eds.), *Clinical Management of Bowel Endometriosis*,
https://doi.org/10.1007/978-3-030-50446-5_11

of outcome variables and our technical preferences before describing our concept of deep endometriosis surgery today.

11.2 Deep Endometriosis: Definition

Deep endometriosis was defined in 1992 as endometriosis infiltrating more than 5 mm under the peritoneum [8]. Realising in 1990 that 'deep endometriosis lesions' were a separate entity associated with severe pain [9] the definition of 5 mm was suggested based on two observations. First the frequency distribution of depth of endometriosis was biphasic with a nadir around 5 mm suggesting two populations. In addition, the histologic observation that the deeper lesions were more in phase with the endometrium and more active than the more superficial typical lesions seemed compatible with the concept that deeper lesions had 'escaped' from the inhibitory effect of peritoneal fluid with a high progesterone content [10]. An effect by diffusion of the hormonal content in peritoneal fluid, up to some 5 mm of depth seemed logic. Unfortunately, a full histological exploration of endometriotic glands and stroma at different depths has not been performed until today. One of the difficulties to do this is the necessity to cut lesions perpendicularly to the surface. Although the

biphasic frequency distribution has been confirmed recently [2], the important overlap between the two populations has rarely been taken into account. If we would use depth of invasion as a predictive test for deep endometriosis, a depth of invasion of 6–7 mm would hardly reach an accuracy of 60% and a depth of invasion of 8–9 mm would not exceed 80% since at these depths deep endometriosis lesions are strongly contaminated with somewhat deeper typical lesions. Only depths deeper than 10 mm would achieve a higher accuracy. Searching for a better definition, adenomyosis externa was considered. However, also this definition was not considered adequate (Dan Martin, personal communication, 2019).

These comments on the definition of deep endometriosis are necessary to understand the apparent discrepancy between this chapter and the literature. In this chapter, we will discuss only the larger deep endometriosis lesions present clinically as glandular spherical lesions during excision or as half-moon glandular nodules in the bowel wall (Fig. 11.1). We will not discuss the deeper typical lesions and the larger fibrotic plaques in the pelvis and on the bowel. Although they fit the criterium of 'deeper than 5 mm' these plaque lesions are rarely deeper than 7–8 mm. They are rarely invasive in the muscularis or only in a small area. They generally can be rather easily excised.

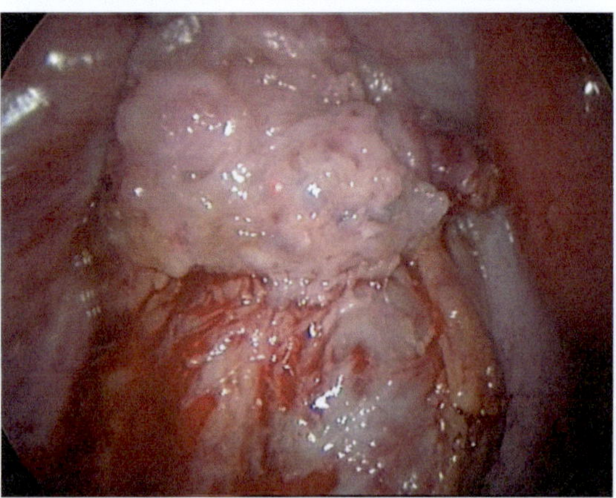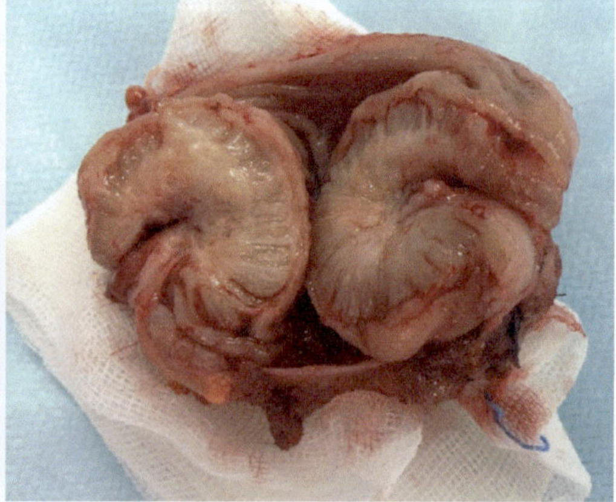

Fig. 11.1 Larger deep endometriosis lesions in the bowel present as glandular spherical lesions during excision (left) or as half-moon glandular nodules in the bowel wall (right)

11.3 History of Deep Endometriosis Surgery

Large severe deep rectovaginal endometriosis was described more than 100 years ago [11–13], even before the description of cystic ovarian endometriosis [14], and was considered a rare pathology.

Laparoscopic deep endometriosis surgery started in the early 1990s with endometriosis excision with a CO_2 laser in women with infertility [8, 9, 15, 16]. Following the borders of endometriosis lesions during excision we realised that some lesions were deeper than the usual typical lesions, that these lesions were associated with severe pain and histologically more active and different from typical lesions [9]. Over the following years we realised that some of these lesions were much bigger, that severity increased with age [16] and that some were triangular lesions, what today we would call deeper typical lesions, in contrast with others which were spherical lesions looking like adenomyosis externa [8, 17]. With excision of progressively larger bowel lesions, we were confronted with muscularis lesions and full thickness resections, which were sutured with one- or two-layer sutures. It should be understood that these were the early days of laparoscopy in abdominal surgery, and that in Leuven, gynecology and abdominal surgery were helping each other, the former teaching bowel surgery to the gynecologists and the latter teaching laparoscopic surgery to the surgeons [18]. With more extensive excisions, we encountered our first ureter lesions [19] and late bowel perforations which were initially not readily recognised [20]. In order to deal with the exponentially growing amount of work, we decided in 1996 that gynecology would continue to perform and explore the limits of conservative excisions or endometriosis with bowel suturing if necessary. The (rare) bowel resections for the very large, especially sigmoid, endometriosis lesions would be performed by abdominal surgery, since this was technically easier surgery and since the abdominal surgeons were still in their learning phase of laparoscopic surgery. During the same period, although two separate universities with little contact at that moment, a similar situation had developed at the University of Louvain with J. Donnez.

This experience of a fast-increasing severity and number of deep endometriosis lesions in Leuven, was repeated in Radcliffe, Oxford UK after 1996 and in Gemelli, Rome, Italy after 2003. We therefore consider this increase a recognition and referral bias, much more than a real epidemiologic increase in severity and incidence [21]. As a consequence of the increasing numbers and with the fast adoption of laparoscopy in abdominal surgery, endometriosis surgery was rapidly introduced in all major hospitals in Belgium and France and by the beginning of the twenty-first century bowel resections performed by abdominal surgeons had become the most frequently performed intervention for larger deep endometriosis lesions. Indeed, without the blessing of the local abdominal surgeon, conservative excision, a more difficult and time-consuming procedure, could not be developed by the gynecologists. Only when deep endometriosis surgery had been initiated before the introduction of laparoscopy in abdominal surgery conservative excisions continued to be performed. After 2000 the concept of the pelvic surgeon resulted at the international level in a revival of conservative excisions and a progressive decrease in bowel resections [22], especially after the introduction of the circular [23, 24] and linear staplers [25, 26] to perform full thickness discoid resections.

11.4 Radicality of Deep Endometriosis Surgery

In the beginning, excision of deep endometriosis was guided by the principle of complete eradication of all endometriotic cells, a rule derived from cancer surgery. However this concept was challenged by the observation that subtle endometriosis which was not necessarily a disease but a normal physiologic phenomenon occurring intermittently in all women [27], and by microscopical endometriosis which was found in over 10% of normal looking peritoneum [28, 29]. Also the observation that endometriosis was found in the lymph nodes of the bowel in over 15% of women with a bowel resection for deep endometriosis [30], raised the question whether all endometrium-like tissue outside the uterus was pathologic. More recently it was demonstrated that bowel deep endometriosis had clusters of endometrium like cells in the bowel wall at least up to 5 cm from the lesions [31, 32].

"The proof of the pudding is in the eating" and radicality of endometriosis surgery should be judged by recurrence rates. Discussing the completeness of deep endometriosis surgery at the mixed surgery-gynecology meetings in Deauville, France and after reviewing mutual videos of surgery, we realised as early as 1998 that the radicality of conservative excisional surgery varied from very complete (with more bowel openings) to much less complete with a rim of endometriosis/fibrosis remaining on the bowel. However, as suggested back then, until today recurrence rates seem not to be obviously different between very complete and less complete excisions [33], between conservative excisions and segmental bowel resections and between small and large bowel resections.

These observations can be explained by the genetic-epigenetic pathophysiology of endometriosis [2] (Fig. 11.2). As suggested in 1999 by the endometriotic disease theory [34], subtle lesions are considered normal endometrium implanted outside the uterus [35], whereas typical, cystic and deep endometriosis, then called endometriotic disease, developed when a threshold of genetic and epigenetic incidents had been reached. This explains that each endometriotic disease lesion is clonal [36, 37], different and originated from a specific incident in adult or neonatal endometrial or stem or bone marrow cells. This explains the heterogeneity of lesions [38], and the association with cancer [39]. The menstrual bleedings in the lesions moreover, risk causing additional incidents and thus influence the growth and severity of the lesions [40].

Whereas genetic mutations are clearly permanent and transmissible, this is much less clear for epigenetic changes. It is unclear which and when epigenetic changes become irreversible and although it is easily understood that they are transmitted by cell cleavage it is unclear whether they are transmissible between generations. A similar confusion exists for histologically observed metaplastic changes. We are unable to distinguish normal endometrial cells from cells with reversible epigenetic changes and cells with irreversible genetic-epigenetic changes. As discussed for subtle lesions [35] we are unable to distinguish a normal implanted endometrium, from metaplastic endometrium like cells following mesenchymal–mesothelial transition and cells with irreversible genetic-epigenetic changes on their way to develop more severe endometriosis lesions. It seems likely that reversible metaplastic changes are caused by reversible epigenetic changes [41–43]. Tumor cells, similarly, can cause metaplastic changes in the surrounding cells which acquire a tumor looking aspect through cell-cell interaction.

In order to explain the similar low recurrence rates of deep endometriosis after a less complete nodulectomy than after a (large) bowel resection for deep endometriosis, our hypothesis today is that the periphery of endometriosis lesions and the fibrosis around these lesions are reversible metaplastic changes without irreversible epigenetic incidents, but induced by the central endometriotic cells with G-E incidents. Although consistent with clinical observations, this hypothesis is speculative today and needs biological confirmation.

Surgically, however, this hypothesis is fundamental since it also can explain that the nests of endometriotic looking cells in the bowel at distance from a nodule and in the lymph nodes do not develop clinically into a symptomatic disease. We even wonder whether following surgical excision of deep endometriosis these endometriotic looking cell at distance return to normal. Unfortunately, this cannot be investigated for obvious ethical reasons. Clinically important is the thickness of these metaplastic changes surrounding the core of deep endometriosis lesions. For surgery, it is important to know whether the metaplastic zone is thin, whether it comprises the

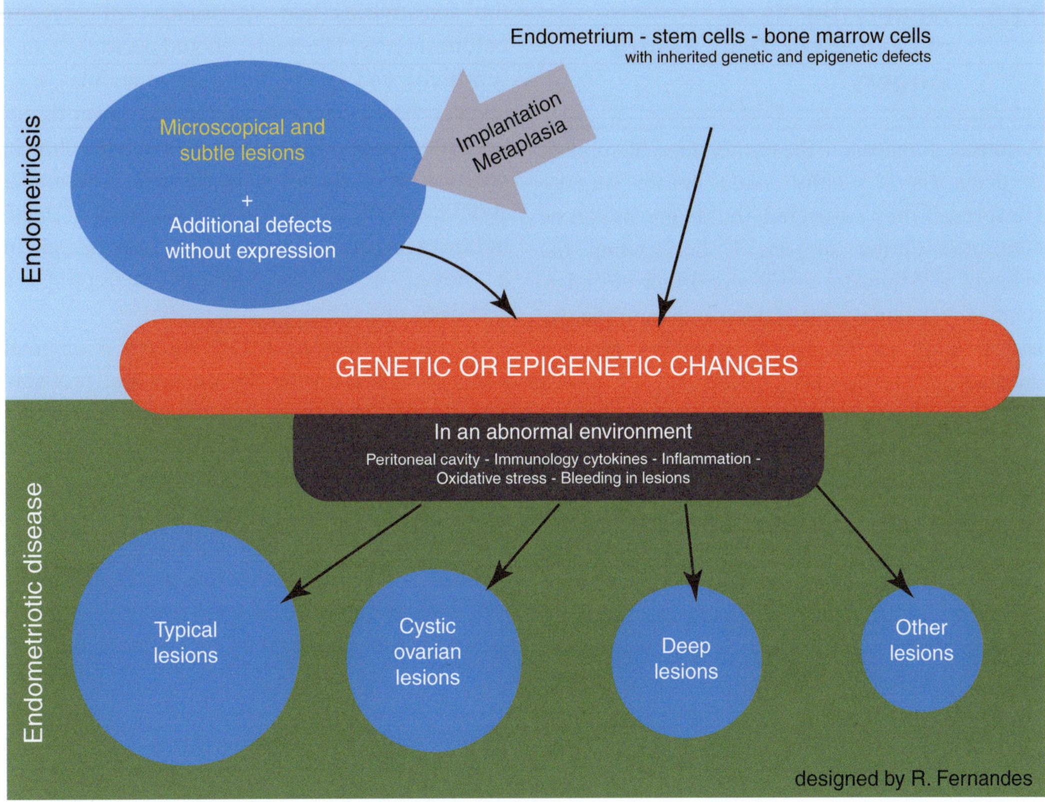

Fig. 11.2 The genetic-epigenetic theory of endometriosis [2]

Fig. 11.3 A deep endometriosis nodule: our hypothesis. The periphery of an endometriotic nodule is composed of metaplastic endometrium like cells without genetic and irreversible epigenetic changes. After excision of the core with genetic and epigenetic changes, the metaplastic cells will return to normal

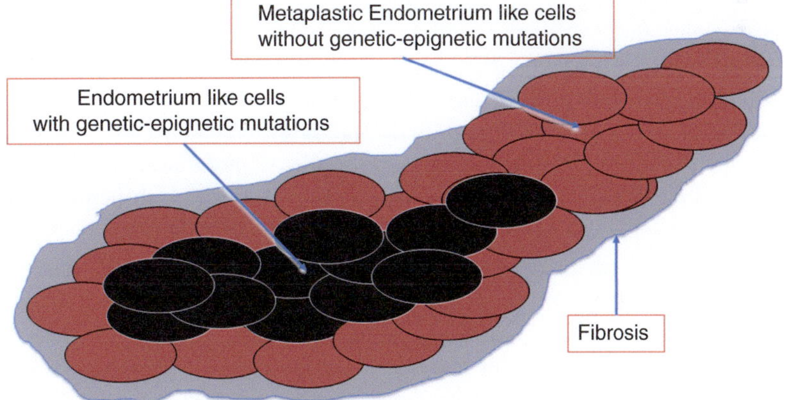

growing columns of cells or whether this layer is much thicker. This indeed will determine the necessary radicality of excision, since after excision of the core, these peripheral metaplastic cells will return to normality—"after cutting the head the snake dies" (Fig. 11.3).

11.5 What Is the Place of Diagnostic Tests Before Surgery?

A correct diagnosis is the cornerstone of surgery. A diagnosis is ideally made before surgery. However, if only suspected, the diagnosis can be confirmed during surgery. Understanding the value of a diagnostic test is important to understand why the treatment of deep endometriosis by nodulectomy or by bowel resection remains debated.

The accuracy of any preoperative test is judged by its sensitivity and its specificity. Sensitivity is the percentage of women with the disease that are detected; specificity is the percentage of women without the disease that are correctly diagnosed as negative. The former thus express the missed diagnoses and the latter the false positives. In addition, when a test is used for a rare condition, specificity should be very high in order to prevent too many false positives. This can best be illustrated with an example of a disease occurring in 1% of the population, or 100 women with the disease in a group of 10,000. A test with 99% sensitivity will find 99 of the 100 women with the disease. A 99% specificity means that 9801 women out of the 9900 will be diagnosed correctly as not having the disease. However, this also means that 99 women will be diagnosed erroneously as having the disease. The test thus will result in 99 true positive and 99 false positive diagnoses. A test with 99% specificity and 99% sensitivity thus will result in as many true positives as false positives for a disease with a prevalence of 1%. This is the well-known reason why screening tests, e.g., for breast cancer, need to be very accurate in order to prevent finding too many false positives.

The clinical usefulness of a test is a clinical decision. For deep endometriosis, a preoperative diagnostic test could help to make the decision to perform surgery and to make the decision which type of surgery should be performed. A full discussion of the clinical usefulness of imaging of deep endometriosis before surgery is beyond the scope of this chapter. However, we invite the readers to check in the other chapters of this book the sensitivities and specificities of imaging before surgery. The reader should decide whether sensitivity and specificity of small nodules, e.g., smaller than 1 cm, and whether the lower detection limit are good enough to overrule the clinical decision to do or not to do surgery. The reader should also decide whether the accuracy of depth of bowel invasion is good enough to decide about a bowel resection without attempting a nodulectomy.

Although imaging before surgery is of great value to discuss with the patient the probable severity of the disease and the type of surgery that will probably be performed, the results should be used with caution. Indeed, with sensitivities and specificities below 99%, and prevalences around 1%, the risk of missing disease and of false positives is high when used as an absolute indication to do surgery or to perform a bowel resection without trying a nodulectomy.

11.6 Outcome of Surgery

A full discussion of the outcome of surgery is far beyond the scope of this chapter. However, the readers are invited to check in the other chapters the results for pelvic pain, for infertility, for recurrence rates, for the quality of life and to check the risks for early and late postoperative complications and functional outcomes [44]. It is not surprising, that because of the complexity, outcomes are invariably given selectively, with a preference of results after a short time. In addition, it is difficult to compare outcomes which are so different. The reader should also realise that describing one outcome while ignoring all the other outcomes can be misleading, something described as "lying with statistics" [45, 46].

Rare events are difficult to judge since solid data are missing, especially for deep endometriosis surgery. A 1% complication, however serious, needs 1000 surgeries to collect ten cases. Any trial thus requires prohibitively large numbers for meaningful conclusions. This is the reason why careful reporting, permitting meta-analysis is important. This has permitted the conclusion (Fig. 11.4) that the incidence of anastomotic

Fig. 11.4 Complications after bowel resection [47]. (L Ret Davalos, de Cicco, D'Hoore, P Koninckx J Min Invas Surg a review of all cases since 1990 ≥10,000)

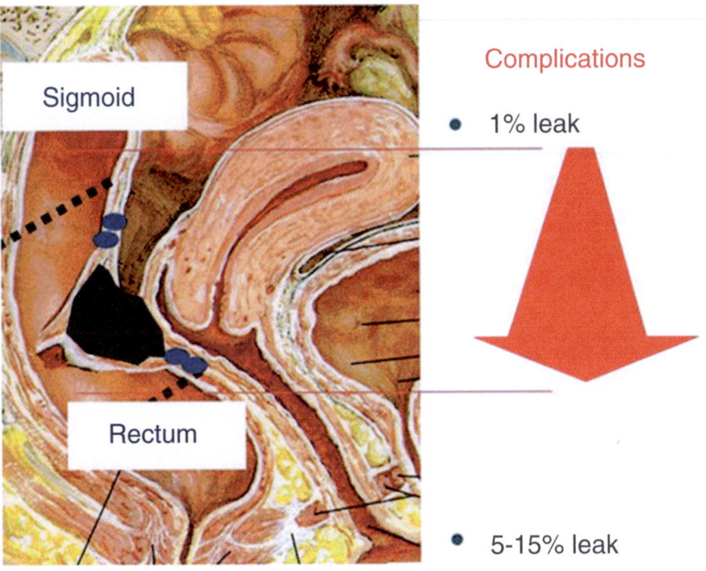

leaks was some 1% for the sigmoid and increased to over 10% for the low rectum [47], with some 30% lifelong bladder, bowel, and 40% sexual problems [47]. It is unfortunate that notwithstanding almost 2000 reported bowel resections for deep endometriosis, solid data on these complications especially sexual problems are not available [48]. A fortiori comparisons between bowel resection versus discoid resection are missing. However, although rarely considered, common sense suggests that sexual problems and anorgasmia are serious complications.

The many different aspects of outcome, the rare events, the inherent variability of the surgery performed in deep endometriosis, and the inherent variability of the skills of the surgeon all contribute to deep endometriosis surgery remaining debated after 30 years.

11.7 Technical Choices

The importance of dissection and of coagulation before cutting, and the choice of energy devices as electrosurgery, sealing devices, CO_2 laser, or ultrasonic devices are highly individual. In addition, few surgeons are equally skilled with all devices.

Deep endometriosis excision from the bowel started in the early 1990s as an extension of CO_2 laser excision of superficial endometriosis. With intermittent pulses at high-power density, CO_2 laser is a precise, fast, cutting instrument through vaporisation of the superficial layers with less than 100 µm tissue damage. "What you see is what you do." The use of the CO_2 laser through the operative laparoscope had the advantage of the surgeon holding the camera. However, the use of the CO_2 laser also has several disadvantages. The CO_2 laser is used at short distance decreasing the overview of the surgical field. Its use requires a high and continuous flow insufflation for smoke evacuation [49], with desiccation and probably adhesion formation as side effects [50]. The CO_2 laser is not suited for dissection and has poor coagulation properties. This requires a specifically well-trained assistant, capable of the immediate coagulation of bleedings. Being not suited for dissection together with the fast cutting, a CO_2 laser is highly suited for fast excision of a deep endometriosis nodule until safety requires dissection. It has some advantages for the excision from the bowel muscularis but not from the mucosa. Other disadvantages are the weight of the coupler and the lower image quality of operative laparoscopes.

Bipolar forceps, cold scissors and electrosurgery are the most versatile instruments for dissection and coagulation of vessels before cutting. However, fat is a poor conductor of electricity and bipolar coagulation is less suited for well irrigated fat, such as bowel fat or omentum. For these tissues sealing and ultrasonic devices are more appropriate.

These comments should explain our personal choices. In Leuven endometriosis surgery was started with CO_2 laser excision assisted with bipolar coagulation and cold scissors dissection before cutting. This combined use of an 80-W CO_2 laser together with bipolar/cold scissors dissection continued to be the basic setting. Whereas the surgeon holding the telescope with the camera and the laser, was considered an advantage in the early years, the increasingly severe endometriosis and the importance of specifically trained assistants resulted in the gradual replacement of registrars by dedicated fellows. In most other centers, dissection surgery was progressively developed since necessary for oncologic and pelvic floor surgery and the CO_2 laser was rarely used. In addition, the introduction of the new generation of telescopes had a much better image quality than the older operative endoscopes. For these reasons, the CO_2 laser has become rarely used for deep endometriosis surgery. It remains however, the preferred instrument for the treatment of superficial endometriosis.

Over the years we have tried many other instruments. With bipolar scissors we had difficulty to follow the plane of cleavage between endometriosis and healthy tissue because of the coagulated tissue. For ultracision and sealing devices we concluded that notwithstanding being superior for transecting bowel fat and epiploon, the dissecting capacities were insufficiently precise for the excision of endometriosis from the bowel wall or the ureter.

11.8 Excision of Deep Endometriosis of the Bowel

Our excision of deep endometriosis of the bowel has been guided by four principles. *First*, we always perform a one bloc resection, without leaving endometriosis to be excised later. To do this the central part of the nodule is left attached to the uterus. The traction by the central endometriosis nodule fixes the tissues and facilitates the judgment of cleaving plane between the endometriosis and the healthy tissue. Leaving endometriosis tissue to be excised later is more difficult when tissues are more mobile. Therefore, *the second principle* is that all lateral endometriosis (ureter, ischial spine, uterosacrals) should be excised first up to the pararectal spaces before starting the excision of the bowel endometriosis. For the same reason, *the third principle* is to keep the bowel attached to the uterus and to dissect the bowel from the endometriosis. This keeps traction on the plane between the nodule and the bowel and permits manipulation by moving the uterus. It avoids the much more difficult dissection of a nodule from a mobile bowel. *Fourth*, we consider the accuracy and predictive value of the estimation of the depth of invasion insufficient to permit the decision that excision of a bowel nodule cannot be done. For this reason, we use the 'try and see' principle and decide during surgery whether excision is feasible. The few exceptions are a bowel obstruction of more than 50% over more than 2 cm diagnosed by contrast enema. Experience has taught us that this is an absolute indication for a (sigmoid) bowel resection. Until today we did not see a single woman with a rectum obstruction after surgery fitting these criteria. However, confronted with a very large spherical nodule of more than 4–5 cm diameter, we learned to be prudent since excision could be long and difficult with the risk that a second intervention because of a late rectum perforation would anyway would be necessary.

11.8.1 The Rectum and Low Rectum

With the principles outlined above, we needed to perform in Leuven over 20 years 5–6 bowel resections only, in more than 1500 deep endometriosis nodules of variable sizes a shown in Fig. 11.5.

According to our principles, before starting the excision of endometriosis from the bowel wall, all lateral endometriosis around ureter, uterosacrals and ischial spine has been taken care

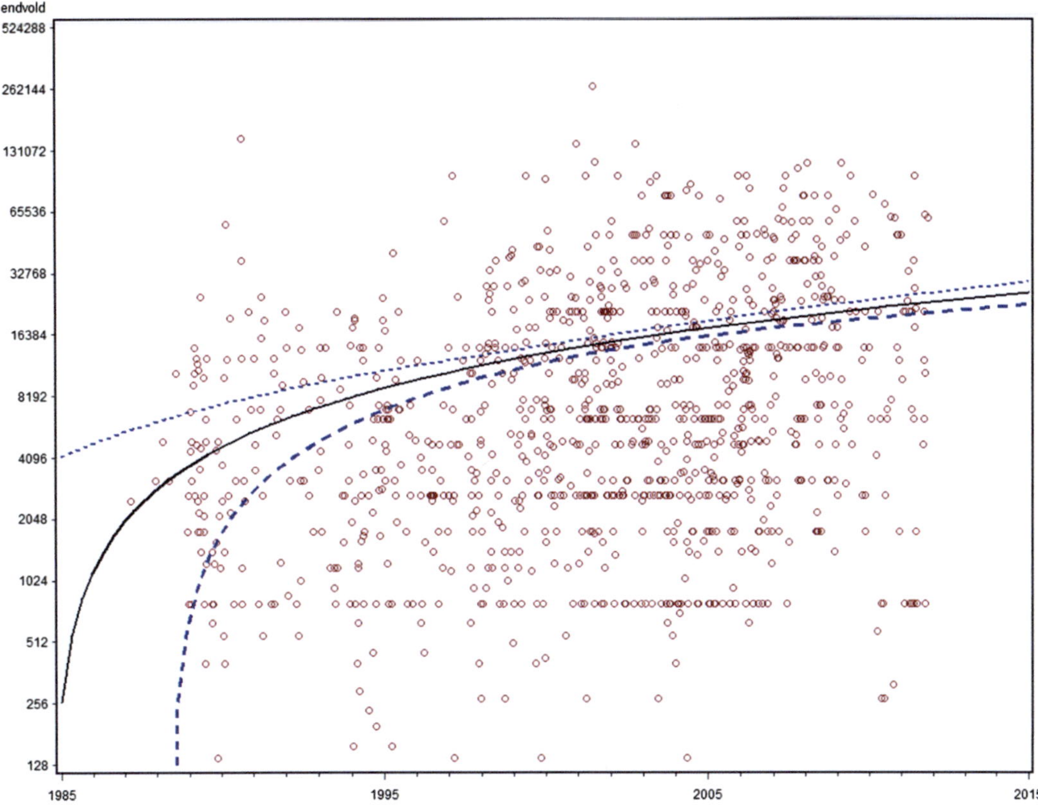

Fig. 11.5 Volume of deep endometriosis nodules in mm³ managed by conservative excision in Leuven between 1989 and 2011. A quadratic regression with 95% confidence limits is shown

of. In addition, both ureters and both pararectal spaces should be clearly identified.

When starting the excision, the endometriosis nodule should remain attached to the uterus/cervix in the central part only (Fig. 11.6). This implies that all lateral dissection up to the uterine arteries and ureters must be performed first. This surgery should respect the sympathetic nerves and it comprises the dissection of the lateral vagina and lateral cervix and the insertion of the uterosacrals. Important in this step is to emphasise the central traction between cervix, nodule and bowel in order to facilitate the visualisation of cleavage plans.

After this, still before starting the dissection between the nodule and the rectum, all bowel fat lateral from the nodule and the bowel is dissected. This can be done with little risks since this fat can be clearly identified, coagulated, and cut. Important is to do this as extensively and as deep as possible since it will increase the focal central traction between cervix, the nodule, and the bowel.

Only thereafter, dissection between the nodule and the bowel wall is started. Opening the peritoneum overlying the bowel is without risks. The difficulty starts when entering and cutting the muscularis. Important is to do this progressively after the lateral dissection of the fat in order to keep the central traction which identifies the plane of cleavage. Whereas 20 years ago, we excised all deep endometriosis lesions including the surrounding fibrosis we became more conservative over the years and left some fibrosis on the bowel. Smaller arteries were coagulated but capillary bleeding are not. The plane of cleavage is dissected with sharp scissors, after the plane of cleave is aligned with the plane of the scissors through uterine manipulation and/or a rectal probe. Only after complete dissection of the bowel from the nodule, the nodule is dissected from the cervix and the vagina. In doubt the posterior fornix of the

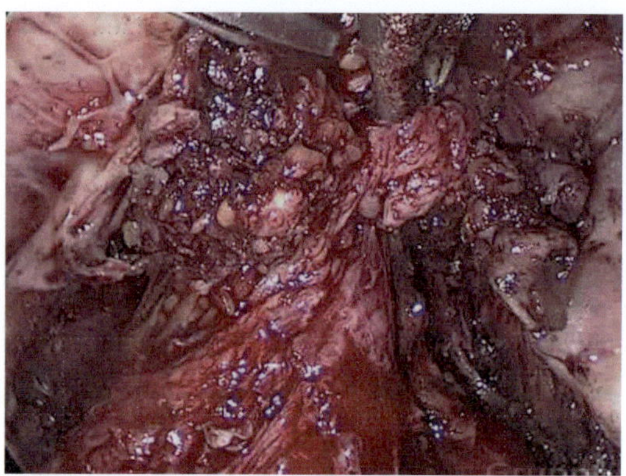

Fig. 11.6 Conservative excision of a 3 × 3 × 3 cm endometriosis nodule from the rectum. Notice the rectum attached centrally to the cervix and the partial dissection of the damaged muscularis which has to be sutured

vagina is resected since all recurrences we have seen were all at in the vaginal cuff.

With this technique over 95% of bowel endometriosis nodules were excised without the need to perform a bowel resection. An eventual small mucosa lesion, occurring in some 10% is sutured immediately in order to prevent prolonged leakage. Although the mucosa is rarely involved, it becomes tricky when the bowel is entered repetitively, and a wedge resection of the bowel is necessary. After excision of the nodule, the bowel is sutured in one layer for muscularis lesions only and in two layers for full thickness resections. It is unclear whether interrupted or running sutures should be preferred. Important is to suture healthy muscularis to healthy muscularis and it is unclear which distance of damaged muscularis can be bridged. Considering the semilunar configuration of bowel nodules (Fig. 11.1), distances up to 5–6 cm seem acceptable.

Today we think that for larger nodules the technique as described can be simplified by leaving some endometriosis on the bowel wall and to use a circular stapler to excise the remaining anterior bowel wall with the remaining endometriosis. However, the technique as described keeps its full importance since it permits a maximal reduction of the nodule volume prior to excision with a circular stapler. Although we never should say never in medicine, today the large majority of rectum endometriosis nodules can be excised conservatively without the need to perform a bowel resection. When nodules are very big and a lengthy excision over a long distance is anticipated, a much faster small bowel resection should be considered.

11.8.2 The Sigmoid

Endometriosis nodules in the sigmoid (Fig. 11.7) are generally much larger than their macroscopic appearance during laparoscopy. Often the strongly distorted anatomy is the only indication of a severe deep endometriosis together with a solid harder mass on palpation.

After been dissected from its physiologic adhesions to the side wall, the sigmoid becomes very mobile. This together with the localisation almost vertically under the umbilicus makes excision of a sigmoid nodule and the suturing of the frequent muscularis defect, or of a full thickness resection technically difficult.

Over the last 30 years we have explored the technical feasibility of excision of sigmoid nodules. The sigmoid was sutured to the round ligaments of the uterus permitting to pull the sigmoid down. This in addition, stabilised the sigmoid somewhat and facilitated the angle of surgery. Fairly rapidly, it was evident that excision of lesions with an occlusion of more than 50% over more than 2 cm on contrast enema almost systematically ended with a bowel resection with end-to-end anastomosis. Therefore the 5% nodules with 'more than 50% occlusion over more than 2 cm on contrast enema' became around 1996 an indication for elective bowel resection. For all other nodules, we started excision but another 5% ended with a bowel resection. It should be noticed that adhesions and spasms can mimic severe bowel stenosis over a short distance, as experienced in 5–10 cases over 30 years.

To the best of our knowledge there are no comparative studies which permit to judge the degree of bowel obstruction with other imaging methods than a contrast enema. The exact predictive value of ultrasound, virtual colonoscopy, and MRI with contrast remains to be established.

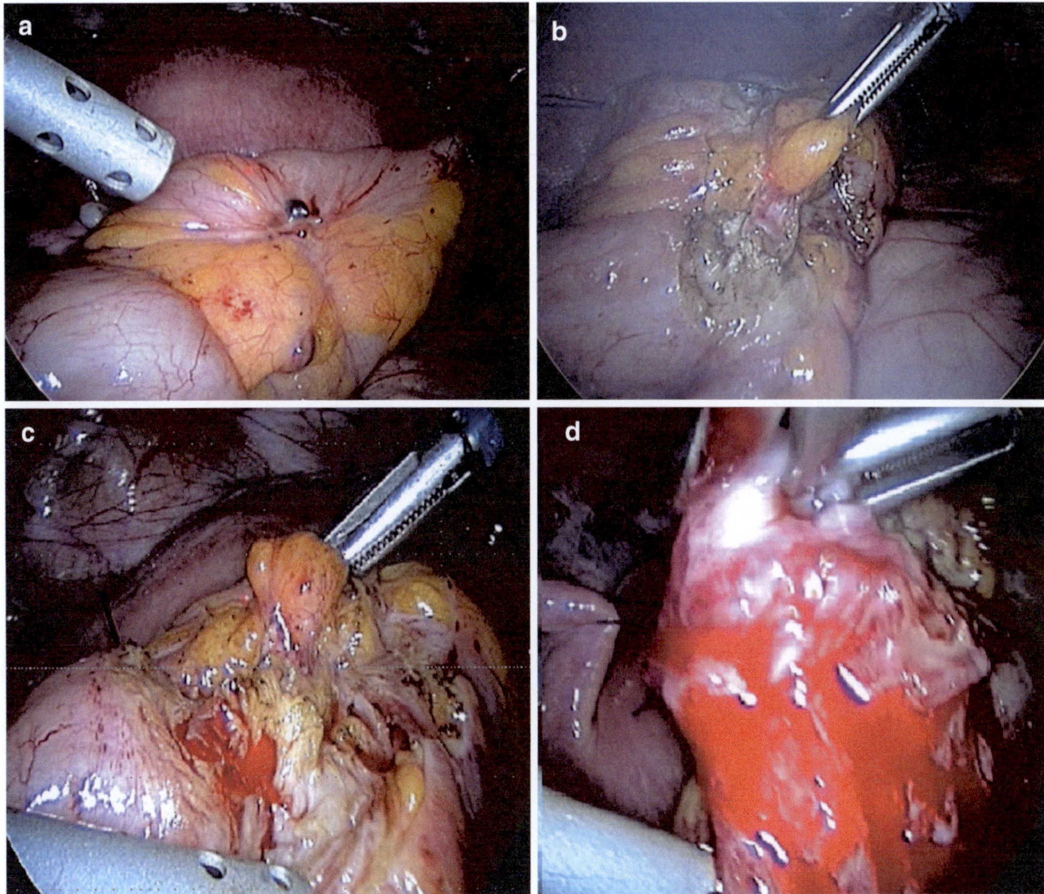

Fig. 11.7 Conservative excision of deep endometriosis from the sigmoid is feasible although no longer recommended. The nodule is more important than judged by inspection (**a**). A CO_2 laser is used up to the muscularis (**b**). Sharp dissection is used thereafter (**c** and **d**)

11.9 Conclusions and Discussion

11.9.1 Conclusions

Looking back at the historical evolution of deep endometriosis bowel surgery and considering newer techniques as (double) discoid excision with a circular or linear stapler, and the short 'economic' bowel resections as developed by A Wattiez, we conclude that (short) segmental bowel resections should be used liberally for sigmoid nodules, whereas conservative excision without bowel resection is the preferred technique for the large majority of deep endometriosis nodules of the rectum. A segmental resection of the sigmoid has a low risk of postoperative leaks and of long-term functional problems of bladder, bowel and sexuality. On the other hand, a conservative excision of a sigmoid nodule is long and technically difficult surgery with frequent muscularis lesions, full thickness resections and at least 5% bowel resections. Therefore, although feasible, excision of sigmoid endometriosis lesions should be reserved for small nodules with a liberal conversion to a bowel resection. Low rectum deep endometriosis nodules can be excised conservatively in most women. In order to do so, it is mandatory to identify the ureters, the pararectal spaces, to free the lateral attachment of the nodule from the cervix up to the vagina, to keep the central attachment to the cervix permitting mobilisation and traction on the nodule and to dissect the bowel from the nodule. If the aim is to suture the muscularis defect or an eventual full thickness defect, we suggest leaving a rim of fibrosis on the bowel wall since this will reduce the risk of opening the bowel without increasing the recurrence risk. If the aim is to use a circular stapler to perform a full thickness resection of the bowel wall excision of the nodule can even be less complete. It is unclear whether the outcome of a conservative excision with discoid resection with a circular stapler is superior to suturing. However, a discoid excision with a circular stapler has the advantages of being technically easier and faster, permitting a more superficial and less complete dissection of the nodule from the bowel. It is unclear until which size the feasibility of conservative excision should be tried. We suggest that when nodules are very big, i.e., more than 4 cm in all directions or a volume of more than 20 ml, a small bowel resection should be considered, given the difficulty and duration of a conservative excision. It is also unclear whether the rare women with two deep endometriosis nodules, one in the sigmoid and another one in the rectum should be treated with a long segmental bowel resection and a high risk of persisting functional disturbances or whether the rectum nodule should be conservatively excised in a first procedure followed later by a small sigmoid resection.

The liberal use of low bowel resections can no longer be recommended. First it is no longer necessary, since conservative excision can be done for most nodules with postoperative complications which are similar to rectum resections [1, 48]. Second, rectum resections are associated with the long-term functional complications of the bladder, bowel, and sexuality. Until proven otherwise this is a major argument to avoid low rectum resections and to prefer conservative excision. Anorgasmia indeed should be considered a serious complication.

Technical considerations suggest that the use of a CO_2 laser belongs to the past. Important is that the CO_2 laser is less suited for the precise dissection of a deep endometriosis nodule from the muscularis and mucosa of the bowel. The proper use of a CO_2 laser moreover requires a continuous flow to prevent blooming of the laser

beam in the telescope and for smoke evacuation, and a trocar with a large side opening [51]. The use of a CO_2 laser needs additional training to learn the technique of the surgeon holding the telescope, working at short distance and relying on a trained assistant for coagulation. Finally, the image quality of the operating telescopes is less than for straight telescopes whereas 4K operative telescopes even do not exist today.

Considering the similar tissue effects of superficial vaporisation with limited tissue damage of a CO_2 laser and of pure cutting current electrosurgery when used with intermitted pulses, both techniques can advantageously be used to speed up the lateral dissection of the nodules up to the muscularis. Looking back, it is surprising to realise that in the early 1990s I used this type of electrosurgery when resecting deep endometriosis nodules when a CO_2 laser was not available, and that over the subsequent years bipolar coagulation and cold scissors dissection became used exclusively. Only recently observing the Brazilian use of electrosurgical hook [52] we think that this technique should be considered to speed up the lateral dissection of the nodule up to the muscularis, in a similar fashion as done with the CO_2 laser previously.

11.9.2 Discussion

We limited our discussion to the larger lesions which seem spherical and glandular during resection of which have the typical semilunar retractive aspect after bowel resection (Fig. 11.1). We excluded slightly deeper typical lesions and larger fibrotic plaques which seem a different pathology although fitting the diagnosis of 'more than 5 mm under the peritoneum'.

Understanding the accuracy and clinical usefulness of diagnostic methods is important to judge whether decisions as an elective bowel resection can be taken before surgery. This has organisational advantages when the presence of an abdominal surgeon has to be planned. The risk however is that bowel resections are too frequently used. Much of the confusion stems from the pitfalls and the poor understanding of the diagnostic accuracy of a diagnostic method.

A first pitfall is that for rare diseases the sensitivities and specificities need to be much higher. Indeed, for a disease with a prevalence of 1%, 99% specificity, and 99% sensitivity will result in unacceptable 50% false positives. A second pitfall is the confusion resulting from extrapolating statistically significant differences as a diagnostic test. Although men are significantly taller than women, height is a poor predictor of gender. The third pitfall is that the clinical usefulness of a diagnostic test is a clinical judgment and that the required accuracy will vary with the pathology. The acceptable risk of missing the diagnosis (sensitivity) of a cancer, and the risk of a false diagnosis of cancer (specificity) with severe consequences of surgery and chemotherapy, should obviously be less than for conditions which are not life-threatening. A fourth pitfall is circular conclusions. The conclusion that this size or the circumference of a nodule is an indication for a bowel resection requires that conservative resection has been tried. A fifth last pitfall is the absence of diagnostic sensitivity and specificity stratified for nodules of different sizes.

Surgery should be judged by its results, which should comprise postoperative complications, permanent bladder, bowel and sexual complications, and improvement of pain, infertility, quality of life, and absence of adhesion formation. With that many variables a comprehensive multivariate analysis does not exist. Moreover, many variables as postoperative complications are rare events requiring prohibitively large groups for meaningful conclusions. Unfortunately, lifelong bladder, bowel and sexual problems are poorly investigated since considered 'unavoidable' and minor side effects.

Confusion is fuelled in addition by the varying interpretation of words. It is unclear when metaplasia, and by extension epigenetic changes, are reversible or irreversible. 'Shaving' sounds as a progressive removal layer by layer which is not what is done during deep endometriosis excision. For this reason, we prefer excision.

It was beyond the aim of this chapter to discuss nerve sparing in deep endometriosis bowel surgery. However, for the rest of the life bowel bladder and sexual problems after traditional rectum resections, and the dissection required to do a bowel resection strongly suggest that a nodulectomy should be preferred if possible and to perform the smallest bowel resection possible if necessary.

In conclusion, to discuss the management of deep endometriosis of the bowel we need a clear understanding and definition of deep endometriosis, we need to understand the accuracy and pitfalls of a diagnostic test and a comprehensive understanding of complications and results. Considering the available evidence today we suggest a liberal use of bowel resection for sigmoid endometriosis. Provided a correct technique, almost all rectal deep endometriosis lesions can be treated conservatively by excision, eventually by discoid excision. Low rectum bowel resections should progressively become obsolete except for the very large lesions, and if performed a short or minimal resection should be performed.

Acknowledgments We thank Marco Bassi, Sao Paulo, Brazil, Paulo Ribeiro Ayrosa, Sao Paulo Brazil, and William Kondo, Curitiba Brazil, for lengthy discussions on deep bowel endometriosis surgery. We thank Dan Martin, Memphis, USA for discussions on pathophysiology and definitions of deep endometriosis. We thank Muna Tahlak, Latiffa, Dubai for facilitating this collaboration.

Conflict of Interest: None of the authors have a conflict of interest to declare.

Financial support: None.

References

1. Donnez O, Roman H. Choosing the right surgical technique for deep endometriosis: shaving, disc excision, or bowel resection? Fertil Steril. 2017;108:931–42.
2. Koninckx PR, Ussia A, Adamyan L, Wattiez A, Gomel V, Martin DC. Pathogenesis of endometriosis: the genetic/epigenetic theory. Fertil Steril. 2019;111:327–39.
3. Koninckx PR, Ussia A, Adamyan L, Wattiez A, Donnez J. Deep endometriosis: definition, diagnosis, and treatment. Fertil Steril. 2012;98:564–71.
4. Di Giovanni A, Casarella L, Coppola M, Iuzzolino D, Rasile M, Malzoni M. Combined transvaginal/transabdominal pelvic ultrasonography accurately predicts the 3 dimensions of deep infiltrating bowel endometriosis measured after surgery: a prospective study in a specialized center. J Minim Invasive Gynecol. 2018;25:1231–40.

5. Exacoustos C, Zupi E, Piccione E. Ultrasound imaging for ovarian and deep infiltrating endometriosis. Semin Reprod Med. 2017;35:5–24.

6. Abrao MS, Andres MP, Barbosa RN, Bassi MA, Kho RM. Optimizing perioperative outcomes with selective bowel resection following algorithm based on pre-operative imaging for bowel endometriosis. J Minim Invasive Gynecol. 2020;27(4):883–91.

7. Muzii L, Miller CE. The singer, not the song. J Minim Invasive Gynecol. 2011;18:666–7.

8. Koninckx PR, Martin DC. Deep endometriosis: a consequence of infiltration or retraction or possibly adenomyosis externa? Fertil Steril. 1992;58:924–8.

9. Cornillie FJ, Oosterlynck D, Lauweryns JM, Koninckx PR. Deeply infiltrating pelvic endometriosis: histology and clinical significance. Fertil Steril. 1990;53:978–83.

10. Koninckx PR, Heyns W, Verhoeven G, Van BH, Lissens WD, De MP, et al. Biochemical characterization of peritoneal fluid in women during the menstrual cycle. J Clin Endocrinol Metab. 1980;51:1239–44.

11. Cullen TS. Adenoma-myoma uteri diffusum benignum. J Hopkins Hosp Bull. 1896;6:133–7.

12. Lockyer C. Adenomyoma in the recto-uterine and recto-vaginal septa. Proc R Soc Med. 1913;6: 112–20.

13. Cullen TS. The distribution of adenomyomata containing uterine mucosa. Am J Obstet Gynecol. 1919;80:130–8.

14. Sampson JA. Perforating hemorrhagic (chocolate) cysts of the ovary. Their importance and especially their relation to pelvic adenomas of the endometrial type. Arch Surg. 1921;3:245–323.

15. Cornillie FJ, Koninckx PR. Morphologic aspects of endometriosis. In: Martin D, editor. Appearances of endometriosis. London: Gower Medical Publishing; 1992. p. 1–6.

16. Koninckx PR, Meuleman C, Demeyere S, Lesaffre E, Cornillie FJ. Suggestive evidence that pelvic endometriosis is a progressive disease, whereas deeply infiltrating endometriosis is associated with pelvic pain. Fertil Steril. 1991;55:759–65.

17. Koninckx PR, Martin D. Treatment of deeply infiltrating endometriosis. Curr Opin Obstet Gynecol. 1994;6:231–41.

18. Penninckx F, Aerts R, Kerremans R, Koninckx PR. Laparoscopic cholecystectomy: some advantages or just an artifice of new technology? HPB Surg. 1991;3:291–4.

19. Neven P, vandeursen H, Baert L, Koninckx PR. Ureteric injury at laparoscopic surgery : the endoscopic management. Case review. Gynaecol Endosc. 1993;2:45–6.

20. Koninckx PR, Timmermans B, Meuleman C, Penninckx F. Complications of CO_2-laser endoscopic excision of deep endometriosis. Hum Reprod. 1996;11:2263–8.

21. Koninckx PR, Ussia A, Keckstein J, Wattiez A, Adamyan L. Epidemiology of subtle, typical, cystic, and deep endometriosis: a systematic review. Gynaecol Surg. 2016;13:457–67.

22. Nassif J, Trompoukis P, Barata S, Furtado A, Gabriel B, Wattiez A. Management of deep endometriosis. Reprod Biomed Online. 2011;23:25–33.

23. Kondo W, Ribeiro R, Zomer MT, Hayashi R, Ferreira LR, Martin RL. Double discoid resection in deep intestinal endometriosis. J Minim Invasive Gynecol. 2015;22:S140.

24. Kondo W, Ribeiro R, Zomer MT, Hayashi R, Ferreira L, Martin R. Surgical techniques for the treatment of bowel endometriosis. J Minim Invasive Gynecol. 2015;22:S131.

25. Ribeiro PA, Rodrigues FC, Kehdi IP, Rossini L, Abdalla HS, Donadio N, et al. Laparoscopic resection of intestinal endometriosis: a 5-year experience. J Minim Invasive Gynecol. 2006;13:442–6.

26. Ohara F, Abdala-Ribeiro HS, Rodrigues FC, Aldrighi JM, Ribeiro PA. Outcomes of laparoscopic treatment of rectosigmoid endometriosis: the linear nodulectomy and the segmental resection. J Minim Invasive Gynecol. 2015;22:S95.

27. Koninckx PR. Is mild endometriosis a condition occurring intermittently in all women? Hum Reprod. 1994;9:2202–5.

28. Nisolle M, Paindaveine B, Bourdon A, Casanas F, Donnez J. Peritoneal endometriosis: typical aspect and subtle appearance. Acta Endosc. 1992;22:15–23.

29. Schenken RS. Microscopic endometriosis. Contrib Gynecol Obstet. 1987;16:7–12.

30. Rossini R, Monsellato D, Bertolaccini L, Pesci A, Zamboni G, Ceccaroni M, et al. Lymph nodes involvement in deep infiltrating intestinal endometriosis: does it really mean anything? J Minim Invasive Gynecol. 2016;23:787–92.

31. Roman H, Hennetier C, Darwish B, Badescu A, Csanyi M, Aziz M, et al. Bowel occult microscopic endometriosis in resection margins in deep colorectal endometriosis specimens has no impact on short-term postoperative outcomes. Fertil Steril. 2016;105:423–9.

32. Badescu A, Roman H, Aziz M, Puscasiu L, Molnar C, Huet E, et al. Mapping of bowel occult microscopic endometriosis implants surrounding deep endometriosis nodules infiltrating the bowel. Fertil Steril. 2016;105:430–4.

33. Koninckx P. Recurrence rate of deep endometriosis. In: Lemay A, Maheux R, editors. Understanding and managing endometriosis: advances in research and practice. New York: Parthenon; 1999. p. 251–9.

34. Koninckx PR, Kennedy SH, Barlow DH. Pathogenesis of endometriosis: the role of peritoneal fluid. Gynecol Obstet Investig. 1999;47(Suppl 1):23–33.

35. Koninckx PR, Donnez J, Brosens I. Microscopic endometriosis: impact on our understanding of the disease and its surgery. Fertil Steril. 2016;105: 305–6.

36. Wu Y, Basir Z, Kajdacsy-Balla A, Strawn E, Macias V, Montgomery K, et al. Resolution of clonal origins for endometriotic lesions using laser capture microdissection and the human androgen receptor (HUMARA) assay. Fertil Steril. 2003;79(Suppl 1):710–7.

37. Mayr D, Amann G, Siefert C, Diebold J, Anderegg B. Does endometriosis really have premalignant potential? A clonal analysis of laser-microdissected tissue. FASEB J. 2003;17:693–5.
38. Koninckx PR, Ussia A, Adamyan L, Wattiez A, Gomel V, Martin DC. Heterogeneity of endometriosis lesions requires new approaches to research, diagnosis and treatment. Facts Views Vis Obgyn. 2019;11(1):57–61.
39. Guo SW. Cancer driver mutations in endometriosis: variations on the major theme of fibrogenesis. Reprod Med Biol. 2018;17(4):369–97.
40. Guo SW. Fibrogenesis resulting from cyclic bleeding: the Holy Grail of the natural history of ectopic endometrium. Hum Reprod. 2018;33:353.
41. Eelen G, de Zeeuw P, Treps L, Harjes U, Wong BW, Carmeliet P. Endothelial cell metabolism. Physiol Rev. 2018;98:3–58.
42. Scutiero G, Iannone P, Bernardi G, Bonaccorsi G, Spadaro S, Volta CA, et al. Oxidative stress and endometriosis: a systematic review of the literature. Oxidative Med Cell Longev. 2017;2017:7265238.
43. Giroux V, Rustgi AK. Metaplasia: tissue injury adaptation and a precursor to the dysplasia-cancer sequence. Nat Rev Cancer. 2017;17:594–604.
44. Roman H, Milles M, Vassilieff M, Resch B, Tuech JJ, Huet E, et al. Long-term functional outcomes following colorectal resection versus shaving for rectal endometriosis. Am J Obstet Gynecol. 2016;215:762.
45. Connor J. How to lie with statistics. Lenexa, KS: Unlimited Press Works LLC; 2015.
46. Huff D. How to lie with statistics. New York: WW Norton & Company; 1982.
47. Ret Davalos ML, De Cicco C, D'Hoore A, De DB, Koninckx PR. Outcome after rectum or sigmoid resection: a review for gynecologists. J Minim Invasive Gynecol. 2007;14:33–8.
48. De Cicco C, Corona R, Schonman R, Mailova K, Ussia A, Koninckx PR. Bowel resection for deep endometriosis: a systematic review. BJOG. 2011;118:285–91.
49. Koninckx PR, Vandermeersch E. The persufflator: an insufflation device for laparoscopy and especially for CO_2-laser-endoscopic surgery. Hum Reprod. 1991;6:1288–90.
50. Koninckx PR, Gomel V, Ussia A, Adamyan L. Role of the peritoneal cavity in the prevention of postoperative adhesions, pain, and fatigue. Fertil Steril. 2016;106:998–1010.
51. Koninckx P, Vandermeersch E. Gas insufflation system for use in endoscopy and a surgical endoscope therefor. Google Patents; 1992.
52. Fernandes LF, Bassi MA, Abrao MS. Surgical principles for disc resection of deep bowel endometriosis. J Minim Invasive Gynecol. 2020;27(2):262.

Laparoscopic Segmental Bowel Resection

12

Marcello Ceccaroni, Roberto Clarizia, and Giovanni Roviglione

12.1 Definition of the Technique

Segmental bowel resection is defined as the removal of an intestinal portion (more frequently rectosigmoid) with subsequent termino-terminal anastomosis with or without ileostomy or protective colostomy. The most commonly used surgical technique involves a minimally invasive surgical phase (laparoscopy, robot-assisted laparoscopy) and a mini-laparotomic or transvaginal phase.

12.2 Historical Curiosities

George Arnaud de Ronsil performed the first right hemicolectomy in 1732. The patient had an incarcerated scrotal hernia with scattered areas of gangrene of the ileum, cecum, and ascending colon. Two Frenchmen, Lisfranc in 1826, and Maurin in 1831, and an Englishman, Herbert Mayo, about the same time, reported successful resection of the rectum for cancer [1].

The French surgeon Henri Hartmann, born in 1860, performed over 30,000 operations, and published extensively in the areas of surgery and gynecology.

Although the Hartmann operation, firstly described in 1923, was performed for cancer, it has been commonly used almost exclusively for acute diverticular disease of the rectosigmoid and sigmoid colon.

Hartmann performed a two-stage operation on two patients with obstructing cancers of the pelvic colon. At the first procedure, he created a sigmoid colostomy, and at the second, he resected the tumor-containing bowel, leaving the sigmoid colostomy, and closing the upper end of the rectum. Hartmann never planned to reestablish intestinal continuity.

Over the years, the Hartmann technique was further developed and underwent technical evolution leading to a single-step technique with colorectal anastomosis in most cases of colorectal cancer, with ileostomy or colostomy meant only to be protective in selected patients at high risk of complications. The first laparoscopic bowel resection was performed by Jacobs in Miami [2] in 1991 and separately by Fowler [3] in Kansas.

Laparoscopic segmental resection for surgical treatment of intestinal endometriosis was firstly described in 1991–1992, by Nezhat, Redwine and Sharpe [4–6]. Since then, the technique has spread to all the major world centers that deal with endometriosis and has evolved and perfected in recent years in order to minimize complications and to improve the impact on the patient's quality of life.

M. Ceccaroni (✉) · R. Clarizia · G. Roviglione
Department of Obstetrics and Gynecology, Gynecologic Oncology and Minimally-Invasive Pelvic Surgery, International School of Surgical Anatomy—IRCCS "Sacro Cuore-Don Calabria" Hospital, Negrar, Verona, Italy

© Springer Nature Switzerland AG 2020
S. Ferrero, M. Ceccaroni (eds.), *Clinical Management of Bowel Endometriosis*,
https://doi.org/10.1007/978-3-030-50446-5_12

Even if rectosigmoid endometriosis accounts for the most cases of intestinal endometriosis, with rectosigmoid junction as the most common reported localization (range, 52.0–65.7%), followed by the sigmoid colon (range, 17.4–19.4%), also ileum (range, 4.1–16.9%), cecum (range, 4.7–6.2%), and appendix (range, 5.0–6.4%) might affected even in the same patients, requiring segmental multiple bowel resections [7, 8].

12.3 Surgical Anatomy Remarks

Knowledge of anatomy is the roadmap allowing the radical pelvic surgeon to move in safe avascular spaces in an extremely complex and puzzling disease such endometriosis is, particularly when visceral and parametrial infiltrations are present (Fig. 12.1).

Following simple embryological rules, apparently labyrinthic distortions of the pelvic anatomy caused by infiltrative diseases may be unraveled.

The golden rule of Toldt's, also called the coalescence's law [9], says that embryologically developed organ may be separated from the other by means of development of an avascular plane between sheaths of fasciae covering the viscera.

The retroperitoneal pelvic spaces are anatomical areas obtained after surgical dissection and separation of structures and fasciae which are naturally in a relationship of contiguity [10–13].

The dissection of the pelvic spaces is usually obtained in a blunt way, separating avascular structures, and is carried out until the caudad limit of the pelvis represented by the levator ani (Fig. 12.2).

We will have a glimpse to the pelvic spaces needed to be opened and developed in a segmental bowel resection for endometriosis.

12.3.1 Pararectal Spaces (PRSs)

The PRSs are the keypoint for the access to the posterior compartment of the pelvis, which is essential to the approach of the retroperitoneum for the isolation of the ureter, for the dissection of the posterior and lateral parametrium in course of radical hysterectomy [10–14], in case of eradication of deep infiltrating endometriosis affecting the parametrial ligaments, and for the medialization of the ureter in course of pelvic lymphadenectomy. Moreover, the dissection of the PRSs is propaedeutic to the latero-dorsal mobilization of the rectosigmoid, in order to better skeletonize the rectovaginal ligaments, the lateral rectal pillars and to dissect and lateralize the hypogastric nerves (for nerve-sparing procedures).

The PRSs are classified in medial PRS (MPRS, Okabayashi's) and lateral PRS (LPRS, Latzko's). The anatomical landmark which divides the PRSs in MPRS and LPRS is the ureter, together with the meso-ureter [10–14].

The MPRS is obtained by dissecting the retroperitoneal areolar tissue between the ureter and the uterosacral ligament and the mesorectum, caudally toward the hypogastric nerves (usually at 1.5–2 cm caudad to the ureter, in the context of the mesoureter) the rectovaginal ligaments and the rectal pillars.

The LPRS is developed between the mesoureter, the hypogastric vessels, caudally to the hypogastric fascia and the pelvic splanchnic nerves (PSNs).

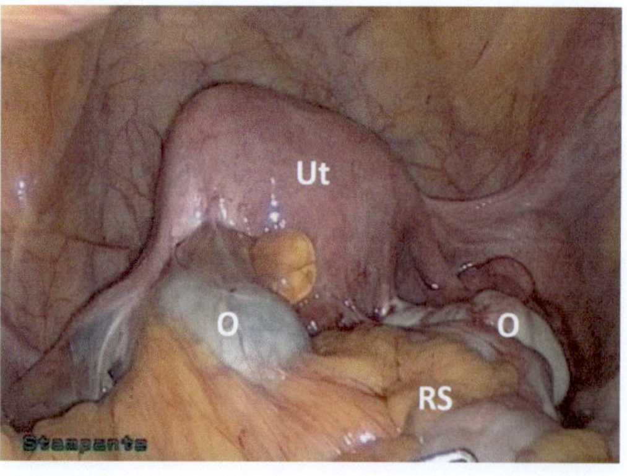

Fig. 12.1 Laparoscopic view of a "frozen pelvis." The initial surgical field of severe DIE with parametrial involvement and rectal wall infiltration with 70% of stenosis. *Ut* uterus, *RS* rectosigmoid, *O* ovary

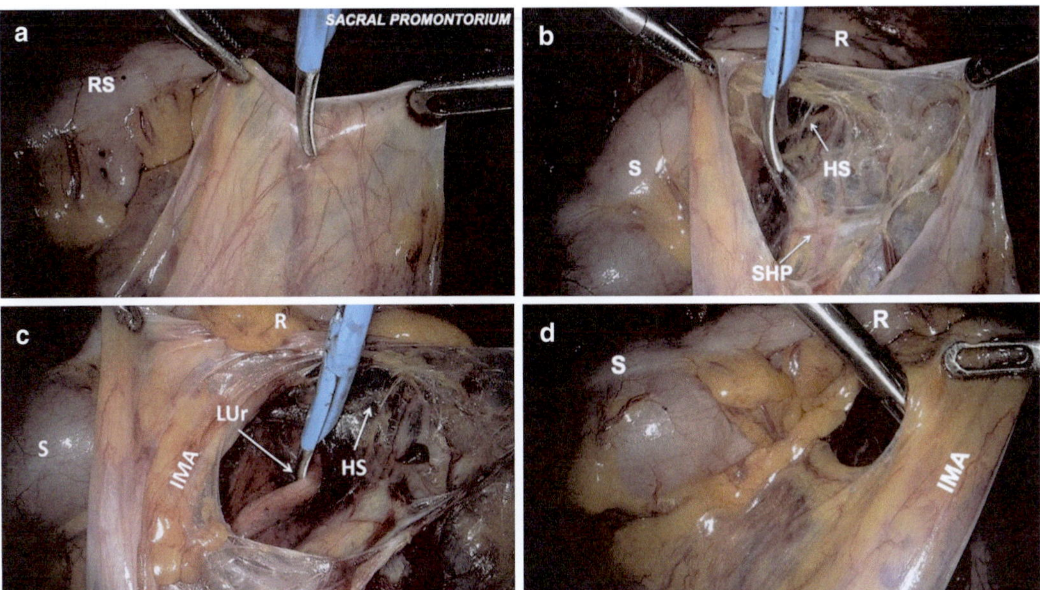

Fig. 12.2 Laparoscopic steps of cranial presacral space development for posterior rectal mobilization. (**a**) Laparoscopic view of peritoneal incision at right sacral promontorium performed in order to initially mobilize the rectosigmoid. *RS* rectosigmoid. (**b**) Laparoscopic view of dissection of the retroperitoneum at right sacral promontorium, with development of retrorectal Heald's "holy" space. *HS* Heald's "holy" space, *R* rectum, *S* sigmoid, *SHP* superior hypogastric plexus. (**c**) Laparoscopic view of dissection of the retroperitoneum at right sacral promontorium, with opening of the so-called "mesocolic window" and exposure of the left ureter. *HS* Heald's "holy" space, *R* rectum, *S* sigmoid, *LUr* left ureter, *IMA* inferior mesenteric artery. (**d**) Laparoscopic view of the fenestration of the mesosigmoid performed in order to skeletonize the inferior mesenteric artery. *R* rectum, *S* sigmoid, *IMA* inferior mesenteric artery

The anatomical limits of the PRSs are:

- Medial: fascia propria recti, rectal pillars; ureter and mesoureter for the LPRS.
- Lateral: PPF, pelvic plexus (PP) with pelvic splanchinc nerves (PSNs), hypogastric artery (HA), piriformis muscle; ureter and mesoureter for the MPRS.
- Dorsal: presacral fascia, sacral bone.
- Ventral: lateral parametrium (i.e., cardinal Mackenrodt's ligament).
- Caudad: sacral bone concavity, after dissecting the presacral Waldeyer' or retro-rectal space (RRS) and the so-called "Heald's Holy plane" [15] at the midline (Fig. 12.2).

12.3.2 Retrorectal Space (RRS) (or Presacral Waldeyer's Space)

The RRS is an avascular space delimited dorsally by the sacral bone, covered by the presacral fascia, and ventrally by the posterior rectal wall which is enveloped in its visceral sheet, called *fascia propria recti*. The dissection of the RRS is carried out separating a loose areolar connectival tissue between these two fasciae (Figs. 12.2 and 12.3), called *tela adiposa retrorectalis*, so defined by Waldeyer [16]. The RRS is obtained by gentle blunt separation of this tissue in a cranio-caudad and mediolateral direction, along the sacral concavity until the coccyx. The cranial starting point of this dissection is at the level of the sacral promontorium and of the superior orthosympathetic hypogastric plexus, and corresponds to the opening of the so-called Heald's holy plane [15], which is developed during the procedures of mobilization of the rectosigmoid for bowel resection.

The anatomical limits of the RRS are:

- Dorsal: the sacrum, covered by the presacral fascia (ventral reflection of the PPF), strictly adherent to the periostium, which covers the

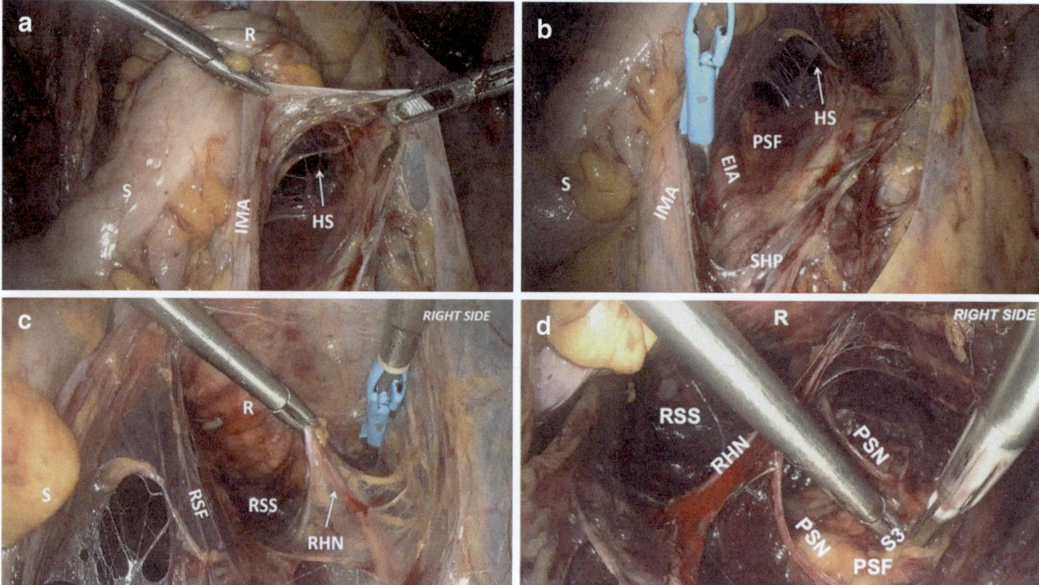

Fig. 12.3 Laparoscopic steps of caudad presacral space development for posterior rectal mobilization. (**a**) Laparoscopic view of dissection of the retroperitoneum at right sacral promontorium, with development of Heald's "holy" space. *HS* Heald's "holy" space, *R* rectum, *S* sigmoid, *IMA* inferior mesenteric artery. (**b**) Laparoscopic view of dissection of the retropertitoneum at right sacral promontorium, with identification of the superior hypogastric plexus. *HS* Heald's "holy" space, *S* sigmoid, *EIA* external iliac artery, *IMA* inferior mesenteric artery, *PSF* presacral fascia, *SHP* superior hypogastric plexus. (**c**) Laparoscopic view of dorsal dissection of the rectosigmoid with identification of the right hypogastric nerve. *RSS* Waldeyer's rectosacral space, *R* rectum, *S* sigmoid, *RSF* Waldeyer's rectosacral fascia, *RHN* right hypogastric nerve. (**d**) Laparoscopic view of the dissection of the right presacral area with decompression of the sacral roots (S3) and exposure of the right pelvic splanchnic nerves. *RSS* Waldeyer's rectosacral space, *R* rectum, *RHN* right hypogastric nerve, *PSN* pelvic splanchnic nerves, *S3* third sacral root, *PSF* presacral fascia

middle sacral artery and vein with the respective artero-venous anastomoses.

- Ventral: the posterior rectal wall, enveloped in the *fascia propria recti* (part of the VPF).
- Lateral: common iliac vessels hypogastric nerves, mesoureters, and ureters.
- Cranial: abdominal peritoneum.
- Caudad: rectosacral Waldeyer's fascia [16], which reflects from the presacral fascia (part of the PPF) to the *fascia propria recti*; (part of the VPF); it represents the posterior support of the rectum, keeping the sacrococcygeal angle during the defecation. The most caudad limit is represented by the anococcygeal raphe, also described by Havenga et al. [17] as rectosacral fascia. It is composed by the merging of the presacral fascia and pelvic parietal fascia fibers caudad to S4 (sacrococcygeal joint).

The rectosacral fascia has been previously described by Crapp and Cuthbertson [18] and by Sato [19] with the probable role of anchoring the rectum to the sacral curvature, preventing rectal prolapse. Nevertheless, its cut may be needed if an ultralow rectal resection is needed (Figs. 12.2 and 12.3).

12.3.3 The Posterior Parametrium

Knowledge of the tissue connecting the uterus (and vagina) to the rectum is the milestone of its dissection, resection, or sparing in a procedure where the goal is to remove an infiltrating disease sticking the rectum itself to the uterus and infiltrating it. In most cases, rectal infiltration comes from a posterior parametrial infiltration rising from a caudo-dorsal spread of a retrocervical nodule.

The parametrium (from the Greek etymology, παρα-μετρος: the region siding the uterus) is properly a layer of connective tissue and extends between the parietal and visceral pelvic fascia (from which it is covered) to the lateral pelvic wall. It contains afferent/efferent lympho-vascular and nervous connections from/to the pelvic viscera and can be anatomically divided into an anterior, lateral, and posterior portion. Many radical procedures required for deep infiltrating endometriosis removal may need extensive parametrectomies, also involving the lateral and anterior parametrium. Below we quickly describe the most commonly parametrial compartment involved when a segmental bowel resection is performed for endometriosis (Fig. 12.4), as to say the posterior parametrium [20].

The posterior parametrium is represented by a set of three key anatomical structures:

1. The uterosacral ligaments, which extend from the cranial portion of the retroperitoneum at the cervico-isthmic level of the uterus, dorsally, to the most ventral portion of the sacrum.
2. The rectovaginal ligaments, which extend retroperitoneally in the most ventral and caudad portion of the rectum up to the most dorsal and caudad portion of the posterior vaginal wall, at the level of the pelvic floor.
3. The lateral ligaments of the rectum (also called "rectal wings" or rectal pillars—LLR), which originate from the lateral portion of the rectum (where the mesorectum joins the fascia propria recti), up to latero-caudad portion of the pelvic wall (from the most lateral portion of S2–S4, to the parietal pelvic fascia covering the obturator muscle and the piriformis).

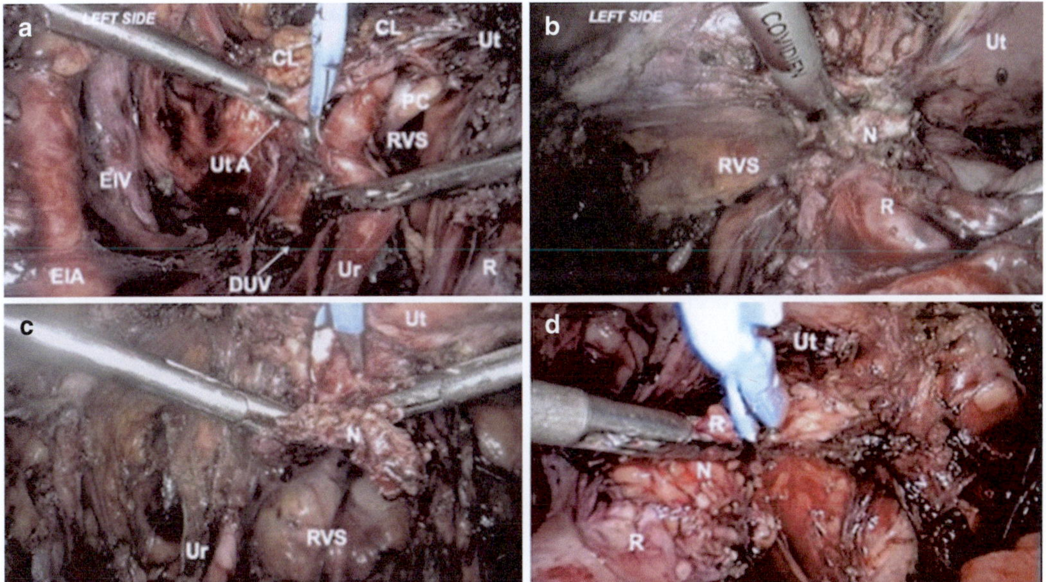

Fig. 12.4 Laparoscopic surgical steps of eradication of DIE of the postero-lateral compartments. (**a**) Laparoscopic view of left ureterolysis during left parametrectomy in course of eradication of DIE with parametrial infiltration. *EIV* external iliac vein, *EIA* external iliac artery, *Ut A* uterine artery, *DUV* deep uterine vein, *Ur* ureter, *R* rectum, *Ut* uterus, *RVS* rectovaginal septum, *CL* cardinal ligament, *PC* paracervix. (**b**) Laparoscopic view of the section of the retrocervical/rectal nodule after development of the rectovaginal septum. *N* DIE nodule, *R* rectum, *RVS* recto-vaginal septum, *Ut* uterus. (**c**) Laparoscopic view of the resection of the retrocervical nodule after complete detachment of the rectum and development of the recto-vaginal septum. *N* DIE nodule, *Ur* ureter, *RVS* rectovaginal septum, *Ut* uterus. (**d**) Laparoscopic view of the transection of the mesorectum in course of eradication of DIE with segmental bowel resection according to the so-called "classical technique". *R* rectum, *N* DIE nodule, *Ut* uterus

The parasympathetic innervation of the pelvic viscera, the rectosigmoid tract and the anal canal is given by the pelvic splanchnic nerves (PSNs) that rise up from the anterior branches of the sacral roots S2–S4, then pierce the PPF covering the pyriformis muscle (also called *fascia hypogastrica sacralis*) to join the orthosympathetic fibers of the HN, then traveling across the parametria.

12.3.4 The Rectovaginal Space (RVS)

In order to perform radical surgery on vaginal or rectal infiltrations brought by deep infiltrating endometriosis or gynecological malignancies, development of the rectovaginal septum is a keypoint. The anterolateral rectum is connected to the vagina by two longitudinal rows of fibrovascular tissue, the so-called rectal pillars, which form the posterior parametrium along with the uterosacral and rectovaginal ligaments (Fig. 12.4). Among these parallel structures is located the rectovaginal space, which is covered by a thickening of the visceral endopelvic fascia. The anterior layer of this fascia constitutes the rectovaginal septum (Denonvilliers fascia) which adheres more to the vagina than to the rectum. The back layer is the rectal fascia, which can be dissected and separated from the rectum, but a rectal lesion is more likely to occur while dissociating in this plane compared to a dissection in the true rectovaginal space. The rectovaginal space has a thin apex while it opens dorsally to the point where the adipose tissue is located, allowing at this level an easy dissection of the posterior vaginal wall from the middle third of the anterior rectum.

12.3.5 The Sigmoid Colon

It represents the distal portion of the descending colon and begins in the left iliac fossa, lateral to the common iliac vessels, ending at the level of the third sacral vertebra [10, 11, 14].

It is S-shaped, is intraperitoneal, has a completely variable mobility and length (usually around 40 cm), and is covered by numerous epiploic appendixes. The distal anatomical limit of the sigmoid is generally referred as the rectumsigmoid junction. The mesosigmoid completely surrounds the colon and does not directly attach dorsally to the pelvic wall. Thanks to this it is able to maintain a certain mobility and at this level the Toldt fascia (the abdominal equivalent of rectal visceral endopelvic fascia, here called fascia propria recti) is not present. The mesosigmoid contains the inferior mesenteric vessels, the inferior mesenteric plexus, the superior hypogastric plexus and other nervous and lymphatic structures. A fundamental surgical step in colorectal surgery is the opening of the "mesocolic" or "mesosigmoid" window, a virtual space developed between the inferior mesenteric artery and the sacral promontory, which allows the identification of the left ureter from the right side in a middle-lateral direction. This is a crucial step for achieving a proper skeletonization of the inferior mesenteric vessels and a proper lateralization of the ureter from them, avoiding ureteral injuries during the vascular transection before rectosigmoid transection.

The characteristics that indicate the anatomical passage between sigma and rectum are: (1) the end of the mesosigmoid, (2) the disappearance of the epiploic appendixes and of the haustra coli, (3) the coalescence of the tenia coli that forms a complete longitudinal muscular layer in the rectum, (4) a narrowing at the level of the rectum-sigmoid joint (functional valve), (5) the level of division of the superior rectal artery. The vasculature of the sigma is guaranteed by 2–4 arteries, the first of which are larger in size and originate from the left colic artery (30% of cases) or from the inferior mesenteric artery. The latter, once entered into the pelvis immediately after the sacral promontory, becomes the superior rectal artery (or superior hemorrhoidal), which is caudally anastomosed with the middle rectal artery, the terminal branch of the hypogastric artery.

12.3.6 The Rectum

The rectum is a continuation of the sigmoid colon, at the third sacral vertebra S3, and extends to the most cranial limit of the anal canal, the so-called "anorectal ring." It measures about 10–15 cm in length and is formed by an antero-posterior curve (sacral flexure), following the profile of the sacrum, and by the *levator ani* muscle. The rectum is wrapped in a layer of endopelvic fascia, the fascia propria recti, which continues with the endopelvic fascia covering the *levator ani*. It is divided into a cranial or pelvic rectum (peritoneal and subperitoneal) and a more caudad perineal portion, corresponding to the anal canal. The proximal third of the rectum is intraperitoneal in its anterolateral portion, where the peritoneum continues with tissue covering pararectal spaces. The anterior peritoneal reflection is located approximately 5–7 cm from the anal margin. The middle third of the rectum is covered by the peritoneum only in the anterior portion, where it continues with the peritoneum of the Douglas' pouch, while in the most caudad third it is completely retroperitoneal. At the level of the pelvic floor, at the middle third of the vagina, the rectum in its most caudad third forms at a 90° angle, in a dorsal direction to form the perineal flexure. Subsequently, it penetrates the pelvic diaphragm and continues caudally with the anus. The rectum in its perineal portion corresponds surgically to the anal canal, extending from the anorectal ring to the anal margin. It is surrounded by the *levator ani* muscle and the anal sphincter, and is fixed dorsally to the coccyx, by the anococcygeal ligament. The mesorectum contains lymphatic vessels, branches of division of rectal vessels, and nerves. It covers the subperitoneal rectum by surrounding approximately three-fourth of it, becoming thinner at the elevator muscle of the anus, caudally. The retroperitoneal space located between the peritoneum and the pelvic diaphragm separates the rectum from the lateral pelvic wall and the elevator muscle of the anus.

The middle rectal artery (with numerous anatomical variations) originates from internal iliac, as well as umbilical, inferior gluteal and lateral sacral artery, or as a branch of the pudendal artery. By a cadaveric specimen study on 30 subjects [21], it is present only in 56.7% of subjects and it is symmetric in 36.7% and monolateral in 20% of cases. It has a variable diameter, extending caudally and medially toward the lateral portion of the rectum, in close proximity to the lateral ligaments of the rectum (or rectal wings). It branches out in two directions, the first posterior feeds the medial portion of the rectum, anastomizing itself with the superior rectal artery; the anterior portion has a larger diameter and reaches the vagina through the more lateral portion of the rectovaginal septum.

12.3.7 The Ileocecal Region

The cecum, is a large tube-like structure considered the first region of the large intestine. It is separated from the ileum (the final portion of the small intestine) by the ileocecal valve (also called Bauhin valve), which is a muscular sphincter limiting the rate of food passage into the cecum and preventing material from returning to the small intestine.

Vascularization to the cecum comes from the upper mesenteric artery through the ileocolic artery, which gives origin to an ileal branch, a colic branch, and an appendicular branch.

The ileocecal sphincter also provides a mechanical barrier to bacterial migration into the small intestine. Loss of the ileocecal sphincter can lead to small-bowel bacterial overgrowth, a condition associated named small-bowel syndrome (SBS), associated with diarrhea and fat and vitamin (B12) malabsorption, both resulting from bile salt deconjugation, along with fluid loss, abdominal cramps, and liver injury [22, 23].

12.4 Laparoscopic Bowel Resection for Deep Infiltrating Endometriosis

In the presence of endometriotic nodules which infiltrate the intestinal wall (with involvement of the internal musculature and/or mucosa) in full thickness for more than 30 mm, in cases of symptomatic, tightened bowel stenosis, in the presence of multiple nodules the segmental resection represent the one of the safest to radically remove the disease [4–6, 24–28].

The "classical" technique has been employed since many years and still represents a surgical option offering satisfactory outcomes on pelvic pain and acceptable intra and perioperative safety. Its steps have been standardized by Redwine and colleagues [4, 5]. Monopolar scissors are employed to make incisions in normal peritoneum lateral and parallel to the involved uterosacral ligaments. The uterosacral ligaments are then bluntly undermined. A transverse incision is created across the posterior cervix above the point of adherence of the bowel, then intrafascial dissection down the posterior cervix toward the rectovaginal septum allows transection of the uterosacral ligaments. Thus, all nodular fibrotic disease to begin to fall away from the posterior cervix still attached to the bowel wall.

If the vaginal wall is involved by endometriosis, the rectovaginal septum is initially approached laparoscopically from the right or left side, avoiding the infiltrated area which lies in the midline, and so also avoiding the risk of an iatrogenic rectal lesion. Once the lateral aspects of the rectovaginal septum have been revealed, dissection follows down the posterior cervix until the rectovaginal septum is encountered, with the help of a vaginal vault. The normal rectovaginal septum is then developed distally, leading to visualize a normal bowel wall being present on all sides of the nodular mass. All the pathology is left on the anterior wall of the mobilized rectum, which is then treated with a segmental resection.

Redwine reported to perform a presacral neurectomy in some of the treated patients as a measure to possibly prevent pelvic pain relapse.

In the last years, also considering increasing number of women undergoing surgery due to a more precise diagnosis, the risk of postoperative visceral nerve dysfunction brought by classical resective technique was considered as an unaffordable burden for this technique.

## 12.5	The Nerve-Sparing Laparoscopic Bowel Resection for Deep Infiltrating Endometriosis: Surgical Steps

Following the good manners of radical oncological surgery, 'nerve-sparing' segmental intestinal resection techniques have been developed in recent years and are now standardized and recognized by the international scientific community [29] as the "Negrar Method."

The goal of the "nerve-sparing" approach is to identify and to spare visceral nerve fibers and surgical landmarks, thus reducing the risk of iatrogenic damage to the pelvic nervous system. This technique, performed in specialized centers, guarantees adequate surgical radicality, albeit with a significantly lower rate of postoperative bladder, rectum, and sexuality dysfunctions, significantly improving patients' quality of life [30–35].

The procedure was standardized in six steps [29, 30] (Figs. 12.5 and 12.6):

- **Step 0: adhesiolysis, ovarian surgery, removal of peritoneal endometriosis.**
- The surgical procedure begins with the evaluation of all the abdominal peritoneal surfaces and with the adhesiolysis. Adhesions may be the result of previous surgical operations or of the extension of the disease. Following is the mobilization of the ovaries and the removal of any ovarian endometriomas with the stripping technique. The ovaries are temporarily suspended on the abdominal wall making it easier to access to Douglas in order to obtain better exposure of the pelvic surgical field. The surgical approach to the obliterated rectovaginal septum is performed after the bilateral isolation of the ureters by retroperitoneal route and completed with the identification and removal of the uterosacral ligaments infiltrated by the disease. Ureteral course in endometriosis of the posterior compartment, is quite always stretched medially by the fibrotic retraction caused by the disease. Ureterolysis consist in freeing the ureter from the affected peritoneum,

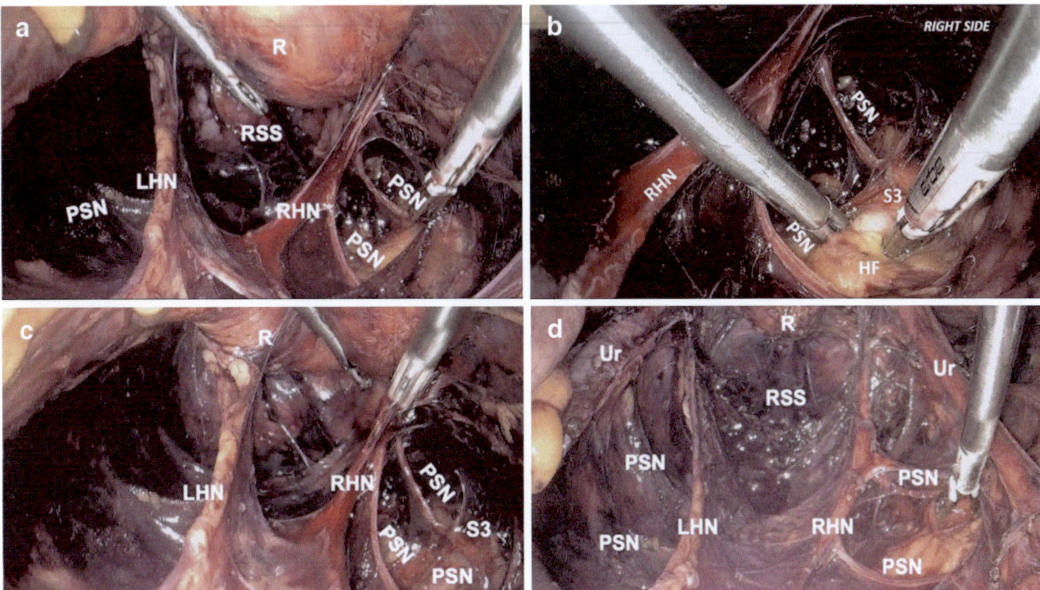

Fig. 12.5 Laparoscopic steps of nerve identification and sparing in course of nerve-sparing eradication of DIE according to the "Negrar Method." (**a**) Laparoscopic view of the dissection of the retrorectal space with identification and preservation of the hypogastric nerves and pelvic splanchnic nerves. *RSS* Waldeyer's rectosacral space, *R* rectum, *RHN* right hypogastric nerve, *LHN* left hypogastric nerve, *PSN* pelvic splanchnic nerves. (**b**) Laparoscopic view of the dissection of the right hypogastric area with decompression of the sacral roots (S3) and exposure of right pelvic splanchnic nerves. *RHN* right hypogastric nerve, *PSN* pelvic splanchnic nerves, *S3* third sacral root, *HF* hypogastric fascia. (**c**) Laparoscopic view of the dissection of the retrorectal space with decompression of the sacral roots (S3) and exposure of the hypogastric nerves and right pelvic splanchnic nerves. *RHN* right hypogastric nerve, *LHN* left hypogastric nerve, *PSN* pelvic splanchnic nerves, *S3* third sacral root, *R* rectum. (**d**) Laparoscopic view before rectal transection with exposure of the hypogastric nerves and pelvic splanchnic nerves. *RHN* right hypogastric nerve, *LHN* left hypogastric nerve, *PSN* pelvic splanchnic nerves, *RSS* rectosacral space, *R* rectum, *Ur* ureter

dissecting it along its course, without dissecting its mural layers.

- **Step I: development of the presacral space, development of retroperitoneal avascular spaces, identification and conservation of the pelvic sympathetic fibers of the inferior mesenteric plexus, superior hypogastric plexus and hypogastric nerves.**
- The inferior mesenteric plexus (IMP) is a network of sympathetic fibers, which follows the inferior mesenteric artery from its aortic origin to the sacral promontory, joining with the superior hypogastric plexus (SHP), which is a triangular-shaped network of sympathetic fibers located in the presacral space at the promontory level. Both plexuses are covered by a peritoneal leaflet and wrapped by the visceral pelvic fascia. The SHP gives rise to the right and left hypogastric nerves (HN), which branch off for about 8 cm along the lateral sides of the mesorectum, in the visceral pelvic fascia following the ureteral course in a dorsal and caudad direction.
- The identification of the SHP and HN fibers is obtained after the opening of Waldeyer's presacral space, following the incision of the peritoneum that covers the promontorium and dissecting the so-called *tela adiposa retrorectalis* up to the coccygeal bone, at the level of the presacral Waldeyer's fascia [16]. The nerves are then pushed caudally to the rectum and to the utero-sacral and rectovaginal ligaments allowing a safe "nerve-sparing" dissection.
- In order to obtain a more precise identification of the hypogastric nerves and the ureters and in order to completely mobilize the rectosig-

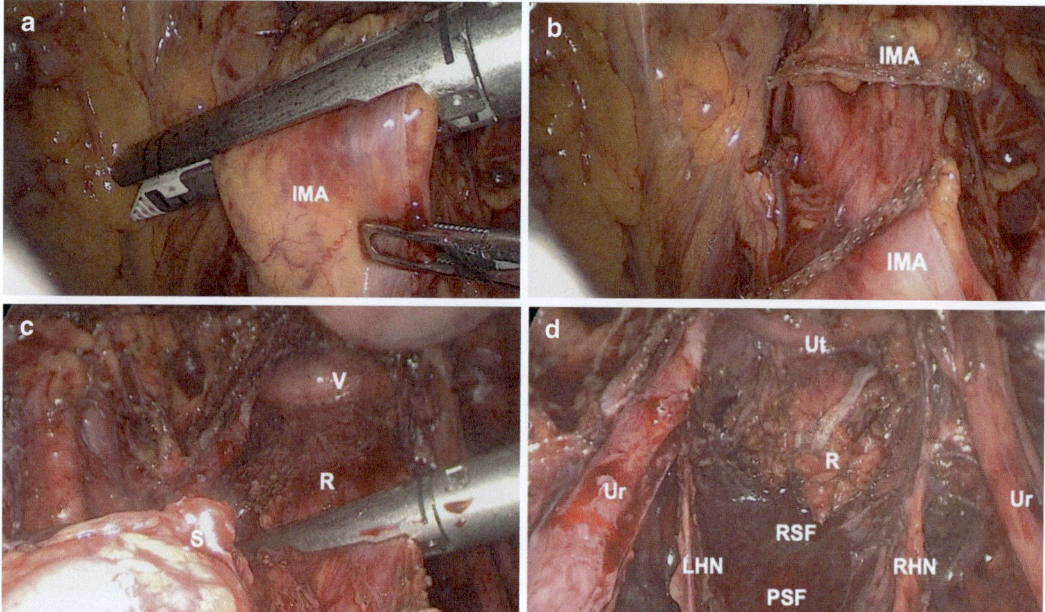

Fig. 12.6 Laparoscopic steps of rectal and mesorectal resection in course of nerve-sparing eradication of DIE according to the "Negrar Method." (**a**) Laparoscopic view of the transection of the inferior mesenteric artery with the 45-mm linear laparoscopic stapler (Endopath). *IMA* inferior mesenteric artery. (**b**) Laparoscopic view after the transection of the inferior mesenteric artery. *IMA* inferior mesenteric artery. (**c**) Laparoscopic view of the transec- tion of the rectum with the 60-mm linear stapler (Endo- GIA) in course of segmental bowel resection for DIE. *R* rectum, *V* posterior vaginal wall, *S* sigmoid. (**d**) Laparoscopic view of the retrorectal area after rectal tran- section with exposure of the hypogastric nerves. *RHN* right hypogastric nerve, *LHN* left hypogastric nerve, *PSN* pelvic splanchnic nerves, *RSF* rectosacral fascia, *PSF* pre- sacral fascia, *R* rectum, *Ur* ureter, *Ut* uterus

moid, a key step is represented by the develop- ment of the pararectal retroperitoneal spaces of Okabayashi and Latzko and the retro-rectal spaces of Heald [10–15]:

– Medial pararectal (Okabayashi space) has the ureter and the mesoureter as the lateral limit and the mesorectum and the rectum as the medial limit; allows a complete ureter- olysis, following of the hypogastric nerves pelvic course, identification of the pelvic splanchnic nerves and pelvic plexuses, medial communication with the retrorectal space of Heald.

– Lateral pararectal (Latzko space) whose lateral limit is the internal iliac artery and, as a medial limit, has the ureter and the mesoureter; allows a complete unroofing of the ureter toward the parametrial tunnel and separation of its course from the vascu- lar branches of the hypogastric artery (that in some cases of parametrectomy might require vascular resections).

– Retrorectal (or presacral of Waldeyer's) which has as a ventral limit the mesorec- tum and as the dorsal limit the sacrum; its dissection is completely avascular and can be achieved toward the coccygeal bone sur- face if the rectosacral fascia (anococcygeal raphe) is cut. Allows identification and sparing of the inferior mesenteric plexus, of the superior hypogastric plexus and both hypogastric nerves. Moreover, allows a complete mobilization of the rectum that will be resected.

• Once the dissection of these anatomical spaces is complete, the rectovaginal ligaments are resected where they are infiltrated by the disease.

• **Step II: dissection of the parametrial planes, isolation of the ureteral course, of**

the hypogastric nerves and of the inferior hypogastric plexus or pelvic plexus.

- In this phase the identification and isolation of the posterior parametria (uterosacral ligaments, rectovaginal ligaments and lateral ligaments of the rectum) and of the lateral parametria (cardinal ligament, paracervix) are of the keystone. This procedure is followed by ureteral isolation up to the parametrial tunnel and up to the intersection with the uterine artery with subsequent identification of the hypogastric nerves and the inferior hypogastric plexus.

- **Step III: posterior parametrectomy, identification of the deep uterine vein, sparing of the pelvic splanchnic nerves and of the cranial and medial portion of the inferior hypogastric plexus.**

- The pelvic viscera (rectosigmoid, anal canal) receive innervation from the parasympathetic fibers of the pelvic splanchnic nerves emerging from the sacral roots S2–S4. These parasympathetic fibers, after piercing the PPF covering the sacral roots, join the orthosympathetic component (hypogastric nerves) forming the inferior hypogastric plexus or pelvic plexus (PP). In order to preserve a woman's rectal, bladder, and sexual functions, nerve-sparing surgery aims to save these nerve fibers by using precise anatomical references. In this consciousness, the deep uterine vein represents the anatomical-surgical landmark that distinguishes the parametrial vascular portion (*pars vasculosa*, ventral and cranial) from the parametrial nerve portion (*pars nervosa*, dorsal and caudad). This step is completed with the posterior and lateral parametrectomy where necessary, and the complete lateralization of the nerve bundles.

- **Step IV: development of the rectovaginal septum and sparing of the caudad portion of the inferior hypogastric plexus.**

- This surgical phase is characterized by the complete development of the rectovaginal septum following a line of incision that is directed in a lateromedial fashion. The dissection goes on medially to the uterosacral ligament and laterally to the mesorectum and continues dorsally to the uterine cervix and ventrally with respect to the anterior wall of the rectum. With this surgical procedure, it is possible to medialize and isolate the endometriotic nodule of the rectovaginal septum and/or the rectal nodule. In the event of infiltration of the vaginal wall, a portion of the same is resected and the vaginal margins sutured by laparoscopy or vaginally.

- **Step V: saving the caudad portion of the inferior hypogastric plexus in the paravaginal spaces.**

- The pelvic plexus crosses the posterior part of the vesicouterine ligament, laterally and caudally with respect to the ureter before it enters the bladder. To perform a "nerve-sparing" surgery it is required a partial or complete opening of the tunnel of the ureter otherwise called "Morrow space" (medially and ventrally to the ureter) as to separate the medial vascular portion of the vesicouterine ligament from its lateral portion in which nerves run. In the presence of an involvement of the anterior parametrium (vesicouterine ligament) a complete unroofing of the ureter to the bladder and the development of the so-called fourth space of Yabuki [10] may be necessary. This is obtained by connecting the medial pararectal space with the lateral paravesical space, thus obtaining the necessary radicality along the paravaginal portions of the paracervix.

- **Step VI: rectal resection and colon-rectal anastomosis.**

- This last phase is characterized by the initial mobilization of the involved bowel tract using a bipolar, ultrasound or combined energy device. In respect of the vascularization of the residual colon, the inferior mesenteric vessels can be isolated and resected in their sigmoid branches using a 45 mm mechanical laparoscopic stapler; this procedure is mainly carried out to obtain a termino-terminal tension-free anastomosis according to the Knight-Griffen technique. The healthy distal part of the intestinal wall is isolated from the surrounding mesorectum in order to expose the serosa at the point where the mechanical stapler must be positioned. A linear laparo-

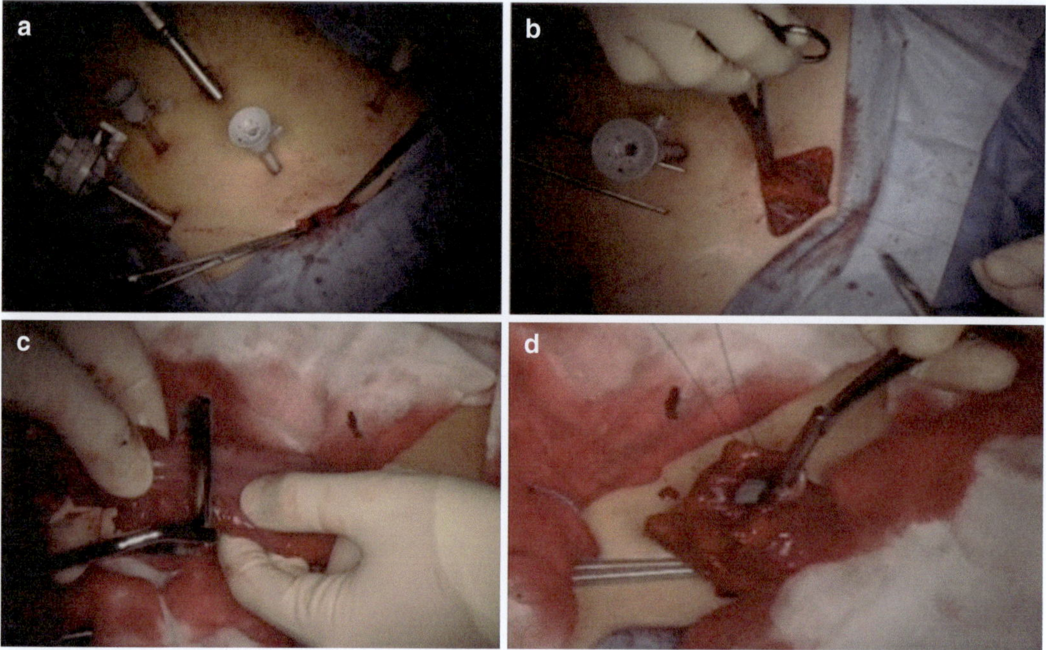

Fig. 12.7 Surgical steps of the extracorporeal proximal bowel transection and closure. (**a**) Abdominal view of the trocars position and of the suprapubic transverse mini-laparotomy. (**b**) Abdominal view of the suprapubic transverse mini-laparotomy for the extraction of the rectosigmoid after distal transection. (**c**) Abdominal view of the proximal transection of the rectosigmoid. (**d**) Abdominal view of the closure of the proximal sigmoid segment with a purse-string suture after insertion of the anvil of the circular endoscopic stapler

scopic stapler is positioned on the distal margin of the resection (1–2 cm distal to the nodule) and is angled to maximize the exposure margin and optimize the ergonomics of the transection (Figs. 12.7, 12.8, and 12.9).

- The affected intestinal segment is exteriorized through an ultralow midline incision in the pubic symphysis (approximately 4 cm in length), or through the vagina, if resection of the infiltrated posterior fornix has been performed. The proximal margin of resection is considered as safe at 1–2 cm from the endometriotic nodule. After the removal of the specimen, the head of a circular endoscopic stapler is fixed with a suture at the distal end of the resected intestine. Finally, this tract is brought back into the abdominal cavity. The abdominal wall is closed (both peritoneal and fascial layers) in order to regain a valid pneumoperitoneum. A 29 or 31 mm end-to-end circular stapler is inserted transanally and, under direct laparoscopic vision, is connected to the previously positioned stapler head. A termino-terminal colorectal anastomosis is then completed, according to the Knight-Griffen technique. The integrity of the anastomosis is checked by rectoscopic evaluation and a hydropneumatic test (see above). If there is a poor resistance to the test (leakage) or if the intestinal resection is very low (4–6 cm from the anal margin according to the studies) or in the presence of a further vaginal, ureteral and/or bladder suture a protective ileostomy or temporary colostomy should be considered. In these cases the recanalization occurs after about 40–60 days from segmental resection after evaluation of the integrity of the suture by double contrast barium enema, or in some cases with a rectoscopy.

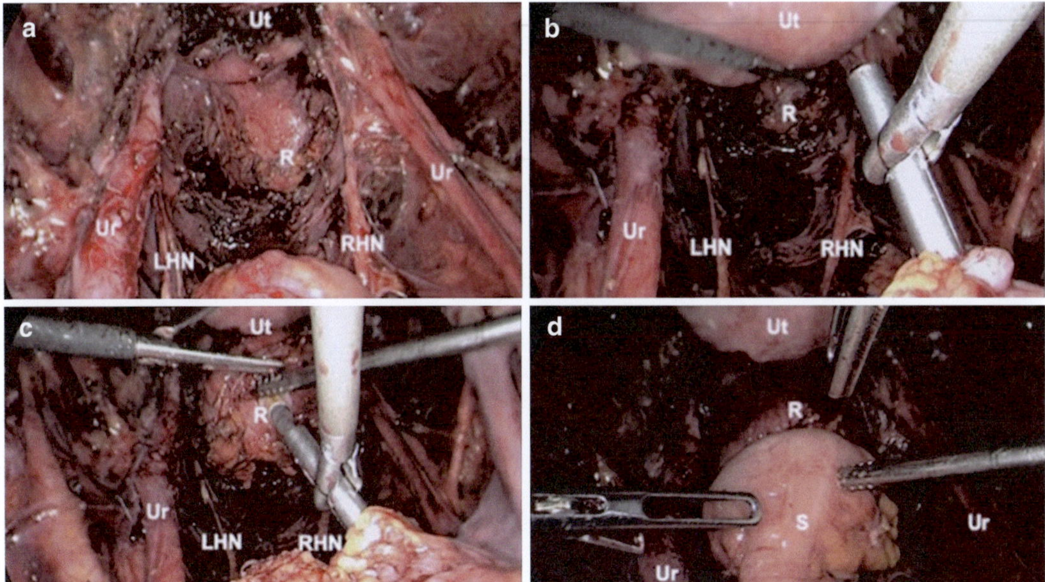

Fig. 12.8 Laparoscopic surgical steps of rectal anastomosis in course of nerve-sparing eradication of DIE according to the "Negrar Method." (**a**) Laparoscopic view of the surgical field after rectal transection with exposure of the hypogastric nerves. *RHN* right hypogastric nerve, *LHN* left hypogastric nerve, *R* rectal stump, *Ur* ureter, *Ut* uterus. (**b**) Laparoscopic view of the initial phase of Knight-Griffen's end-to-end rectosigmoid anastomosis with trans-anal introduction of the laparoscopic circular stapler. *RHN* right hypogastric nerve, *LHN* left hypogastric nerve, *R* rectal stump, *Ur* ureter, *Ut* uterus. (**c**) Laparoscopic view of the Knight-Griffen's end-to-end rectosigmoid anastomosis with connection of the anvil of the circular stapler. *RHN* right hypogastric nerve, *LHN* left hypogastric nerve, *R* rectal stump, *Ur* ureter, *Ut* uterus. (**d**) Laparoscopic view of the final phase of the Knight-Griffen's end-to-end rectosigmoid anastomosis, after closure of the circular stapler. *R* rectal stump, *S* sigmoid, *Ur* ureter, *Ut* uterus

12.6 Ileocecal Resection

In our case-series of over 2500 bowel resections for deep infiltrating endometriosis, we report a 8% of associated ileocecal endometriosis [7].

Inversely, if only the total number of ileocecal endometriosis is considered, 80% of those patients were also bearing rectosigmoid endometriosis.

Resective procedure is considered after evaluating the risk of ileocecal valve mutilation and subsequent small-bowel syndrome, so it has to be guided by severe preoperative symptoms complaint or risk of occlusion.

This procedure might be performed all by laparoscopy or employing an accessory mini-laparotomy [8]. After visualization of the infiltrated area (often a pelvic right sidewall nodule extending caudally to the right adnexa and parametrium and cranially to the ileocecal region), mobilization of the cecum and right colon is performed using a combined energy device (Thunderbit, Olympus, Tokyo, Japan or Ultracision harmonic scalpel LCS 10; Ethicon Endosurgery, Cincinnati, OH, USA). This allows de-rotation of the right bowel from pelvic sidewall according to which in laparotomy is known as the "Kocher" maneuver. Ileocolic vessels are isolated, clipped, and divided. The segment affected is isolated and resected and then a side-to-side or end-to-side ileocecal anastomosis is performed by laparoscopy or open. To exteriorize the bowel, a mini-laparotomy in the right iliac region or suprapubic incision is performed. Mechanical anastomosis is realized with Covidien Circular Stapler with DST Series Technology (25 mm). When only the ileum is involved an extracorporeal ileal resection with end-to-end manual anastomosis is performed with simple extra mucosal interrupted suture (Fig. 12.10).

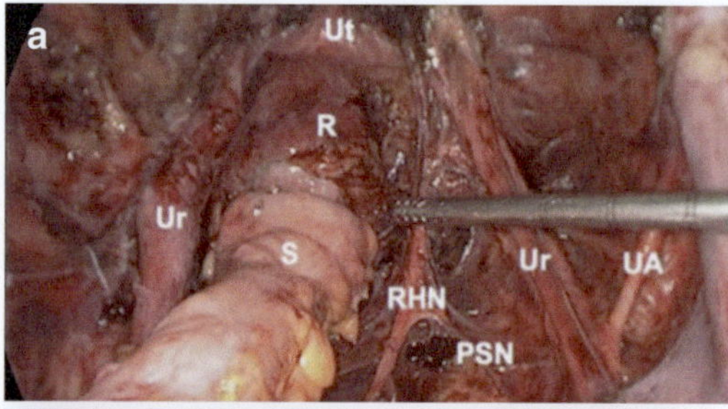

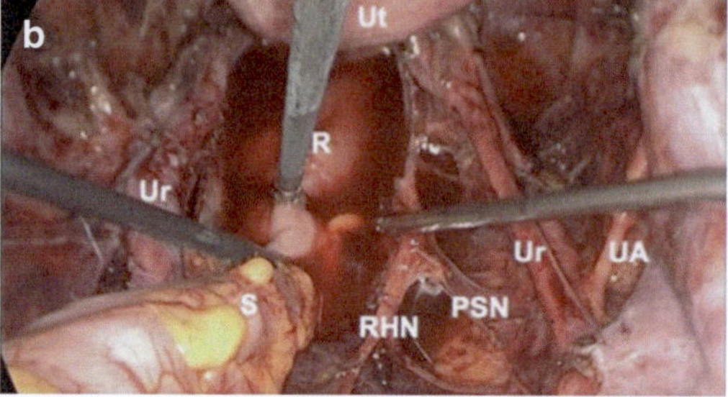

Fig. 12.9 Final view after a nerve-sparing laparoscopic eradication of DIE with rectal and parametrial resection according to the "Negrar Method". (**a**) Laparoscopic view of the surgical field after Knight-Griffen's end-to-end rectosigmoid anatomosis. *PSN* pelvic splanchnic nerves, *RHN* right hypogastric nerve, *R* rectal stump, *S* sigmoid, *Ur* ureter, *Ut* uterus, *UA* umbilical artery. (**b**) Laparoscopic view of the surgical field after Knight-Griffen's end-to-end rectosigmoid anatomosis in course of pneumatic rectal integrity test. *PSN* pelvic splanchnic nerves, *RHN* right hypogastric nerve, *R* rectal stump, *S* sigmoid, *Ur* ureter, *Ut* uterus, *UA* umbilical artery

12.7 Appendectomy and Typhlectomy

In all case of gross abnormalities of the cecal appendix, such as enlargement, dilation, tortuosity, or discoloration, or presence of suspected endometriotic implants appendectomy is performed, isolated, or associated with ileocecal resection. In case of isolated appendectomy after the cecum and appendix were mobilized, the mesoappendix was secured and cut, and the appendicular artery is isolated, coagulated, and transected. Three endoloops are introduced through the right lower quadrant trocar and applied to the junction where the appendix extends into the cecum. Two ligatures are located at the base of the appendix 2 mm apart. The final ligature is placed approximately 7 mm above the

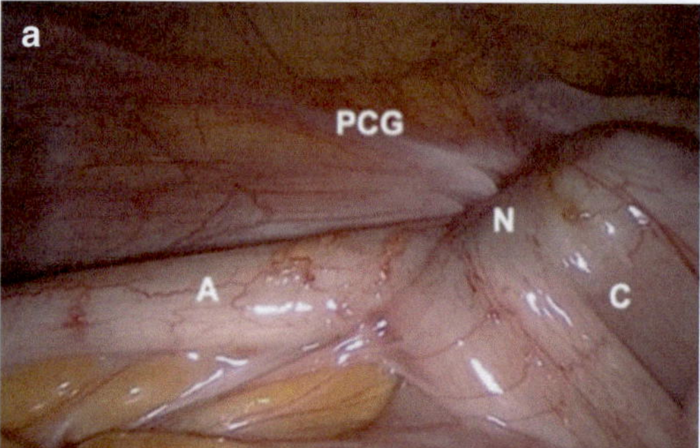

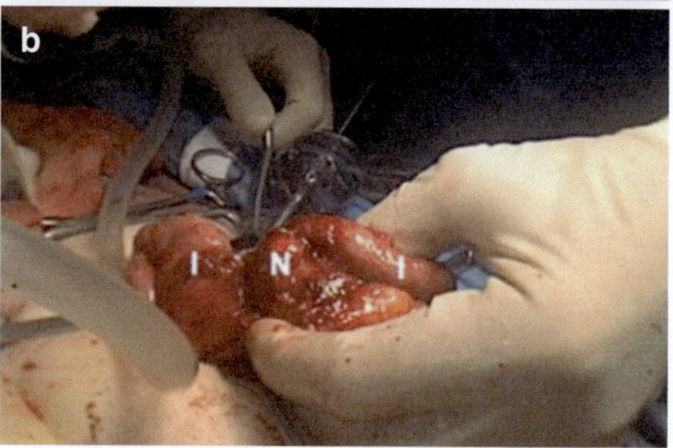

Fig. 12.10 Surgical steps of management of ileocecal endometriosis. (**a**) Laparoscopic view of DIE infiltrating the appendix and cecum. *A* appendix, *C* cecum, *N* DIE nodule, *PCG* paracolic gutter. (**b**) Abdominal view of DIE infiltrating the ileum. *I* ileum, *N* DIE nodule

last ligature, and then the area between the second and third ligature is coagulated and cut. If also the cecal fundus seems to be affected by endometriosic infiltration, en-bloc removal is performed with a linear laparoscopic stapler (Endo-GIA) (Autosuture Co., Norwalk CT, USA) placed across the distal margin of the resection (1–2 cm distal to the nodule), angled to maximize the exposure and resection margin, closed and activated for transection.

12.8 Conclusions

The standardization of the segmental resection technique and the use of minimally invasive and nerve-sparing techniques have made it possible to reduce the incidence of neurological dysfunctions by up to 5–6% and to improve the impact on the quality of life of the patient candidate for this kind of surgery [29–35].

This advanced radical surgery should therefore only be performed in reference centers and by gynecologists and colorectal surgeons experienced in pelvic neuroanatomy, nerve-sparing techniques, and oncological radical procedures [36–47].

References

1. Cotlar AM. Historical landmarks in operations on the colon—surgeons courageous. Curr Surg. 2002;59(1):91–5.
2. Jacobs M, Verdeja JC, Goldstein HS. Minimally invasive colon resection (laparoscopic colectomy). Surg Laparosc Endosc. 1991;1:144–50.
3. Fowler DL, White SA. Laparoscopy-assisted sigmoid resection. Surg Laparosc Endosc. 1991;1:183–8.
4. Redwine DB, Koning M, Sharpe DR. Laparoscopically assisted transvaginal segmental resection of the rectosigmoid colon for endometriosis. Fertil Steril. 1996;65(1):193–7.
5. Redwine DB, Sharpe DR. Laparoscopic segmental resection of the sigmoid colon for endometriosis. J Laparoendosc Surg. 1991;1(4):217–20.
6. Sharpe DR, Redwine DB. Laparoscopic segmental resection of the sigmoid and rectosigmoid colon for endometriosis. Surg Laparosc Endosc. 1992;2(2):120–4.
7. Scioscia M, Bruni F, Ceccaroni M, Steinkasserer M, Stepniewska A, Minelli L. Distribution of endometriotic lesions in endometriosis stage IV supports the menstrual reflux theory and requires specific preoperative assessment and therapy. Acta Obstet Gynecol Scand. 2011;90(2):136–9. https://doi.org/10.1111/j.1600-0412.2010.01008.x. Epub 2010 Dec 2.
8. Ruffo G, Stepniewska A, Crippa S, Serboli G, Zardini C, Steinkasserer M, Ceccaroni M, Minelli L, Falconi M. Laparoscopic ileocecal resection for bowel endometriosis. Surg Endosc. 2011;25(4):1257–62.
9. Toldt C. Anatomischer Atlas für Studierende und Ärzte. Berlin: Urban & Schwarzenberg; 1919.
10. Yabuki Y, Asamoto A, Hoshiba T, et al. Radical hysterectomy: an anatomic evaluation of parametrial dissection. Gynecol Oncol. 2000;77:155–63.
11. Kamina P. Anatomie Clinique. Paris: Maloine; 2009.
12. Ceccaroni M, Fanfani F, Ercoli A, Scambia G. Innervazione viscerale e somatica della pelvi femminile. Testo-Atlante di anatomia chirurgica. Rome: CIC editions; 2006.
13. Ercoli A, Delmas V, Fanfani F, Gadonneix P, Ceccaroni M, Fagotti A, Mancuso S, Scambia G. Terminologia Anatomica versus unofficial descriptions and nomenclature of the fasciae and ligaments of the female pelvis: a dissection-based comparative study. Am J Obstet Gynecol. 2005;193(4):1565–73.
14. Einarsson JI, Wattiez A. Minimally invasive gynecologic surgery: evidence-based laparoscopic, hysteroscopic and robotic surgeries. London: Jp Medical Pub; 2016.
15. Heald RJ. The 'Holy Plane' of rectal surgery. J R Soc Med. 1988;81(9):503–8.
16. Waldeyer W. Das Becken. Bonn: Cohen; 1899.
17. Havenga K, DeRuiter MC, Enker WE, Welvaart K. Anatomical basis of autonomic nerve-preserving total mesorectal excision for rectal cancer. Br J Surg. 1996;83(3):384–8.
18. Crapp AR, Cuthbertson AM. William Waldeyer and the rectosacral fascia. Surg Gynecol Obstet. 1974;138(2):252–6.
19. Sato K, Sato T. The vascular and neuronal composition of the lateral ligament of the rectum and the rectosacral fascia. Surg Radiol Anat. 1991;13(1):17–22.
20. Ceccaroni M, Clarizia R, Roviglione G, Ruffo G. Neuro-anatomy of the posterior parametrium and surgical considerations for a nerve-sparing approach in radical pelvic surgery. Surg Endosc. 2013;27(11):4386–94. https://doi.org/10.1007/s00464-013-3043-z. Epub 2013 Jun 20.
21. DiDio LJ, Diaz-Franco C, Schemainda R, Bezerra AJ. Morphology of the middle rectal arteries. A study of 30 cadaveric dissections. Surg Radiol Anat. 1986;8(4):229–36.
22. Goulet OJ, Revillon Y, Jan D, et al. Neonatal short bowel syndrome. J Pediatr. 1991;119:18–23.
23. Lichtman SN, Sartor RB, Keku J, Schwab JH. Hepatic inflammation in rats with experimental small intestinal bacterial overgrowth. Gastroenterology. 1990;98(2):414–23.
24. Abrão MS, Petraglia F, Falcone T, Keckstein J, Osuga Y, Chapron C. Deep endometriosis infiltrating the recto-sigmoid: critical factors to consider before management. Hum Reprod Update. 2015;21(3):329–39. https://doi.org/10.1093/humupd/dmv003. Epub 2015 Jan 24. Review.
25. Minelli L, Fanfani F, Fagotti A, Ruffo G, Ceccaroni M, Mereu L, Landi S, Pomini P, Scambia G. Laparoscopic colorectal resection for bowel endometriosis: feasibility, complications, and clinical outcome. Arch Surg. 2009;144(3):234–9; discussion 239.
26. Vercellini P, Frattaruolo MP, Rosati R, Dridi D, Roberto A, Mosconi P, De Giorgi O, Cribiù FM, Somigliana E. Medical treatment or surgery for colorectal endometriosis? Results of a shared decision-making approach. Hum Reprod. 2018;33(2):202–11. https://doi.org/10.1093/humrep/dex364.
27. Vercellini P, Buggio L, Somigliana E. Role of medical therapy in the management of deep rectovaginal endometriosis. Fertil Steril. 2017;108(6):913–30. https://doi.org/10.1016/j.fertnstert.2017.08.038. Review.
28. Vercellini P, Giudice LC, Evers JL, Abrao MS. Reducing low-value care in endometriosis between limited evidence and unresolved issues: a proposal. Hum Reprod. 2015;30(9):1996–2004.
29. Ceccaroni M, Clarizia R, Bruni F, D'Urso E, Gagliardi ML, Roviglione G, Minelli L, Ruffo G. Nerve-sparing

laparoscopic eradication of deep endometriosis with segmental rectal and parametrial resection: the Negrar method. A single-center, prospective, clinical trial. Surg Endosc. 2012;26(7):2029–45. https://doi.org/10.1007/s00464-012-2153-3. Epub 2012 Jan 26.

30. Ceccaroni M, Clarizia R, Tebache L. Role and technique of nerve-sparing surgery in deep endometriosis. J Endometr Pelvic Pain Disord. 2016;8(4):141–51.

31. Ceccaroni M, Fanfani F, Ercoli A et al. Nerve-sparing radical hysterectomy: an anatomical evaluation of middle rectal artery and deep uterine vein as surgical landmarks during parametrial dissection. Proceedings of the International Symposium on Radical Hysterectomy, dedicated to Hidekazu Okabayashi, Kyoto, 2007; p 12, 155.

32. Ceccaroni M, Fanfani F, Ercoli A et al. Anatomo-surgical principles and feasibility for a true Type III laparoscopic nerve-sparing Radical Hysterectomy. Proceedings of the International Symposium on Radical Hysterectomy, dedicated to Hidekazu Okabayashi, Kyoto; 2007. p 89.

33. Ceccaroni M, Pontrelli G, Scioscia M, et al. Nerve-sparing laparoscopic radical excision of deep endometriosis with rectal and parametrial resection. J Minim Invasive Gynecol. 2010;17(1):14–5.

34. Ceccaroni M, Clarizia R, Roviglione G. Nerve-sparing surgery for deep infiltrating endometriosis: laparoscopic eradication of deep infiltrating endometriosis with rectal and parametrial resection according to the negrar. Method Minim Invasive Gynecol. 2020;27(2):263–4. https://doi.org/10.1016/j.jmig.2019.09.002. Epub 2019 Sep 10.

35. Landi S, Ceccaroni M, Perutelli A, et al. Laparoscopic nerve-sparing complete excision of deep endometriosis: is it feasible? Hum Reprod. 2006;21:774–81.

36. Ford J, English J, Miles WA, Giannopoulos T. Pain, quality of life and complications following the radical resection of rectovaginal endometriosis. BJOG. 2004;111(4):353–6.

37. Pereira RM, Zanatta A, Serafini PC, Redwine D. The feasibility of laparoscopic bowel resection performed by a gynaecologist to treat endometriosis. Curr Opin Obstet Gynecol. 2010;22(4):344–53. https://doi.org/10.1097/GCO.0b013e32833beae0. Review.

38. Remorgida V, Ferrero S, Fulcheri E, Ragni N, Martin DC. Bowel endometriosis: presentation, diagnosis, and treatment. Obstet Gynecol Surv. 2007;62(7):461–70. Review.

39. Remorgida V, Ragni N, Ferrero S, Anserini P, Torelli P, Fulcheri E. How complete is full thickness disc resection of bowel endometriotic lesions? A prospective surgical and histological study. Hum Reprod. 2005;20(8):2317–20. Epub 2005 May 5.

40. Minelli L, Fanfani F, Fagotti A, et al. Laparoscopic colorectal resection for bowel endometriosis: feasibility, complications, and clinical outcome. Arch Surg. 2009;144(3):234–9; discussion 239.

41. De Cicco C, Corona R, Schonman R, Mailova K, Ussia A, Koninckx P. Bowel resection for deep endometriosis: a systematic review. BJOG. 2011;118(3):285–91.

42. Ruffo G, Scopelliti F, Scioscia M, Ceccaroni M, Mainardi P, Minelli L. Laparoscopic colorectal resection for deep infiltrating endometriosis: analysis of 436 cases. Surg Endosc. 2010;24(1):63–7.

43. Dubernard G, Piketty M, Rouzier R, Houry S, Bazot M, Darai E. Quality of life after laparoscopic colorectal resection for endometriosis. Hum Reprod. 2006;21(5):1243–7.

44. Bassi MA, Podgaec S, Dias JA Jr, D'Amico Filho N, Petta CA, Abrao MS. Quality of life after segmental resection of the rectosigmoid by laparoscopy in patients with deep infiltrating endometriosis with bowel involvement. J Minim Invasive Gynecol. 2011;18(6):730–3.

45. Mangler M, Herbstleb J, Mechsner S, Bartley J, Schneider A, Köhler C. Long-term follow-up and recurrence rate after mesorectum-sparing bowel resection among women with rectovaginal endometriosis. Int J Gynaecol Obstet. 2014;125(3):266–9.

46. Abrão MS, Borrelli GM, Clarizia R, Kho RM, Ceccaroni M. Strategies for management of colorectal endometriosis. Semin Reprod Med. 2017;35(1):65–71. https://doi.org/10.1055/s-0036-1597307.

47. Roman H, Bubenheim M, Huet E, Bridoux V, Zacharopoulou C, Daraï E, Collinet P, Tuech JJ. Conservative surgery versus colorectal resection in deep endometriosis infiltrating the rectum: a randomized trial. Hum Reprod. 2018;33(1):47–57. https://doi.org/10.1093/humrep/dex336.

Simone Ferrero, Fabio Barra, Emad Mikhail, and Stefano Tamburro

13.1 Introduction

Standard laparoscopy (SL) is commonly used to treat endometriosis-related pain symptoms when conservative therapy fails [1]. In fact, when compared with laparotomy, SL is associated with less postoperative pain, decreased requirement for analgesics, a shorter hospital stay, and earlier return to normal activity [2]. Furthermore, when surgery for colorectal endometriosis is necessary, the SL has been demonstrated to increase the chances of spontaneous conception and successful pregnancy if compared to laparotomy [3]. However, SL has several intrinsic technical limitations such as ergonomic limitations, reduced degrees of freedom, and an unstable camera platform that is totally dependent on the assistant surgeon. Moreover, in pelvic endometriosis the operating field is rather narrow. Robotic-assisted laparoscopy (RAL) is an implementation of SL and it may overcome some limitations of the SL [4].

13.2 Robotic-Assisted Treatment of Deep Endometriosis: Non comparative Studies

In the last ten years several retrospective studies investigated the feasibility and safety of RAL in the treatment of deep infiltrating endometriosis (DIE). A case report published in 2006 described for the first time a case of DIE of the bladder (4 cm) that was treated by partial cystectomy using a combined transurethral and RAL [5]. Subsequently, another case report published in 2008 confirmed the feasibility of RAL partial bladder resection for endometriosis [6]. Four trocars were used; one with a 12 mm umbilical port for the robotic camera, two lateral 8 mm ports were placed for the right and left arm of the robot, and a 10 mm trocar to assist the surgeon. The surgical time was 297 min and the intraoperative blood loss was approximately 100 mL. In 2011, Nezhat et al. reported a case series of five patients with bowel, bladder, and ureteral endometriosis treated by RAL [7]. All the patients had favorable outcomes, thus suggesting that RAL is feasible and safe in the treatment of DIE. An American

S. Ferrero (✉) · F. Barra
Academic Unit of Obstetrics and Gynecology, IRCCS Ospedale Policlinico San Martino, Genova, Italy

Department of Neurosciences, Rehabilitation, Ophthalmology, Genetics, Maternal and Child Health (DiNOGMI), University of Genova, Genova, Italy
e-mail: fabio.barra@icloud.com

E. Mikhail
Department of Obstetrics and Gynecology, Morsani College of Medicine, University of South Florida, Tampa, FL, USA
e-mail: emikhail@usf.edu

S. Tamburro
Grosseto Hospital, Grosseto, Italy

© Springer Nature Switzerland AG 2020
S. Ferrero, M. Ceccaroni (eds.), *Clinical Management of Bowel Endometriosis*,
https://doi.org/10.1007/978-3-030-50446-5_13

retrospective study analyzed the perioperative outcomes of 80 patients with rASRM stage IV endometriosis who underwent RAL [8]. Twenty-three (28.9%) patients had previous surgery for endometriosis. Sixty-seven patients (84%) underwent hysterectomy (with bilateral salpingo-oophorectomy or completion of bilateral salpingo-oophorectomy). Ureterolysis was performed in 29 (36.3%) patients. No patient had bowel surgery (discoid resection or segmental resection). The mean (± SD) operative time was 115 (±46) min. The mean estimated blood loss was 88 (±67) ml and no patient required transfusion. The mean length of hospital stay was 1.0 (±0.37) days. Four conversion to laparotomy occurred during the first 15 cases and none thereafter. There were four (5%) perioperative complications: one ureteral transection (repaired by laparotomic uretero-neocystostomy), a vaginal cuff abscess requiring drainage under anesthesia, a vaginal cuff hematoma that did not require surgical treatment, and one patient readmitted on postoperative day 2 because of nausea and vomiting secondary to narcotic use. Seventy-nine (98.8%) patients were pain-free at 2-month follow-up. Only one patient had second surgery after hysterectomy and bilateral salpingo-oophorectomy because of dyspareunia, she underwent resection of the vaginal cuff and uterosacral ligament. However, the major limitation of the study was the lack of long-term follow-up for recurrence of pain and endometriosis. Another American retrospective study examined the safety and feasibility of RAL hysterectomy and unilateral or bilateral oophorectomy in 43 patients with histologically confirmed ASRM stage III and IV endometriosis [9]. Patients who underwent conservative treatment of endometriosis with uterine preservation were excluded from the study. The median total operative time was 190 min (range, 97–368 min); while the median actual operative time was 145 min (range, 67–325 min). There was one conversion to laparotomy because of the presence of multiple fibroids; another patient required vaginal assistance to complete the hysterectomy. Ninety-five of the patients were discharged on the day after surgery. There were two postoperative complications: one postoperative ileus and one vaginal cuff abscess. A multicentric international retrospective study investigated the use of RAL in the treatment of DIE [10]. The study included only patients with stage IV endometriosis; patients who underwent simultaneous hysterectomy were also included in the study. Patients were treated by RAL depending on the choice of the surgeon and the availability of the robot. One hundred and sixty-four patients were included in the study. Thirty-three of the patients had undergone previous surgery (29.8% had history of ovarian surgery for endometriosis). The number of robotic arms were varied depending on the operator and type of surgery, with most cases managed using three robotic arms. The robot was side-docked on the left side in 78.5% of the patients. The mean (±SD) operative time was 180 (±77.2) min; the time with the console was 137.6 (±80.6) min. Eighty-eight patients requiring rectal surgery, there was a conversion to laparotomy in a patient undergoing segmental rectal resection. There were two rectal injuries during rectal shaving: one was sutured and the other required segmental rectal resection without need for a stoma. The median blood loss in patients undergoing rectal surgery was 127.5 ml (range, 5–2300 ml); one patient required blood transfusion. In patients undergoing bladder surgery ($n = 23$), there were two complications: one vesicovaginal hematoma after a partial cystectomy and one case of prolonged (6-month) intermitted self-catheterization after surgery. In patients undergoing surgery on the ureter and uterosacral ligaments ($n = 115$), there were two ureteral fistulae. One fistula occurred after rectal shaving and ureterolysis. The other fistula occurred after partial cystectomy and ureterovesical reimplantation; in this patient, a wound dehiscence required a second ureterovesical reimplantation. Twenty-eight patients underwent hysterectomy; there was no major complication. The overall reoperation was rate was 1.8% ($n = 3$); the surgeries involved drainage of an abscess wall, two ureterovesical reimplantations, and a ureteric fistula. The mean (±SD) follow-up period was 10.2 (±8.5) months. 86.7% of the patients had complete recovery, 12.3% had persistent postoperative pain, 3.5% had postoperative urinary symptoms, and 5.3% had postoperative gastrointestinal symptoms.

28.2% of the patients desiring pregnancy conceived after surgery. Based on these results, the authors concluded that RAL seems to have a place in the surgical treatment of stage IV endometriosis. A case series study including 35 patients assessed the feasibility of RAL for the treatment of DIE [11]. There was no conversion to open surgery or to laparoscopy. Rectal shaving was performed in 25 patients (71.43%), colorectal anastomosis in four patients (11.43%) and disc excision in three patients (8.57%). Eleven patients had hysterectomy. Three patients had partial cystectomy for bladder nodules with diameter >3 cm. Two patients required resection of the ureter followed by reimplantation into the bladder. There was one major complication: a large fistula of the ureter probably caused by thermal injury; it was managed by open surgery with resection of the ureter and reimplantation. At 1-year follow-up there was no recurrence of endometriosis; there was a significant improvement in pain symptoms, intestinal complains and quality of life. Recently, Giannini et al. retrospectively reported a case series of patients with DIE involving the ureter [12]. Thirty-one patients were included in the study. Mean operating time was 184.8 ± 81 min (range 70–330 min) and estimated blood loss 207 ± 142 ml (range 35–430 ml). None of the patients required an intraoperative blood transfusion. In 28 cases (90.3%) surgeons preferred three robotic arms whereas in three (9.7%) cases the fourth arm was used. Ureterolysis was successfully completed in all the patients and the resection of the endometriotic nodule was considered to be complete. Five patients (16%) reported immediate intraoperative or postoperative complications; four out of five involved the urinary tract.

13.3   Robotic-Assisted Versus Standard Laparoscopy in the Treatment of Deep Endometriosis

Several studies compared RAL and SL in the treatment of DIE. A retrospective cohort study based on a prospectively collected database compared the perioperative outcomes of patients undergoing RAL versus SL for ASRM stage III or IV endometriosis [13]. All the procedures were performed by an experienced surgeon. The surgeon decided the route of each procedure based on obesity, expected complexity of disease, previous and planned surgical procedures, and availability of the robotic platform. The study included 118 patients, 32 treated by RAL. Patients treated by RAL had significantly higher body mass index (BMI) than those treated by SL (27.36 kg/m^2 vs. 24.53 kg/m^2). The median operative time was significantly higher in the RAL group (250 min) than in the SL group (174 min). The difference in the operative time was observed in obese patients (283 min in RAL vs. 174 min in SL) but not in normal weight or overweight patients. There was no significant difference between the two study groups in the hysterectomy rate, in the estimated blood loss, in the length of stay, in the rate of intraoperative or postoperative complications. There was no conversion to laparotomy. A retrospective controlled study compared 40 RAL with 38 matched SL performed using the CO_2 laser [14]. The stage of endometriosis was evenly distributed between the two study groups. The blood loss was minimal, without significant differences between the two study groups (RAL, 60 ml, range 0-350; SL, 65 ml, range 0.500). There was no intraoperative or postoperative complication. No conversion to laparotomy was required. The operative time was significant longer in the RAL (mean: 191 min; range, 135–295 min) than in the SL (159 min; 85–320 min). The authors concluded that SL and RAL have similar outcomes; however, RAL requires longer surgical and anesthesia time. A retrospective study compared the feasibility of treating patients with suspected endometriosis who were not undergoing hysterectomy using RAL (180 patients) compared with CO_2 SL (100 patients) [15]. All the procedures were performed by a single surgeon. 47.7% of the patients in the robot-assisted cohort and 46.0% of the patients in the CO_2 laser laparoscopy cohort had stage III/IV endometriosis. The biopsy rate was similar in RAL and SL (88.9% vs. 95%), but the rate of biopsy-confirmed endometriosis was significantly higher in the RAL (80.0% vs. 56.8%). The operative time was comparable in the two groups

(77.4 ± 41.6 min in patients treated by RAL vs. 72.3 ± 28.5 min in patients treated by SL). The estimated blood loss was very low and similar in the two study groups (29.2 ± 43.2 ml in patients treated by RAL vs. 24.9 ± 24.3 ml in patients treated by SL). Two complications occurred in the RAL: one intraoperative cystotomy and one postoperative staphylococcus infection. No conversions to laparotomy occurred in either group. Most patients reported improved postoperative pain at the first follow-up visit with no differences between the surgical approaches. A retrospective cohort study including 420 women compared RAL with SL for the treatment of advanced stage deep endometriosis [16]. Patients were selected to undergo RAL or SL on the basis of availability of the patient on the robot operating room day. Patients were excluded if they had stage 1 or 2 endometriosis or if they needed bladder, ureteral, or bowel resection (including disc excision) or hysterectomy, myomectomy, or thoracoscopy. All the procedures were performed by the same surgeon. Two hundred and seventy-three patients underwent SL and 147 underwent RAL. The estimated blood loss was similar in the two study groups (25 ml in the SL and 40 ml in the RAL). The mean operative time was significantly shorter in the SL (135 min) than in the RAL (196 min). All 147 patients in the RAL remained in the hospital overnight, and were discharged on day after surgery; whereas most patients in the SL (76.9%) were discharged to home on the day of surgery. There was no major complication in either group.

A large retrospective study investigated the perioperative outcomes and factors impacting operating time, length of hospital stay, and complications of patients undergoing surgery for stage III or IV endometriosis [17]. Four-hundred and ninety-three patients were included in the study; 331 underwent RAL and 162 SL. Patients in the SL and RAL groups were not comparable, because of the higher number of procedures and more radical operations in the RAL. Significantly more patients in the RAL group underwent simple hysterectomy, modified radical hysterectomy, pelvic peritonectomy, and excision of peritoneal implants. However, the RAL resulted in 16.2% shorter operating time than SL after adjusting for age, blood loss, and number of procedures per patient.

An American multicenter randomized trial (LAROSE) investigated whether RAL is better than SL in the treatment of endometriosis [18]. Seventy-three patients were randomized for mode of surgery type (38 in the SL and 35 in the RAL group); the follow-up was performed at 6 weeks and 6 months after surgery. The mean operative time (primary outcome of the study) was similar in the two study groups (106.6 ± 48.4 min for RAL vs. 101.6 ± 63.2 for SL). There were no statistical differences in operative time, intraoperative blood loss or intraoperative complications between the two surgical approaches. There were no differences in rate of endometriosis confirmation by pathology between the two surgical approaches. There were no differences in intraoperative or postoperative complications, rates of conversion to laparotomy, or type of surgery performed in the two arms. Two patients in the RAL required rehospitalization for pain management: one because of pain associated with pyelonephritis and the other for postoperative pain control because of ileus. Three patients in the SL required rehospitalization: two for pain secondary to ileus and abscess and one patient for postoperative urinary tract infection. Other postoperative complications included wound infection/cellulitis (three patients), urinary retention (one patient), and vaginal bleeding (one patient). Quality of life similarly improved in the two study groups. Unfortunately, for most outcomes, event rates were low, and the sample size was insufficient to detect potential differences between groups [19].

13.4 Robotic Single-Site Treatment of Endometriosis

Robotic single-site surgery (RSSAL) may be superior to multiport procedures not only in cosmetics but also in the postoperative pain (because of the presence of just one wound). Gargiulo et al. described the use of RSSAL for the treatment of bilateral endometriomas [20]. A right endometrioma was removed by stripping. A left endometrioma was partially removed by stripping and the remnant part of the endometrioma was ablated with CO_2 laser. The procedure lasted 127 min, there was no complication and the patient was discharge home on the day of surgery. A case report demonstrated the feasibility of robotic single-site resection of advanced endometriosis in a 36 years old woman [21]. The Firefly technology was used to facilitate the identification and removal of endometriosis. In particular, the patient underwent ureterolysis, adhesiolysis, peritoneal stripping, and a rectal nodule excision. Surgery not only caused complete resolution of pain, but it was also associated with excellent cosmetic results. More recently, a Korean retrospective study compared the perioperative outcomes of RSSAL with conventional single-port laparoscopic surgery (SPSL) for the treatment of advance-stage endometriosis [22]. All the patients underwent cystectomy and adhesiolysis. No patient required conversion to multiport laparoscopic or robotic surgery. The total operation time was significantly longer in the RSSAL group (107.8–37.6 min) compared with the SPSL group (76.9–46.4 min). The estimated blood loss was lower in the SPSL group (57.1–44.9 mL) compared with the RSSAL group (135.6–143.9 mL), but the mean size of endometriosis in the SPSL group (4.37–2.14 cm) was significantly smaller than that of the RSSAL surgery group (5.23–2.53 cm). The rate of deep infiltrating endometriosis was 76.5% in the RSSAL group and 63.5% in the SPSL group. The duration of the hospital stay was similar in the two study groups. The laparoscopic single-port surgery places limits for suturing; in contrast, the RSSAL (with flexible and rotated instruments) allows a precise suturing of the ovarian tissue after cystectomy. However, single-site surgery has some limitations; in fact, both RSSAL and SPSL have limited range of motion compared with multisite procedures. In a recent prospective observational study, 20 patients were treated with RSSAL [23]. No hemorrhage, blood transfusions, allergic reactions, or any other form of intraoperative complications were reported. There were no conversions to laparotomy. Surgery caused a significant improvement of endometriosis-related pain.

13.5 Robotic-Assisted Treatment of Intestinal Endometriosis

In 2008 Chammas et al. described a case of a 23-year-old patient who had a 4 cm bladder nodule and a rectal endometriotic lesion [24]. Partial cystectomy and the resection of the rectal nodule were performed by RAL. Four trocars were used, two of them 10 mm and the other two 12 mm. The rectum was repaired in two layers using running 3.0 Vycril sutures. The total operative time was 197 min, the intraoperative blood loss was approximately 100 ml and there was no complication. In 2010 Averbach et al. reported a case of rectosigmoidectomy for DIE performed by RAL in a 35-year-old woman with infertility, rectal bleeding, and painful defecation [25]. Five trocars were used; two of 8 mm were used for the left and right robot arms; two 12 mm trocars were placed, one at the right iliac fossa, and the other at the right hypochondrium. The umbilical incision at 12 mm was enlarged to around 4 cm for bowel resection. Surgery lasted 5 h (90 min used for setting up the robotic system). Surgery was uneventful and there was no postoperative complication. The patient was discharged on the fifth postoperative day. In 2011, Nezhat et al. described two cases of bowel endometriosis treated by RAL [7]. A 41-year-old patient underwent segmental rectosigmoid resection, hysterectomy, and bilateral salpingo-oophorectomy. The procedure was uneventful, and the patient was discharged on the third postoperative day. The second patient underwent RAL disc excision of a rectal nodule. The lesion was excised using grasper and scissors. The intestinal defect was repaired with multiple interrupted 2-0 Vicryl sutures. Following these case reports, several retrospective studies reported the surgical outcomes of patients with bowel endometriosis treated by RAL. Lim et al. compared morbidity and outcome of patients treated by RAL low anterior resection with primary sigmoid rectal anastomosis combined with ureterolysis, hysterectomy, and bilateral salpingo-oophorectomy ($n = 8$) with an historical cohort of patients treated by laparotomy ($n = 10$) [26]. All the patients had previously undergone surgical and hormonal treatment of endometriosis, had stage IV endometriosis and desired definitive surgical treatment of endometriosis. The eight patients who underwent RAL completed the entire procedure intracorporeally, including the anastomosis without requirement of minilaparotomy. The RAL allowed to complete intracorporeal purse string suturing, to place the anvil of the circular staples in the proximal sigmoid colon, and to perform the colorectal anastomosis of the bowel. There was no significant difference in the total operative time between the two study groups (RAL = 238.5 ± 57.8 min vs. laparotomy = 237.4 ± 117.7 min). The overall transfusion rate in the series was 22.2% (4/18); there was no significant difference in the blood loss between the two study groups (RAL = 425 ± 462.1 cc vs. laparotomy = 630 ± 432.2 cc). Also, the length of the hospitalization was similar in the two study groups (RAL = 5.5 ± 2.4 days vs. laparotomy = 6.2 ± 1.6 days). Finally, there was no significant difference in the incidence of complications between the laparotomy group (two blood transfusions and two rectovaginal fistulas) and the RAL group (two complications). Notably, there was no rectovaginal fistula in the RAL group. Therefore, the authors concluded that RAL is a feasible and safe procedure. Subsequently, an Italian retrospective study reported the data of 22 patients who underwent RAL treatment of colorectal endometriosis [27]. The video laparoscope was introduced in the umbilical access or in a right paraumbilical access. Two robotic trocars (8 mm) and two assistant trocars (5 and 12 mm) were used. The procedures were performed with a nerve-sparing approach. When the "shaving technique" was used to excise the intestinal nodule, the reconstruction of the muscular portion of the rectal wall was performed by using 3/0, interrupted, absorbable monofilament sutures placed in the transverse direction to avoid narrowing the lumen. In case of segmental resection, the anastomosis was performed as in classical laparoscopy, a 4 cm suprapubic incision was used to exteriorize the distal bowel end, to cut the proximal end extracorporeally and to create a purse for the anvil. The terminal-to-terminal anastomosis was performed by using a rectally introduced circular stapler (29 mm). Twelve patients underwent segmental resection (median diameter of the largest nodule 35 mm) and ten patients underwent rectal shaving (median diameter of the largest nodule 30 mm). In patients undergoing shaving, there was no inadvertent rectal perforation. No patient had ileostomy or colostomy. There was no conversion to laparotomy. There was no intraoperative complication. No patient required intraoperative or postoperative blood transfusion. One patient who had underwent segmental bowel resection was readmitted because of small bowel occlusion 14 days after surgery; the case was resolved in three days with medical treatment. There was no other major postoperative complication (such as transient or persistent urinary retention, late perforation, anastomotic fistula or leakage or rectovaginal fistula). Postoperatively, there was a statistically significant improvement of patient symptoms. Neme et al. confirmed the feasibility of RAL colorectal resection for endometriosis in ten women [28]. The mean operative time with the robot was 157 min (range, 90–190 min). Docking the robot averaged 12 min (range, 8–19 min). Intraoperative blood loss was insignificant and no patient required blood transfusion. There were no intraoperative or postoperative complications. None of the patients had ileostomy or colostomy. The length of stay was three days in all cases. At 12-month follow-up pain and intestinal symptoms disappeared in all the patients. Vitobello et al. used a hybrid robotic and laparoscopic technique to treat seven symptomatic patients with rectosigmoid endometriosis and ASRM stage IV endometriosis [29]. At the time of docking the robot, a 12-mm trocar used for the camera was introduced in the umbilicus. A 10-mm trocar was placed 8 cm to the left and 15° above the umbilicus for assistance. The right and left robotic working ports consisting of 8-mm trocars were placed 8 cm lateral to the umbilicus. The robotic technique was suspended after completely mobilizing the bowel and prior to resection. The laparoscopy was used to mobilize the descending colon until the splenic flexure, to cut the inferior mesenteric artery (when required), and to perform the intestinal resection. A 4-cm minilaparotomy was carried out to remove the

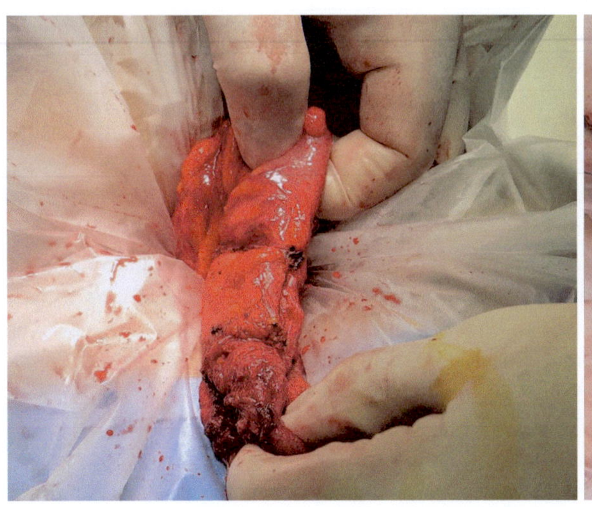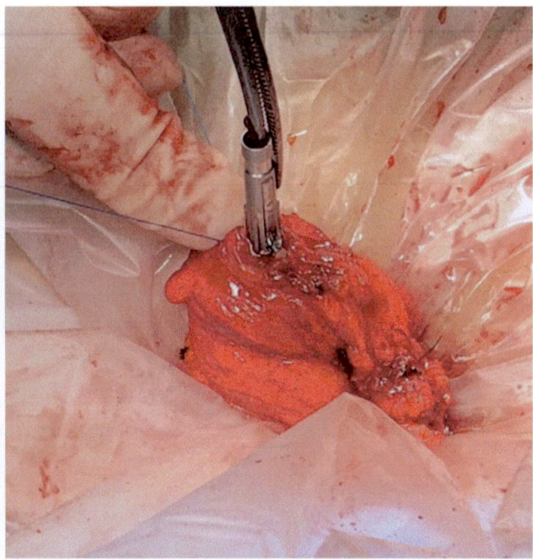

Fig. 13.1 Robotic-assisted laparoscopic segmental resection. A minilaparotomy is carried out to assess the rectosigmoid endometriotic nodule and cut the bowel

intestine, assess the rectosigmoid endometriotic lesions and cut the bowel (Fig. 13.1). The procedure was completed performing a termino-terminal anastomosis with a circular stapler. No patient required a protective stoma. The mean intraoperative blood loss was 250 ml (range, 50–550 ml) and no patient required blood transfusion. The mean operative time was 210 min (range, 180–320 ml). The average hospital stay was 5 days (range, 4–6 days). There was one postoperative complication: one patient required reoperation by SL because of bleeding of an artery branch at the level of the descending colon. A follow-up was performed at 3, 6, and 12 months after surgery and there was a significant improvement in all endometriosis-related symptoms. An Italian retrospective study based on a prospectively collected database confirmed the feasibility of RAL for the treatment of DIE [30]. Forty-three patients were included in the study. All the procedures were performed by the same surgeon. Nineteen women underwent rectosigmoid resection, the mean length of the resected bowel specimen was 11 cm. No temporary ileostomy or colostomy was performed. Twenty-three patients underwent excision of deep infiltrating endometriosis of the rectovaginal septum, with or without rectal shaving. No inadvertent rectal perforation occurred. In addition, five women had

bladder resection for deep endometriosis. There was no intraoperative complication and no conversion to laparotomy. There were two postoperative complications: one patient had hemoperitoneum for bleeding from the inferior mesenteric vessels on postoperative day 1 which required laparoscopic haemostasis and blood transfusion. Another woman had an anastomotic leakage on postoperative day 10 which required temporary colostomy. Another Italian retrospective study investigated the feasibility, limits, and short-term results of patients with deep infiltrating endometriosis with intestinal involvement treated by RAL colorectal resection [31]. The study included 46 procedures were performed by SL (one laparotomy conversion) and 19 by RAL. The criteria for colorectal resection were lesion with diameter >2 cm, multiple lesions involving the bowel wall, and/or circumferential involvement more than 50%. All the procedures were performed by a single colorectal surgeon. The procedures were performed using a nerve-sparing technique. In patients treated by RAL, the intestinal anastomosis was performed as in the SL without using the robot. A 4 cm suprapubic incision was used to exteriorize the distal bowel, to cut the proximal end extracorporeally, and to create a purse for the anvil. The terminal-to-terminal anastomosis was created by using a rectally introduced circular stapler (29 mm). No laparotomic conversion was performed in patients treated by RAL. No intraoperative complication was observed. The mean operative time was 370 min (range = 250–720 min) and the estimated blood loss was 150 ml (range = 50–350 ml). The overall complication rate was 10% (two rectovaginal fistulae, only one requiring temporary ileostomy). In the SL group, the mean operative time was 180 (80–220) min; the blood loss was 320 (100–650) ml. The hospital stay was similar in patients treated by SL and in those treated by RAL. At 1 and 6 months after surgery, intestinal and urinary function showed that there was no severe damage to pelvic nerves and patients had good quality of life. A retrospective multicentric study investigated the role of RAL in the treatment of DIE [32]. Eighty-eight patients with rectal nodules were included in the study. The mean (±SD) operative time was 188.2 (±75.7) min. The mean (±SD) intraoperative blood loss was 127.5 (±293.3) ml. There was a laparotomy conversion, two sutured rectal injuries and a red cells blood transfusion. The mean length of hospitalization was 4.2 (±2.7) days. An Italian prospective cohort study evaluated the feasibility and outcome of RAL shaving of DIE of the rectovaginal space [33]. The patients underwent removal of endometriotic nodules from the rectovaginal septum with rectal shaving alone or in combination with other procedures. All procedures were performed by the same surgeon. The median operating time from skin opening to closure was 174 min (range, 75–300 min). The median docking time was 20 min (range, 5–25 min). The median intraoperative blood loss was 0 mL (range, 0–100 mL). The rectal lumen was opened in one patient. There was one conversion to SL. The median length of stay was three nights. At a median follow-up of 22 months (range, 6–50 months), there were three recurrences of rectovaginal septum endometriosis (diagnosed by vaginal examination and ultrasonography). A case series including ten patients investigated the short- and mid-term surgical and functional outcomes of RAL for the treatment of DIE with colorectal involvement [34]. A nerve-sparing technique was used. The median operating time was 280 min (range 180–420 min), and the median intraoperative blood loss was negligible (range 100–400 ml). No patient required intraoperative blood transfusion. There was no conversion to laparotomy. No patient required a diverting ileostomy. The mean postoperative hospital stay was 6 days (range 4–7 days). One patient reported a wound infection. None of the patients required reintervention. All patients had a statistically significant improvement in symptoms after surgery. The Female Sexual Function Index was used to assess sexual function. Desire, arousal, lubrication, orgasm, and overall sexual satisfaction all worsened significantly 1 month after surgery; but all parameters showed a subsequent progressive improvement, and at 12 months from surgery, the scores were comparable to those measured preoperatively. Dyspareunia was significantly improved 12 months after surgery compared to preoperatively. The International Consultation on Incontinence Female Lower Urinary Tract Symptoms questionnaire was used for the evaluation of lower urinary tract symptoms and their impact on quality of life. Women experienced a significant worsening in the grade of bladder filling and incontinence both 1 and 6 months after surgery. In contrast, voiding symptoms worsened at 1 month postoperatively but started to gradually improve 6 months after surgery. There was a gradual improvement for all parameters one year after surgery. Scores for bladder filling, voiding symptoms, and incontinence 1 year postoperatively were not significantly different to the respective preoperative scores. With respect to the impact of urinary symptoms on quality of life, women experienced a significant worsening both at 1 and 6 months after surgery. However, gradual improvement of urinary symptoms was associated with an amelioration in overall quality of life so that 1 year after surgery, no statistically significant difference was observed compared to the preoperative period.

A case series investigated the role of RAL nerve-sparing rectal nodulectomy in the treatment of 33 consecutive patients with retrocervical-rectal deep infiltrating endometriosis of any diameter not involving the mucosa nor producing rectal stenosis >50% [35]. The resection was performed using monopolar scissors or a hook with extraction through the vagina or into a bag through the optical trocar. One or two layers of 00 Vicryl interrupted sutures were placed in the same direction as the rectal axis to reinforce the rectal wall and help ensuring the hemostasis. Thirty-one patients underwent RAL nodulectomy; two patients with additional not radiologically detected endometriotic nodules involving the sigmoid were excluded from the study; one patient with a nodule with diameter >32 mm was treated by segmental bowel resection because at the end of the nodulectomy there was an extensive devascularization of the rectal wall. No patient required conversion to laparotomy. The patients underwent a variety of associated procedures including ureterolysis and full-thickness resection of the vagina. There was no intraoperative complication and, in particular, no patient had inadvertent rectal perforation during nodulectomy. No patient had temporary ileostomy or colostomy. No patient required blood transfusion intraoperatively or postoperatively. The mean length of the excised nodules measured on the longer axis of the formalin-fixed specimens was 26.6 (±9.4) mm. There were three complications: one hemorrhage with hemoperitoneum owing to a partial uterine artery rupture on the second day after surgery, which required a SL to ensure hemostasis, a periumbilical hematoma and a case of paralytic ileus (both of which resolved with medical therapy). The mean follow-up was 27.6 (±16.7) months. There were two recurrences of intestinal endometriosis, both occurred after at least 12 months from surgery. One patient developed a de novo bladder nodule. In the remaining patients there was a persistent improvement of symptoms. There was no case of postoperative bladder or rectal dysfunction. The most important finding of this study was that RAL nodulectomy was feasible independently from the size of the rectal nodule. A recent American retrospective study described the use of RAL for the treatment of DIE with colorectal involvement [36]. All the procedures were performed by a single colorectal surgeon in conjunction with the gynecological surgical team. The robot was

docked from either the right or left side of the patient depending on the operating room setup and the preference of the gynecologists. Although docking either from right or left does not affect pelvic surgery and mobilization of the sigmoid, docking robot from the left is required if extensive mobilization of the white line of Toldt is required. The shaving technique was used when the nodule did not exceed 30% of the circumference of the lumen. The defects were repaired with a 2-0 V-Loc suture in two layers. Fifty-seven patients had RAL excision of DIE. Fifteen patients had rectosigmoid nodules and required low anterior resection. There was no intraoperative complication and no conversion to laparotomy. Postoperative complications (one superficial wound infection, four patients with pelvic abscesses, a bowel leak, and one rectovaginal fistula) occurred in 5 out of 15 patients, three of which required percutaneous drainage and one required reoperation. Two of the 15 patients were lost to follow up in clinic in the immediate postoperative period. All patients who were followed-up continued on oral contraceptives and had resolution of dysmenorrhea and pain in the immediate postoperative period.

In cases of DIE of the low rectum, low anterior resection might be required depending on size of the lesion. The new robotic technology (Xi) simplifies the docking procedure and makes single docking feasible even for complex multiquadrant procedure with mobilization of splenic flexure is needed [37–40]. This might be beneficial in reducing operative time. On the other hand, the Firefly® technology can be used for intraoperative perfusion assessment of bowel and particularly an anastomosis during colorectal surgery [41] with a proposed benefit of decreasing incidence of postoperative leaks. These added benefits of the robotic technology might be more pronounced in cases that requires intestinal resection and anastomosis. It is worth mentioning there is not enough data to determine the ability of Firefly®-aided ureteral identification in preventing iatrogenic ureteral injuries during surgery for deep infiltrating endometriosis. It is reported that the robotic surgical platform might assist a novice operator to master more complex colorectal procedures through a shorter learning curve [40]; however, there are no studies that looked at the learning curve for robotic bowel surgery for DIE, and whether proficiency in standard laparoscopic management of bowel endometriosis is necessary.

13.6 Conclusion

In the last 15 years, several studies showed that RAL achieve the same operative and postoperative results compared with SL in the treatment of colorectal diseases and rectal cancer [42–44]. The studies described in this chapter demonstrate the feasibility and safety of RAL in the treatment not only of DIE but also of rectosigmoid endometriosis. Notably, RAL has been used to perform all the techniques used to treat bowel endometriosis: shaving [10, 11, 27, 30, 33] (Figs. 13.2 and 13.3), disc excision [7, 11, 35, 45], and segmental resection [7, 27, 29–31, 34]. However, most of these studies are retrospective, they report the surgical outcomes and, sometimes, short-term postoperative follow-up. Unfortunately, long-term postoperative outcomes are not investigated.

The robot has several potential advantages in the treatment of rectosigmoid endometriosis. It is possible to visualize the pelvis at much higher magnification which affords superior visualization of tissue planes with the three-dimensional imaging system. There is a better stability and magnification of the camera. The mobility of robotic instruments is outstanding, as they offer 7 degrees of freedom compared to only 3 in conventional laparoscopy; this enables the surgeon to dissect and skeletonize the tissue better [7, 15, 26, 29, 30, 33, 34]. A final advantage of the robot is that in complex operation it may decrease the fatigue allowing the surgeon to sit [11]. If the initial operative time seems of longer, it is shortened with surgical experience [10]. Although the docking procedure lengthens the setup, the advantages of subsequent robotic surgery decrease the subsequent operative time [10]. In contrast, the robotic system has some drawbacks such as lack of tactile sensation, time required to dock and separate the robotic cart from the patient, large-sized port (8 mm), limited ability to operate in adjacent fields (such as the splenic flexure) without redocking one or more robotic arm, inability to move the surgical table once the robot arms are attached and inability to operate in different quadrants at the same time [9, 29]. Finally, intraoperative examination of the vagina by the surgeon sitting at the console is difficult [11].

Several studies in the literature showed that the surgical robot increases the operative time in patients with deep endometriosis even when the procedures are performed by experienced surgeons [14, 16]. Obviously, the time needed to dock and undock contributes to increasing the operative time. In case of large endometriomas, trocar placement and removal of the specimen may contribute to increase the operative time [16]. In addition, when endometriotic lesions are located in the upper abdomen (such as around the liver and the diaphragm) or on the appendix, there is limited flexibility in changing the locations of the instruments. Finally, in difficult cases, during SL, it is possible to move the camera to different ports much easier than with the

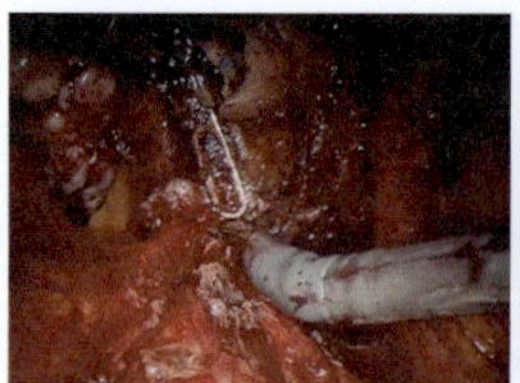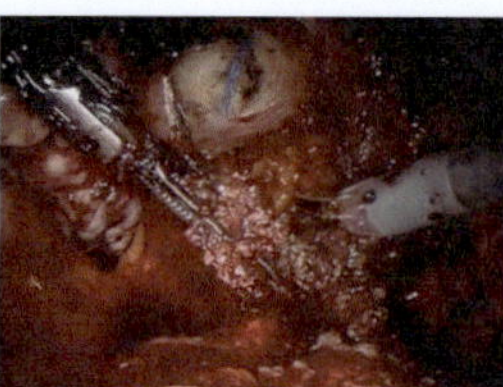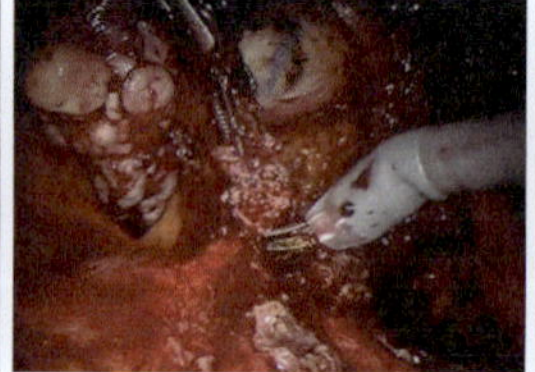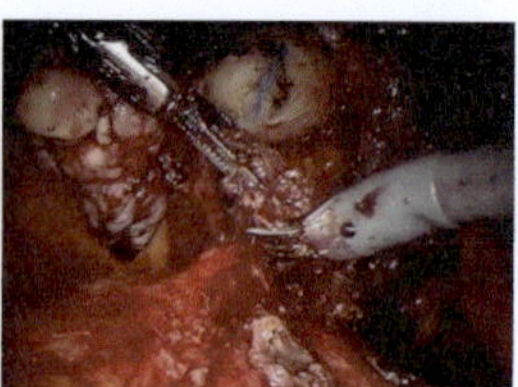

Fig. 13.2 Robotic-assisted laparoscopy shaving

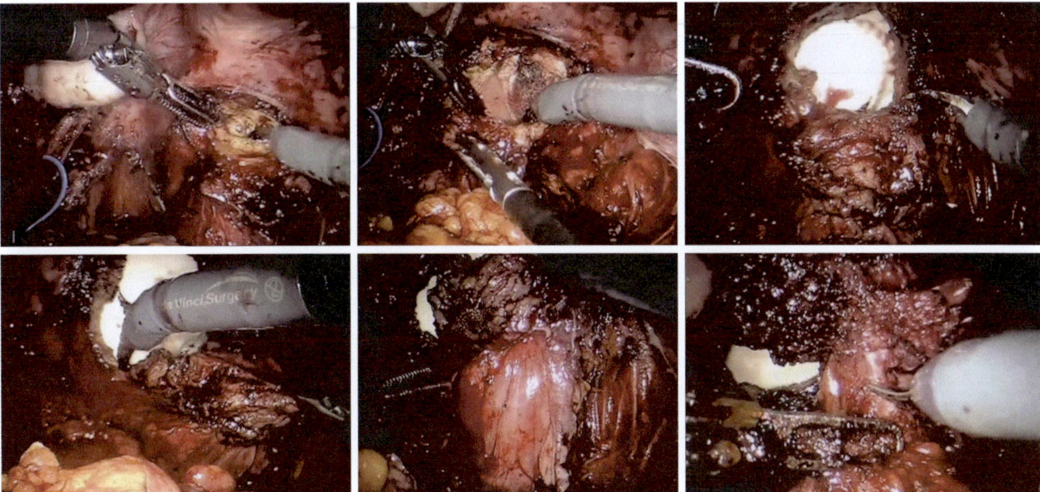

Fig. 13.3 A large rectal endometriotic nodule infiltrating the vagina is excised by robotic-assisted laparoscopy shaving

robotic platform. One study reported similar operative time between RAL and SL [15]. Only one study reported shorted operative time for RAL compared with SL [17]. The rate and severity of complications observed during RAL treatment of DIE are similar to those observed with SL [10]. Similarly, the incidence of complications observed during RAL treatment of rectosigmoid endometriosis is similar to that observed during laparotomy [26].

A systematic review including 17 studies investigated the role of RAL in the treatment of endometriosis [46]. The authors observed that most of the studies report a longer operating time in patients treated by RAL than in those undergoing SL. No study has reported a significant difference in blood loss between RAL and SL. The rate of major complications was 1.5% in the RAL group and 0.3% in the SL group and the rate of conversion to laparotomy was 0.3% in the RAL group and 0.5% in the SL group. Therefore, the authors concluded that RAL treatment of endometriosis dos not provide benefits over SL, overall and among subgroups of women with severe endometriosis, peritoneal endometriosis and obesity. However, the available evidence was of low-quality, and data regarding long-term pain relief and pregnancy rates are lacking.

References

1. Duffy JM, Arambage K, Correa FJ, Olive D, Farquhar C, Garry R, Barlow DH, Jacobson TZ. Laparoscopic surgery for endometriosis. Cochrane Database Syst Rev. 2014;4:CD011031.
2. Chapron C, Fauconnier A, Goffinet F, Breart G, Dubuisson JB. Laparoscopic surgery is not inherently dangerous for patients presenting with benign gynaecologic pathology. Results of a meta-analysis. Hum Reprod. 2002;17:1334–42.
3. Roman H. Endometriosis surgery and preservation of fertility, what surgeons should know. J Visc Surg. 2018;155(Suppl 1):S31–6.
4. Gianardi D, Giannini A. Minimally invasive surgery for deep-infiltrating endometriosis and its impact on fertility: can robotic surgery play a role? J Robot Surg. 2019;13:789–90.
5. Sener A, Chew BH, Duvdevani M, Brock GB, Vilos GA, Pautler SE. Combined transurethral and laparoscopic partial cystectomy and robot-assisted bladder repair for the treatment of bladder endometrioma. J Minim Invasive Gynecol. 2006;13:245–8.
6. Liu C, Perisic D, Samadi D, Nezhat F. Robotic-assisted laparoscopic partial bladder resection for the treatment of infiltrating endometriosis. J Minim Invasive Gynecol. 2008;15:745–8.
7. Nezhat C, Hajhosseini B, King LP. Robotic-assisted laparoscopic treatment of bowel, bladder, and ureteral endometriosis. JSLS. 2011;15:387–92.
8. Brudie LA, Gaia G, Ahmad S, Finkler NJ, Bigsby GE, Ghurani GB, Kendrick JE, Rakowski JA, Groton JH, Holloway RW. Peri-operative outcomes of patients with stage IV endometriosis undergoing robotic-assisted laparoscopic surgery. J Robot Surg. 2012;6:317–22.

9. Bedaiwy MA, Rahman MY, Chapman M, Frasure H, Mahajan S, von Gruenigen VE, Hurd W, Zanotti K. Robotic-assisted hysterectomy for the management of severe endometriosis: a retrospective review of short-term surgical outcomes. JSLS. 2013;17:95–9.

10. Collinet P, Leguevaque P, Neme RM, Cela V, Barton-Smith P, Hebert T, Hanssens S, Nishi H, Nisolle M. Robot-assisted laparoscopy for deep infiltrating endometriosis: international multicentric retrospective study. Surg Endosc. 2014;28:2474–9.

11. Abo C, Roman H, Bridoux V, Huet E, Tuech JJ, Resch B, Stochino E, Marpeau L, Darwish B. Management of deep infiltrating endometriosis by laparoscopic route with robotic assistance: 3-year experience. J Gynecol Obstet Hum Reprod. 2017;46:9–18.

12. Giannini A, Pisaneschi S, Malacarne E, Cela V, Melfi F, Perutelli A, Simoncini T. Robotic approach to ureteral endometriosis: surgical features and perioperative outcomes. Front Surg. 2018;5:51.

13. Nezhat FR, Sirota I. Perioperative outcomes of robotic assisted laparoscopic surgery versus conventional laparoscopy surgery for advanced-stage endometriosis. JSLS. 2014;18(4):e2014.00094.

14. Nezhat C, Lewis M, Kotikela S, Veeraswamy A, Saadat L, Hajhosseini B, Nezhat C. Robotic versus standard laparoscopy for the treatment of endometriosis. Fertil Steril. 2010;94:2758–60.

15. Dulemba JF, Pelzel C, Hubert HB. Retrospective analysis of robot-assisted versus standard laparoscopy in the treatment of pelvic pain indicative of endometriosis. J Robot Surg. 2013;7:163–9.

16. Nezhat CR, Stevens A, Balassiano E, Soliemannjad R. Robotic-assisted laparoscopy vs conventional laparoscopy for the treatment of advanced stage endometriosis. J Minim Invasive Gynecol. 2015;22:40–4.

17. Magrina JF, Espada M, Kho RM, Cetta R, Chang YH, Magtibay PM. Surgical excision of advanced endometriosis: perioperative outcomes and impacting factors. J Minim Invasive Gynecol. 2015;22:944–50.

18. Soto E, Luu TH, Liu X, Magrina JF, Wasson MN, Einarsson JI, Cohen SL, Falcone T. Laparoscopy vs. Robotic Surgery for Endometriosis (LAROSE): a multicenter, randomized, controlled trial. Fertil Steril. 2017;107:996–1002.

19. Lawrie TA, Liu H, Lu D, Dowswell T, Song H, Wang L, Shi G. Robot-assisted surgery in gynaecology. Cochrane Database Syst Rev. 2019;4:CD011422.

20. Gargiulo AR, Feltmate C, Srouji SS. Robotic single-site excision of ovarian endometrioma. Fertil Res Pract. 2015;1:19.

21. Guan X, Nguyen MT, Walsh TM, Kelly B. Robotic single-site endometriosis resection using firefly technology. J Minim Invasive Gynecol. 2016;23:10–1.

22. Moon HS, Shim JE, Lee SR, Jeong K. The comparison of robotic single-site surgery to single-port laparoendoscopic surgery for the treatment of advanced-stage endometriosis. J Laparoendosc Adv Surg Tech A. 2018;28:1483–8.

23. Jayakumaran J, Pavlovic Z, Fuhrich D, Wiercinski K, Buffington C, Caceres A. Robotic single-site endometriosis resection using near-infrared fluorescence imaging with indocyanine green: a prospective case series and review of literature. J Robot Surg. 2019;14(1):145–54.

24. Chammas MF Jr, Kim FJ, Barbarino A, Hubert N, Feuillu B, Coissard A, Hubert J. Asymptomatic rectal and bladder endometriosis: a case for robotic-assisted surgery. Can J Urol. 2008;15:4097–100.

25. Averbach M, Popoutchi P, Marques OW Jr, Abdalla RZ, Podgaec S, Abrao MS. Robotic rectosigmoidectomy – pioneer case report in Brazil. Current scene in colorectal robotic surgery. Arq Gastroenterol. 2010;47:116–8.

26. Lim PC, Kang E, Park do H. Robot-assisted total intracorporeal low anterior resection with primary anastomosis and radical dissection for treatment of stage IV endometriosis with bowel involvement: morbidity and its outcome. J Robot Surg. 2011;5:273–8.

27. Ercoli A, D'Asta M, Fagotti A, Fanfani F, Romano F, Baldazzi G, Salerno MG, Scambia G. Robotic treatment of colorectal endometriosis: technique, feasibility and short-term results. Hum Reprod. 2012;27:722–6.

28. Neme RM, Schraibman V, Okazaki S, Maccapani G, Chen WJ, Domit CD, Kaufmann OG, Advincula AP. Deep infiltrating colorectal endometriosis treated with robotic-assisted rectosigmoidectomy. JSLS. 2013;17:227–34.

29. Vitobello D, Fattizzi N, Santoro G, Rosati R, Baldazzi G, Bulletti C, Palmara V. Robotic surgery and standard laparoscopy: a surgical hybrid technique for use in colorectal endometriosis. J Obstet Gynaecol Res. 2013;39:217–22.

30. Siesto G, Ieda N, Rosati R, Vitobello D. Robotic surgery for deep endometriosis: a paradigm shift. Int J Med Robot. 2014;10:140–6.

31. Cassini D, Cerullo G, Miccini M, Manoochehri F, Ercoli A, Baldazzi G. Robotic hybrid technique in rectal surgery for deep pelvic endometriosis. Surg Innov. 2014;21:52–8.

32. Hanssens S, Nisolle M, Leguevaque P, Neme RM, Cela V, Barton-Smith P, Hebert T, Collinet P. Robotic-assisted laparoscopy for deep infiltrating endometriosis: the Register of the Society of European Robotic Gynaecological Surgery. Gynecol Obstet Fertil. 2014;42:744–8.

33. Pellegrino A, Damiani GR, Trio C, Faccioli P, Croce P, Tagliabue F, Dainese E. Robotic shaving technique in 25 patients affected by deep infiltrating endometriosis of the rectovaginal space. J Minim Invasive Gynecol. 2015;22:1287–92.

34. Morelli L, Perutelli A, Palmeri M, Guadagni S, Mariniello MD, Di Franco G, Cela V, Brundu B, Salerno MG, Di Candio G, Mosca F. Robot-assisted surgery for the radical treatment of deep infiltrating endometriosis with colorectal involvement: short- and mid-term surgical and functional outcomes. Int J Color Dis. 2016;31:643–52.

35. Ercoli A, Bassi E, Ferrari S, Surico D, Fagotti A, Fanfani F, De Cicco F, Surico N, Scambia G. Robotic-

assisted conservative excision of retrocervical-rectal deep infiltrating endometriosis: a case series. J Minim Invasive Gynecol. 2017;24:863–8.

36. Graham A, Chen S, Skancke M, Moawad G, Obias V. A review of deep infiltrative colorectal endometriosis treated robotically at a single institution. Int J Med Robot. 2019;15:e2001.

37. Ozben V, Cengiz TB, Atasoy D, Bayraktar O, Aghayeva A, Erguner I, Baca B, Hamzaoglu I, Karahasanoglu T. Is da Vinci Xi better than da Vinci Si in robotic rectal cancer surgery? Comparison of the 2 generations of da Vinci systems. Surg Laparosc Endosc Percutan Tech. 2016;26:417–23.

38. Tamhankar AS, Jatal S, Saklani A. Total robotic radical rectal resection with da Vinci Xi system: single docking, single phase technique. Int J Med Robot. 2016;12:642–7.

39. Ngu JC, Sim S, Yusof S, Ng CY, Wong AS. Insight into the da Vinci(R) Xi – technical notes for single-docking left-sided colorectal procedures. Int J Med Robot. 2017;13 https://doi.org/10.1002/rcs.1798.

40. Ngu JC, Tsang CB, Koh DC. The da Vinci Xi: a review of its capabilities, versatility, and potential role in robotic colorectal surgery. Robot Surg. 2017;4:77–85.

41. Koerner C, Rosen SA. How robotics is changing and will change the field of colorectal surgery. World J Gastrointest Surg. 2019;11:381–7.

42. D'Annibale A, Morpurgo E, Fiscon V, Trevisan P, Sovernigo G, Orsini C, Guidolin D. Robotic and laparoscopic surgery for treatment of colorectal diseases. Dis Colon Rectum. 2004;47:2162–8.

43. Pigazzi A, Ellenhorn JD, Ballantyne GH, Paz IB. Robotic-assisted laparoscopic low anterior resection with total mesorectal excision for rectal cancer. Surg Endosc. 2006;20:1521–5.

44. Baik SH, Ko YT, Kang CM, Lee WJ, Kim NK, Sohn SK, Chi HS, Cho CH. Robotic tumor-specific mesorectal excision of rectal cancer: short-term outcome of a pilot randomized trial. Surg Endosc. 2008;22:1601–8.

45. Araujo SE, Seid VE, Marques RM, Gomes MT. Advantages of the robotic approach to deep infiltrating rectal endometriosis: because less is more. J Robot Surg. 2016;10:165–9.

46. Berlanda N, Frattaruolo MP, Aimi G, Farella M, Barbara G, Buggio L, Vercellini P. 'Money for nothing'. The role of robotic-assisted laparoscopy for the treatment of endometriosis. Reprod Biomed Online. 2017;35:435–44.

Simone Ferrero, Fabio Barra, Roberto Clarizia,
and Marcello Ceccaroni

14.1   Introduction

Bowel endometriosis can be treated by various techniques. Bowel shaving may find uneven definitions and applications from excision of a nodule within the intestinal muscularis propria to a full-thickness excision of an anterior intestinal wall portion with subsequent sutures. Disc excision is the entire resection of the bowel wall, including the mucosa, and it is followed by the closure of the intestinal defect by suture or using a stapler. Finally, segmental resection is the resection of the colon. The choice of the surgical technique is mainly based on the characteristics of bowel endometriotic nodules, such as the largest diameter of the infiltrating nodule, the presence of multiple nodules in the same bowel segment, the depth of infiltration of endometriosis in the intestinal wall and the degree of stenosis of the intestinal lumen. Furthermore, the experience of the surgeon has an essential role in choosing the type of surgery, and some surgeons are more prone to perform bowel resection, whereas others prefer conservative approaches. Rectosigmoid endometriosis may be associated with lesions infiltrating the vagina and the uterosacral ligaments. Simultaneous resections of these lesions may increase the risk of postoperative complications related to colorectal procedures. The potential risk of complications is a significant obstacle for young women when they consider undergoing surgery.

14.2   Short-Term Complications

Patients undergoing surgery for bowel endometriosis may experience various short-term complications such as rectovaginal fistula, anastomotic leakage, pelvic abscess, and postoperative bleeding.

14.2.1 Rectovaginal Fistula

The rectovaginal fistula is one of the most frequent complications following surgery for rectosigmoid endometriosis (Table 14.1). A fistula is an abnormal communication between two epithelialized surfaces; the rectovaginal fistula develops between the rectum and the vagina. Rectovaginal fistulae may be low (between the

S. Ferrero (✉) · F. Barra
Academic Unit of Obstetrics and Gynecology, IRCCS
Ospedale Policlinico San Martino, Genova, Italy

Department of Neurosciences, Rehabilitation,
Ophthalmology, Genetics, Maternal and Child Health
(DiNOGMI), University of Genova, Genova, Italy

R. Clarizia · M. Ceccaroni
Department of Obstetrics and Gynecology,
Gynecologic Oncology and Minimally-Invasive
Pelvic Surgery, International School of Surgical
Anatomy, IRCCS "Sacro Cuore – Don Calabria"
Hospital, Verona, Italy

© Springer Nature Switzerland AG 2020
S. Ferrero, M. Ceccaroni (eds.), *Clinical Management of Bowel Endometriosis*,
https://doi.org/10.1007/978-3-030-50446-5_14

Table 14.1 Prevalence of rectovaginal fistulas in women undergoing surgery for rectosigmoid endometriosis

Authors	Study design	n	Type of surgery	Prevalence
Laparotomy				
Dousset et al. [19]	Prospective study	100	Colorectal resection	4 (4.0%)
Lim et al. [51]	Retrospective study	10	Colorectal resection	2 (20.0%)
Laparoscopy				
Darai et al. [2]	Prospective study	40	Colorectal resection	3 (7.5%)
Minelli et al. [7]	Prospective study	357	Colorectal resection	14 (3.9%)
Ruffo et al. [18]	Prospective study	436	Colorectal resection	14 (3.2%)
Belghiti et al. [42]	Prospective study	198	Colorectal resection	9 (4.5%)
Akladios et al. [8]	Retrospective study	41	Colorectal resection ($n = 6$) or disc excision ($n = 35$)	1 (2.4%)
Malzoni et al. [9]	Retrospective study	248	Colorectal resection	6 (2.4%)
Roman et al. [10]	Retrospective study	1135	Shaving, disc excision or colorectal resection	31 (2.7%)
Balla et al. [3]	Systematic review	3079	Colorectal resection	74 (2.4%)
Zheng et al. [4]	Retrospective study	104	Shaving, disc excision or colorectal resection	5 (4.8%)
Boudy et al. [49]	Retrospective study	27	Hysterectomy + colorectal resection ($n = 15$) or disc excision ($n = 12$) + prevesical peritoneum interposition	1 (suspected; 3.7%)
Robotic-assisted laparoscopy				
Lim et al. [51]	Prospective study	8	Colorectal resection	0 (0%)
Ercoli et al. [52]	Retrospective study	12	Shaving or colorectal resection	0 (0%)
Neme et al. [53]	Retrospective study	10	Colorectal resection	0 (0%)
Morelli et al. [54]	Retrospective study	10	Colorectal resection	0 (0%)
Ercoli et al. [55]	Prospective study	33	Disc excision	0 (0%)
Graham et al. [56]	Retrospective study	15	Colorectal resection	1 (6.7%)

lower third of the rectum and the lower half of the vagina) or high (between the middle third of the rectum and the posterior vaginal fornix). They can be also classified according to their diameter: small <0.5 cm, medium 0.5–2.5 cm, and large >2.5 cm [1]. The rectovaginal fistula is usually diagnosed between 5 and 16 days after surgery [2]. Patients can experience malodorous vaginal discharge, fever, and lower abdominal pain. A major risk factor for the development of rectovaginal fistula is the concomitant resection of vaginal and rectosigmoid nodules as well as a vaginal cuff suture after hysterectomy close to a colorectal anastomosis. Spontaneous closures of rectovaginal fistulas are rare unless their diameter is very small. Therefore, surgical repair of this fistula is almost always indicated. Surgical correction can be performed by transanal, transperineal, transvaginal, or transabdominal approach and may require more than one operation. Surgical approach and success rate depend on the fistula location, quality of surrounding tissues, and history of previous surgical repairs. Rectovaginal fistulas significantly increase the length of the hospital stay and negatively affects the medical cost.

A systematic literature review, including 3079 patients treated with colorectal resection, demonstrated that rectovaginal fistula occurs in 2.8% of the patients (Table 14.1). Its frequency was found to be 2.8% after open surgery ($n = 210$), 2.2% after laparoscopic surgery ($n = 2651$) and 7.4% after robotic surgery ($n = 54$) [3]. A retrospective study investigated the risk factors for rectovaginal fistula in patients treated for deep infiltrating endometriosis [4]. One hundred and four patients were included in the study; rectovaginal fistula occurred in 4.8% of the patients at 5–16 days postoperatively. The risk factors for rectovaginal fistula were the location of the endometriotic lesions in the cul de sac, the larger size of the nodule, and surgical technique (higher risk with disc excision and bowel resection than with shaving of rectosigmoid nodules).

14.2.2 Bowel Anastomotic Leakage

Anastomotic leakage is the most severe complication after colorectal surgery, and it is associated with a substantial increase in morbidity, mortality, and length of hospital stay [5]. A systematic literature review (3079 patients) showed that anastomotic leakage occurs in 2.1% of patients treated with colorectal resection (Table 14.2) [3]. Patients with anastomotic leakage usually present with the following clinical features: peritonitis caused by the leakage, pelvic abscess, discharge of feces, presence of pus or gas in the abdominal drain, discharge of pus from the rectum, and rectovaginal fistula [6]. When anastomotic leakage is suspected, the diagnosis should be confirmed by one or more of the following techniques: colon barium enema, CT scan, sigmoidoscopy. A leakage may be only a small scar or can extend to the whole anastomosis leading to complete dehiscence and may occur in mechanic as well as in manual anastomoses (Fig. 14.1). The early detection of leakage is a critical factor in performing a timed treatment that may be laparoscopic if the fecal material is limited to the pelvis and if the medical conditions of the patient are not already changed to a septic shock state.

Some intraoperative factors may increase the risk of anastomotic leakage: a positive intraoperative leakage test, anastomotic rings not intact, anastomosis that is considered unsatisfactory by the surgeon, iatrogenic tear in the distal rectum. Ultralow anastomosis (≤ 5 cm from the anal verge) is a well-established risk factor for anastomotic leakage.

Treatment of a leakage quite always requires an intestinal derivation (ileostomy or colostomy).

The affected anastomosis may, in some cases, be repaired with a simple suture (if the leakage is

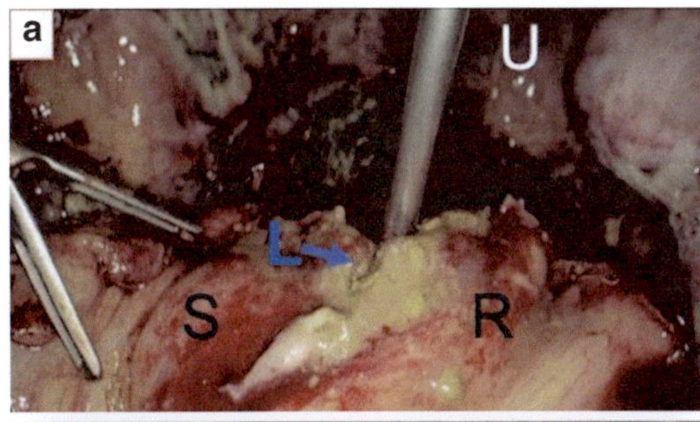

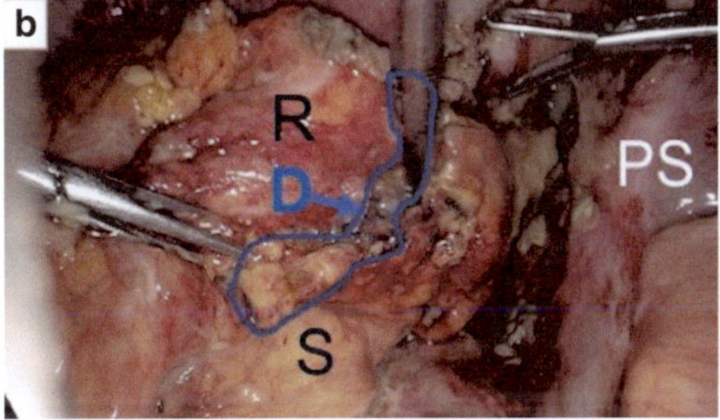

Fig. 14.1 Colorectal anastomosis leakage (**a**) and complete dehiscence (**b**). *S* sigmoid, *R* rectum, *U* uterus, *L* leakage, *D* dehiscence, *PS* pelvic sidewall

Table 14.2 Prevalence of anastomotic leakage in women undergoing surgery for rectosigmoid endometriosis

Authors	Study design	n	Type of surgery	Prevalence
Minelli et al. [7]	Prospective study	357	Colorectal resection	4 (1.1%)
Ruffo et al. [18]	Prospective study	436	Colorectal resection	5 (1.1%)
Dousset et al. [19]	Prospective study	100	Colorectal resection	2 (2.0%)
Belghiti et al. [42]	Prospective study	198	Colorectal resection	6 (3.0%)
Akladios et al. [8]	Retrospective study	41	Colorectal resection ($n = 6$) or disc excision ($n = 35$)	1 (2.4%)
Malzoni et al. [9]	Retrospective study	248	Colorectal resection	4 (1.6%)
Roman et al. [10]	Retrospective study	1135	Shaving, disc excision or colorectal resection	9 (0.8%)
Balla et al. [3]	Systematic review	3079	Colorectal resection	67 (2.1%)

Table 14.3 Prevalence of pelvic abscess in women undergoing surgery for rectosigmoid endometriosis

Authors	Study design	n	Type of surgery	Prevalence
Darai et al. [2]	Prospective study	40	Colorectal resection	1 (2.5%)
Minelli et al. [7]	Prospective study	357	Colorectal resection	3 (0.8%)
Akladios et al. [8]	Retrospective study	41	Colorectal resection ($n = 6$) or disc excision ($n = 35$)	1 (2.4%)
Malzoni et al. [9]	Retrospective study	248	Colorectal resection	2 (0.8%)
Roman et al. [10]	Retrospective study	1135	Shaving, disc excision or colorectal resection	39 (3.4%)
Balla et al. [3]	Systematic review	3079	Colorectal resection	16 (0.5%)
Boudy et al. [49]	Retrospective study	27	Hysterectomy + colorectal resection ($n = 15$) or disc excision ($n = 12$) + prevesical peritoneum interposition	3 (11.1%)

small), but in most cases resection of the anastomotic tract is required and followed by re-anastomosis (associated to protective ileostomy) or terminal colostomy with a re-anastomosis scheduled in the following months.

14.2.3 Pelvic Abscess

Prophylactic antibiotics and washing of the pelvis at the end of the procedure are routine after colorectal surgery for endometriosis. However, pelvic abscess occurs in 0.8–3.4% of patients with colorectal endometriosis treated by segmental resection (Table 14.3) [2, 3, 7–10]. A pelvic abscess is usually treated by second laparoscopy to clean up the abdominopelvic cavity and to place a drain. Less frequently, depending on the accessibility, percutaneous drainage under computed tomography or ultrasound guidance can be performed [6].

14.2.4 Anastomotic Stricture

Anastomotic stricture is a well-known complication of colorectal surgery. It may occur after the treatment of both benign and malignant disease [11–14]. A retrospective analysis of a prospectively collected database evaluated the incidence, risk factors, and treatment of colorectal anastomotic stenosis in 1643 patients who underwent rectosigmoid resection for endometriosis using the Negrar method (without the ligature of the inferior mesenteric artery at its origin and the mobilization of the splenic flexure) [15]. Stenosis was defined

as the lack of passage through the anastomosis of a 12-mm proctoscope. Symptomatic stenosis was defined as the presence of endoscopically confirmed stricture accompanied by at least two of the following symptoms: constipation, need to push, tenesmus, ribbon stools. One hundred and four (6.3%) patients had symptomatic stenosis. The stoma and history of pelvic surgery were the only significant predictors of anastomotic stenosis. Anastomotic strictures were always treated with endoscopic dilatation. Ninety patients (86.5%) underwent three endoscopic dilatations (Fig. 14.2). There was no recurrent stenosis at a 12-month follow-up.

14.2.5 Anastomotic/Suture Bleeding

Occurs in 0.1–1% of cases [16, 17] and is mostly represented in disc resection due to the "bite" of a stapler on the healthy mucosa beside the resected "half-moon" shaped anterior surface of the bowel. Nevertheless, also in segmental bowel resections performed by a circular stapler, bleeding may occur. Treatment is always feasible by the endoscopic placement of clips and local micro-injection of catecholamines (Fig. 14.3).

14.2.6 Other Complications

Several other complications may occur during surgery for bowel endometriosis. Ureteral damages occur in 0.5–3.7% of patients treated for rectosigmoid endometriosis [7, 8, 10, 18]. Urinary retention may occur in up to 20% of

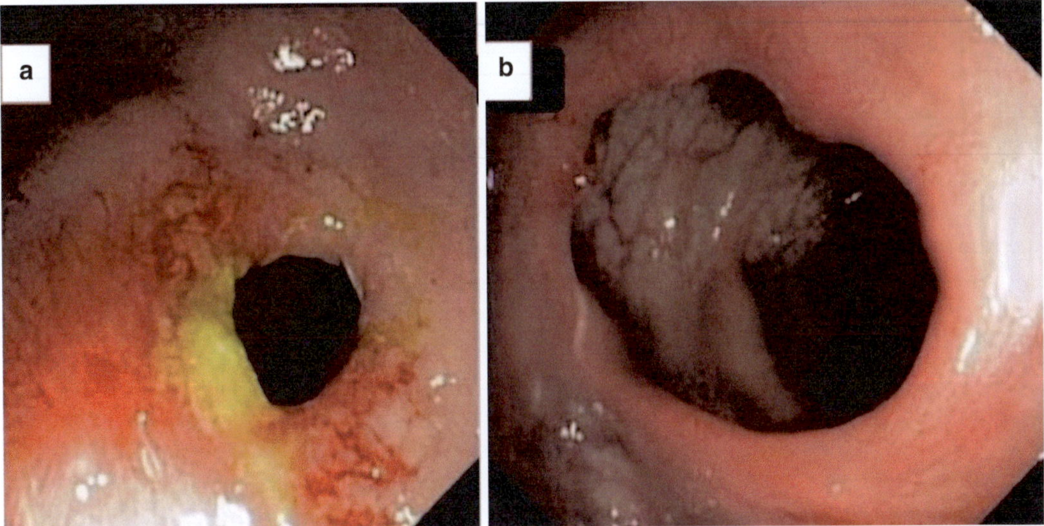

Fig. 14.2 Anastomotic stenosis before (**a**) and after (**b**) endoscopic dilatation

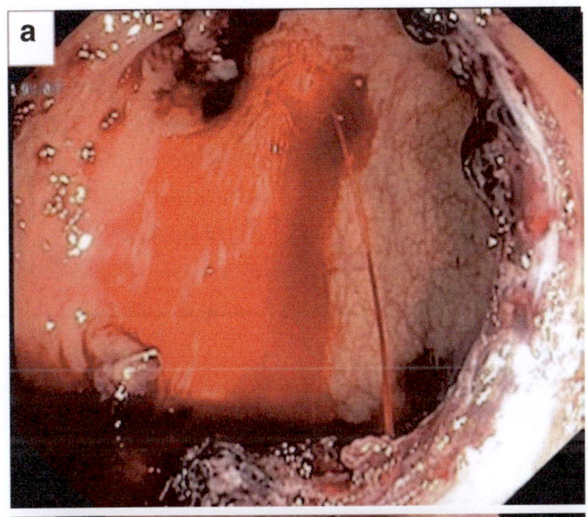

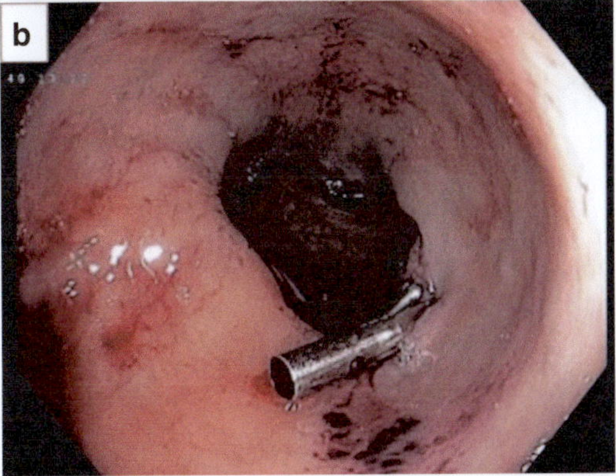

Fig. 14.3 Bleeding from a disc resection (**a**) and endo-clip placed in anastomosis bleeding after a segmental resection (**b**)

patients treated for rectosigmoid endometriosis [3, 7, 8, 18, 19]. Postoperative bleeding that may require second surgery occurs in 1.1–2.4% of patients treated for bowel endometriosis [3, 7, 8, 18, 19].

14.3 Surgical Factors Influencing the Risk of Short-Term Complications

In patients undergoing colorectal segmental resection, some intraoperative factors (such as ischemia and increased tension of the anastomosis) may affect the risk of anastomotic leakage.

14.3.1 Anastomosis Perfusion

The two margins of the bowel segments should have an adequate blood supply to perform a safe anastomosis. Oxygen is essential for intestinal anastomotic healing. Acute postoperative systemic hypoxia may occur following intestinal resection because of complications such as severe intraoperative blood loss, pneumonia, pulmonary edema, or acute respiratory distress syndrome. A study performed in Juvenile male Sprague-Dawley rats investigated the effects of hypoxia on anastomotic healing, showing that systemic hypoxia directly translates into local tissue hypoxia and impairment of anastomotic healing [20]. In agreement with these experimental findings, a prospective study including 55 patients with rectosigmoid cancer showed that blood flow reduction at the rectal stump is associated with an increased risk of anastomotic leak [21].

14.3.2 Anastomotic Tension

Tension at the anastomosis site may increase the risk of leakage. In the case of high-tension anastomosis, some surgeons perform intestinal mobilization even up to the splenic flexure [22–24]. This colonic mobilization may require ligation of the inferior mesenteric artery or its branches. In general, patients with bowel endometriosis do not require extensive resection; however, the importance of anastomotic tension may be considered in patients with a multifocal disease or previous bowel resections [25].

14.3.3 Use of Drain

The use of drain after colorectal surgery for endometriosis is a controversial issue [25]. The general purpose of a drain is to prevent the accumulation of blood and fluid in the pelvis. Furthermore, it may allow early detection of leaks of fecaloid or purulent material in the abdominal cavity. However, a randomized study suggested that the drain does not facilitate the early diagnosis of anastomotic complications [26]. Also, two randomized controlled studies showed that prophylactic pelvic drain after elec-

tive rectal or anal anastomosis increases the risk of abscess and fistula [27, 28].

14.3.4 Leak Tests

Anastomotic leakage must be tested during surgery by injecting air or liquid (usually methylene blue) into the rectosigmoid under pressure in a fluid-filled abdomen, while the bowel is occluded proximally to the anastomosis. An inadequate anastomosis is demonstrated by air or contrast leak. When the leakage is diagnosed intraoperatively, the surgeon can merely suture the anastomosis defect (Fig. 14.4), redo the anastomosis, or perform a protective defunctioning stoma. A study based on a prospective colorectal database investigated the value of anastomotic leak testing in left-sided colorectal anastomoses. Nine hundred ninety-eight colorectal anastomoses were performed without protective stoma [29]. Intraoperative air leaks were noted in 7.9% of the tested anastomoses. When the surgeon merely sutured the anastomotic defect that tested positive for air leakage, the anastomotic leakage rate after surgery was 12.2%. In contrast, no leakage occurred when the anastomosis was completely redone or when a protective stoma was made.

14.4 Surgical Strategies Used to Prevent Short-Term Complications

Several surgical procedures have been proposed to decrease the risk of short-term complications in patients undergoing treatment of colorectal endometriosis.

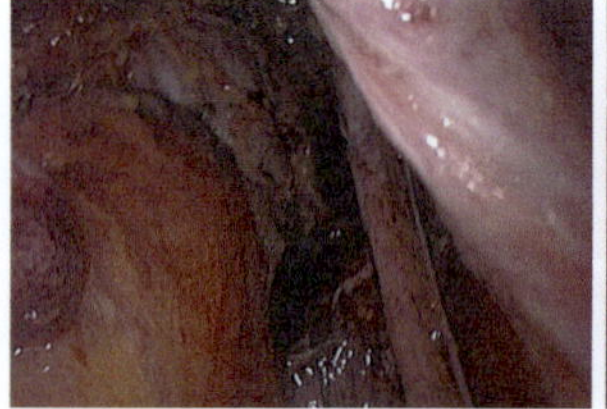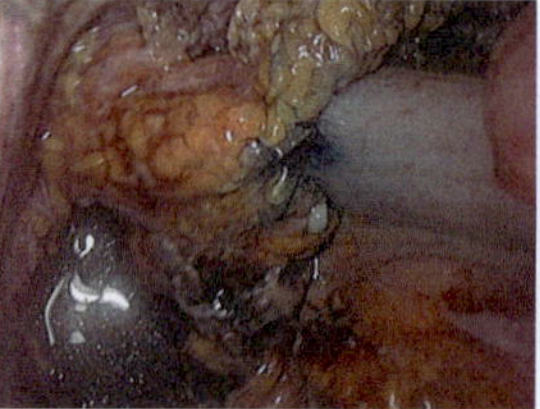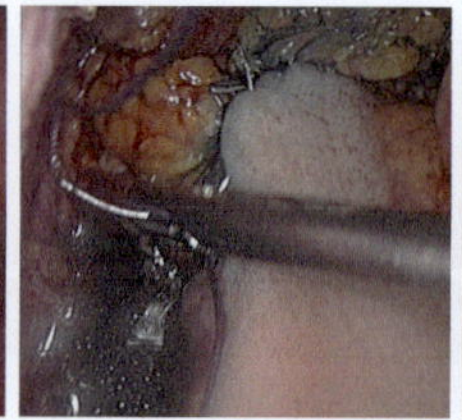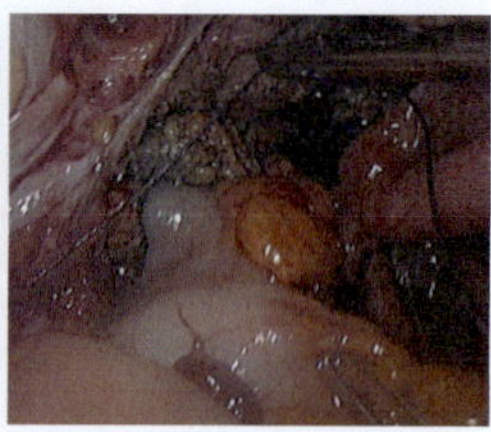

Fig. 14.4 Anastomotic leakage after laparoscopic rectosigmoid resection. Methylene blue is injected into the rectosigmoid under pressure. A leakage is diagnosed intraoperatively, and the anastomosis defect is sutured

14.4.1 Protective Defunctioning Stoma

A stoma involves the exteriorization of a loop of ileum or colon during a lapse of time considered necessary for the complete healing of colorectal sutures (Fig. 14.5). After approximately one week to 3 months from stoma creation, colorectal surgeons perform a second surgical procedure to close the stoma by bowel suture and a suture of the abdominal wall. The purpose of protective diverting ostomy is to decrease the amount of intestinal contents arriving at the area of anastomosis and to allow the patient to feed earlier. A stoma may be performed electively during surgery (primary stoma) or during second surgery performed because of postoperative complications such as a rectovaginal fistula (secondary stoma). The secondary stoma minimizes the impact of peritoneal sepsis following an anastomotic leak by diverting the fecal stream from a distal anastomosis. Several studies support the usefulness of stoma in patients managed for low rectal cancer (up to 5–7 cm above the anal verge) [30–32]. However, extrapolation of these data to women treated for rectosigmoid endometriosis is questionable. Patients with rectosigmoid endometriosis are younger than those treated for rectal cancer, their body mass index is usually low or normal [33], and they are more likely to undergo concomitant large resection of the vagina. Furthermore, a stoma may have a negative impact

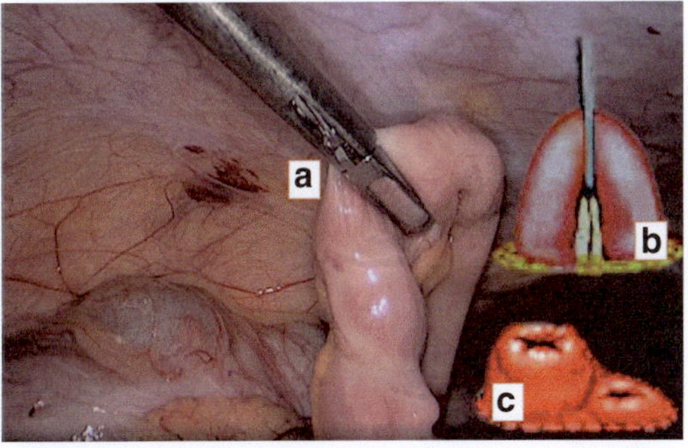

Fig. 14.5 Loop ileostomy. (A) Choosing of the ileal loop at about 30–60 cm from the ileocecal valve; (B) pulling up from a cutaneous wound of the chosen loop; (C) opening of the loop

on the quality of life (especially in body image and self-concept) [34], which may persist after the recanalization. Furthermore, in comparison with endometriosis, rectal resection to treat cancer is associated with a much higher leakage rate (which ranges from 2.8% to 15% in patients with multiple risk factors, such as diabetes and atherosclerosis) in particular after radiotherapy [35–41]. Finally, the need to perform a second surgical procedure may not be easily tolerated by young patients with a gynecological disease. The creation of a protective defunctioning stoma was recommended in all patients requiring partial colpectomy or multiple bowel resections after a preliminary study of laparoscopic colorectal resection, which showed that partial colpectomy was associated with an increased risk of rectovaginal fistula [2]. Subsequently, a French prospective cohort study evaluated the role of a protective defunctioning stoma on the occurrence of intestinal complications after colorectal resection for endometriosis [42]. The creation of a protective defunctioning stoma was recommended in patients requiring partial colpectomy or multiple bowel resections. Omentoplasty was performed when feasible in patients requiring colorectal resection and hysterectomy. One hundred ninety-eight patients were included in the study. Thirty-two percentage of the patients had vaginal endometriosis requiring partial colpectomy. Fifty-three patients (43%) had a protective defunctioning stoma (32 had a colostomy and 21 had an ileostomy). Eighty-four patients had low colorectal anastomosis and 11 patients had mid-colorectal anastomosis. There were 15 (7.5%) digestive tract complications: nine (4.5%) rectovaginal fistulas and six (3%) anastomotic leakages. This study confirmed that two factors are associated with the occurrence of rectovaginal fistula: partial colpectomy and low colorectal anastomosis. Eight of nine (89%) rectovaginal fistulas occurred in patients who underwent colpectomy and all occurred in patients with low colorectal anastomosis. Primary stoma decreased the number of rectovaginal fistulas in women undergoing partial colpectomy and low colorectal resection from 27% to 15%; the difference did not reach statistical significance, possibly because of the sample size. There was no anastomotic leakage in patients with a primary stoma. Six patients (3%) had anastomotic leakage with fever and infection; none of these patients had a primary stoma. No factors were associated with the occurrence of anastomotic leakage. Of 70 patients undergoing en bloc hysterectomy and colorectal resection, 26 (37%) had a low colorectal anastomosis. Thirty-one of the 70 patients (44%) underwent omentoplasty. Nine of the 31 patients (29%) had low colorectal anastomosis. The rate of rectovaginal fistula in patients undergoing en bloc hysterectomy and colorectal resection was similar in patients with and without omentoplasty (respectively, 6% and 5%). Of the 26 patients with low colorectal anastomosis, the rate of rectovaginal fistula in patients with and without omentoplasty was 22% and 12%, respectively ($p = 0.06$). The authors concluded that primary stoma is not necessary for patients with mid-colorectal anastomosis or low anastomosis without colpectomy. In contrast, it may decrease but not eliminate the risk of rectovaginal fistula in patients requiring both partial colpectomy and low colorectal anastomosis [42]. A retrospective study assessed the safety of laparoscopic resection for rectosigmoid endometriosis without primary stoma formation [8]. Forty-one patients were included in the study. Six patients (15%) underwent segmental resection, 21 patients (51%) underwent anterior disc resection of high rectal lesions (>10 cm from the anal verge) and 14 (34%) underwent anterior disc resection of low rectal lesions (<10 cm from the anal verge). There was one anastomotic leak (2.4%) diagnosed on day 4 in a patient with unprotected anastomosis at 6 cm from the anal margin. Four primary ileostomies were created in patients with ultralow anastomosis (<5 cm from the anal verge); one of these patients had postoperative stenosis necessitating early closure of the ileostomy and restoration of bowel continuity after only seven days from surgery. Protective defunctioning stoma carries some risks, such as hernia, stoma retraction, dehydration, prolapse, peristomal skin irritation, and necrosis. A retrospective study assessed the risk of complications related to the use of temporary diverting stoma (primary or secondary) in patients treated for colorectal endometriosis [43]. One hundred sixty-three women with a diverting stoma were included in the study, 158 (96.9%) had a primary stoma and five women (3.1%) with a postoperative bowel fistula had a secondary stoma. Stoma was performed on the ileum in 28 women (17.2%) and on the colon in 135 (82.8%). Colorectal endometriosis was treated by rectal shaving in two women (1.2%), disc excision in 62 (38%), colorectal resection in 87 (53.4%), and combined rectal disc excision and sigmoid colon segmental resection in 12 women with multifocal colorectal endometriosis (7.4%). Clavien–Dindo I stoma-related complications occurred in 23.3% of the patients; stoma scar required specific postoperative care due to subcutaneous infection, dehiscence, or delayed healing. Most Clavien–Dindo II complications were wound or urinary infections following stoma closure. Clavien–Dindo III complications occurred in 8.6% of the patients and were related to leakage, hemoperitoneum, hernia of the abdominal wall, subcutaneous abscess, and bowel obstruction syndrome. Also, the study showed that patients presenting with stoma-related complications were significantly older, had higher AFSr scores, and were more likely to be managed by segmental resection compared with women without stoma-related complications. Recently, Ferreira et al. described the use of ghost ileostomy in a patient undergoing segmental bowel resection for endometriosis [44]. This technique was previously used by general surgeons to prevent complications in patients submitted to low rectal resection [45]. Once the colorectal anastomosis is accomplished, the third from the last ileal loop is identified, and an opening is made in the related mesentery adjacent to the intestine. An elastic tape is passed around the ileal loop and out of the abdomen through a small hole in the right iliac fossa. It is then secured to a gauze pad to avoid intra-abdominal retraction. Given an uneventful postoperative outcome, the tape is simply cut, and the loop dropped back. If an anastomotic leak occurs, the ghost ileostomy is converted into a loop ileostomy by extracting the isolated loop through an adequate abdominal wall incision.

14.4.2 Omentoplasty

Omentoplasty is the transposition of a vascularized pedicle of the omentum to cover the sutures on the vaginal and intestinal walls (Fig. 14.6). Some surgeons believe that this procedure decreases the risk of rectovaginal fistula and anastomotic leak [19]. Theoretically, this technique may give two main benefits: re-enforcement of the anastomotic line during the first postoperative days (acting as a biologically viable plug which can seal microscopic leaks) and increased angiogenesis and neo-vascularization at the anastomotic site. In a prospective study including 100 women, laparotomic colorectal resection was systematically combined with omentoplasty and pelvic drainage [19]. All these patients had total mesorectal excision, including inferior mesenteric artery ligation. Primary ileostomy was performed in 96% of the patients. Anastomotic leakage occurred in 2% of the patients and rectovaginal fistula in 4% of the patients. A systematic review with meta-analysis, including three studies, investigated the use of omentoplasty in colorectal anastomosis [46]. It was found that there was no significant difference in anastomotic leak rate between patients treated with and without omentoplasty (5.0% vs. 8.4%). Also, omentoplasty may sometimes be a challenging procedure because of difficulties in releasing sufficient

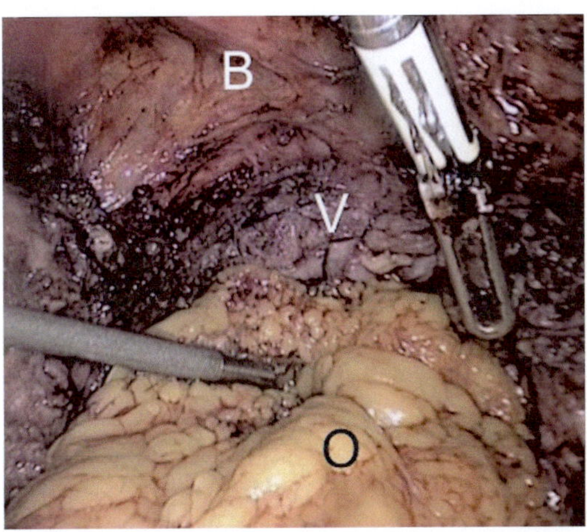

Fig. 14.6 Omental J-flap interposed between the vaginal cuff and the colorectal anastomosis. *V* vaginal suture, *B* bladder, *O* omental flap

omentum. Furthermore, a limitation of the omentoplasty is that it may be the source of adherence in the Douglas.

14.4.3 Mesorectal Flap Interposition

The mesorectum is a fatty lymphovascular structure surrounding the rectum, and it is wrapped by the perirectal fascia. The mesorectum begins at the rectosigmoid junction, where it blends with the connective tissue of the sigmoid mesentery and extends to the end of the rectum at the levator ani muscle. It encloses the rectum, and it is limited superficially by the mesorectal fascia. The mesorectum contains perirectal fat, the superior rectal artery and branches, superior rectal vein and tributaries, lymph nodes, and vessels. The mesorectum can be surgically separated from the rectum and preserved. Hanacek et al. described the interposition of a mesorectal flap in three women undergoing concomitant laparoscopic resection of vaginal and rectosigmoid endometriosis [47]. The mesorectal flap was constructed from the left mesorectum. The mesorectum was mobilized and cut at the level of the distal resection line of the rectum. This vascularized flap was rotated and inserted in between the sutures on the rectum and vagina. The flap was then fixed with an interrupted 2/0 polyglactin suture approximately 2 cm caudally to the vaginal closure. The three patients had no intestinal complications or rectovaginal fistula development. However, the limited data available on the use of mesorectal flap interposition do not allow us to draw a definitive conclusion on its usefulness in preventing short-term complications of patients treated for bowel endometriosis.

14.4.4 Prevesical Peritoneum Interposition

The prevesical peritoneum can be used to protect the vaginal suture in case of concomitant hysterectomy and colorectal resection for endometriosis [48]. This procedure is usually performed with two or three absorbable stitches placed on the posterior vaginal wall. If necessary, the prevesical peritoneum is dissected from the anterior vesical wall to facilitate its mobilization. This technique allows to completely isolate the vaginal suture from the intestinal anastomosis, thus theoretically limiting the risk of rectovaginal fistula. A recent retrospective study investigated the risk of rectovaginal fistula after en bloc hysterectomy and surgical treatment of rectosigmoid endometriosis using prevesical peritoneum interposition while avoiding systematic defunctioning stoma [49]. The study was based on a prospectively collected database, and it included 27 patients. The prevesical peritoneum was mobilized and then sutured to the posterior vaginal wall by absorbable stitches over the vaginal suture. Thus, the prevesical peritoneum was interposed between the vaginal and intestinal scars. Fifty-six percentage of the patients underwent segmental resection and 44% discoid excision. In this study, the only case of suspected rectovaginal fistulae was observed after rectal shaving associated with a segmental colorectal resection complicated by a pelvic abscess with subsequent vaginal dehiscence; no fistula was seen intraoperatively.

14.5 Conclusion

The complication rate is slightly lower in patients undergoing colorectal surgery for deep endometriosis than after bowel surgery for other indications [6, 50]. Bowel surgery in the context of endometriosis is different from that of cancer (no need for radical surgery on the mesorectum and colonic mesentery arteries, and young and healthy patients), and the indication for a protecting stoma even in low rectal resections (<5 cm), in the absence of other intraoperative risk factors, may be questioned. However, there is some evidence that primary stoma may be considered in patients with ultralow anastomosis (<5 cm from the anal verge) [8, 25]. Also, the primary stoma may be considered in patients requiring partial colpectomy that may decrease the risk of rectovaginal fistula [42]. When excising vaginal nodules, the excessive use of electrocoagulation may increase the risk of rectovaginal fistulae and

abscess, due to the risk of necrosis of the vaginal wall [6]. Other surgical techniques may decrease the risk of complications (rectovaginal fistula and anastomotic leakage) such as omentoplasty, mesorectal flap interposition, and prevesical peritoneum interposition in patients undergoing concomitant hysterectomy. However, the usefulness of these techniques is still a matter of debate. When complications occur, a timely diagnosis is necessary, although the clinical presentation may be not specific. A diagnostic delay is associated with increased morbidity, length of hospital stay, and, potentially, mortality.

References

1. Champagne BJ, McGee MF. Rectovaginal fistula. Surg Clin North Am. 2010;90(1):69–82; Table of Contents.
2. Darai E, Thomassin I, Barranger E, Detchev R, Cortez A, Houry S, et al. Feasibility and clinical outcome of laparoscopic colorectal resection for endometriosis. Am J Obstet Gynecol. 2005;192(2):394–400.
3. Balla A, Quaresima S, Subiela JD, Shalaby M, Petrella G, Sileri P. Outcomes after rectosigmoid resection for endometriosis: a systematic literature review. Int J Color Dis. 2018;33(7):835–47.
4. Zheng Y, Zhang N, Lu W, Zhang L, Gu S, Zhang Y, et al. Rectovaginal fistula following surgery for deep infiltrating endometriosis: does lesion size matter? J Int Med Res. 2018;46(2):852–64.
5. Trencheva K, Morrissey KP, Wells M, Mancuso CA, Lee SW, Sonoda T, et al. Identifying important predictors for anastomotic leak after colon and rectal resection: prospective study on 616 patients. Ann Surg. 2013;257(1):108–13.
6. Bouaziz J, Soriano D. Complications of colorectal resection for endometriosis. Minerva Ginecol. 2017;69(5):477–87.
7. Minelli L, Fanfani F, Fagotti A, Ruffo G, Ceccaroni M, Mereu L, et al. Laparoscopic colorectal resection for bowel endometriosis: feasibility, complications, and clinical outcome. Arch Surg. 2009;144(3):234–9; discussion 9.
8. Akladios C, Messori P, Faller E, Puga M, Afors K, Leroy J, et al. Is ileostomy always necessary following rectal resection for deep infiltrating endometriosis? J Minim Invasive Gynecol. 2015;22(1):103–9.
9. Malzoni M, Di Giovanni A, Exacoustos C, Lannino G, Capece R, Perone C, et al. Feasibility and safety of laparoscopic-assisted bowel segmental resection for deep infiltrating endometriosis: a retrospective cohort study with description of technique. J Minim Invasive Gynecol. 2016;23(4):512–25.
10. Roman H, Group F. A national snapshot of the surgical management of deep infiltrating endometriosis of

the rectum and colon in France in 2015: a multicenter series of 1135 cases. J Gynecol Obstet Hum Reprod. 2017;46(2):159–65.

11. Polese L, Vecchiato M, Frigo AC, Sarzo G, Cadrobbi R, Rizzato R, et al. Risk factors for colorectal anastomotic stenoses and their impact on quality of life: what are the lessons to learn? Color Dis. 2012;14(3):e124–8.

12. Ambrosetti P, Francis K, De Peyer R, Frossard JL. Colorectal anastomotic stenosis after elective laparoscopic sigmoidectomy for diverticular disease: a prospective evaluation of 68 patients. Dis Colon Rectum. 2008;51(9):1345–9.

13. Bannura GC, Cumsille MA, Barrera AE, Contreras JP, Melo CL, Soto DC. Predictive factors of stenosis after stapled colorectal anastomosis: prospective analysis of 179 consecutive patients. World J Surg. 2004;28(9):921–5.

14. Lee SY, Kim CH, Kim YJ, Kim HR. Anastomotic stricture after ultralow anterior resection or intersphincteric resection for very low-lying rectal cancer. Surg Endosc. 2018;32(2):660–6.

15. Bertocchi E, Barugola G, Benini M, Bocus P, Rossini R, Ceccaroni M, et al. Colorectal anastomotic stenosis: lessons learned after 1643 colorectal resections for deep infiltrating endometriosis. J Minim Invasive Gynecol. 2019;26(1):100–4.

16. Meuleman C, Tomassetti C, D'Hooghe TM. Clinical outcome after laparoscopic radical excision of endometriosis and laparoscopic segmental bowel resection. Curr Opin Obstet Gynecol. 2012;24(4):245–52.

17. Meuleman C, Tomassetti C, Wolthuis A, Van Cleynenbreugel B, Laenen A, Penninckx F, et al. Clinical outcome after radical excision of moderate-severe endometriosis with or without bowel resection and reanastomosis: a prospective cohort study. Ann Surg. 2014;259(3):522–31.

18. Ruffo G, Scopelliti F, Scioscia M, Ceccaroni M, Mainardi P, Minelli L. Laparoscopic colorectal resection for deep infiltrating endometriosis: analysis of 436 cases. Surg Endosc. 2010;24(1):63–7.

19. Dousset B, Leconte M, Borghese B, Millischer AE, Roseau G, Arkwright S, et al. Complete surgery for low rectal endometriosis: long-term results of a 100-case prospective study. Ann Surg. 2010;251(5):887–95.

20. Attard JA, Raval MJ, Martin GR, Kolb J, Afrouzian M, Buie WD, et al. The effects of systemic hypoxia on colon anastomotic healing: an animal model. Dis Colon Rectum. 2005;48(7):1460–70.

21. Vignali A, Gianotti L, Braga M, Radaelli G, Malvezzi L, Di Carlo V. Altered microperfusion at the rectal stump is predictive for rectal anastomotic leak. Dis Colon Rectum. 2000;43(1):76–82.

22. Thum-umnuaysuk S, Boonyapibal A, Geng YY, Pattana-Arun J. Lengthening of the colon for low rectal anastomosis in a cadaveric study: how much can we gain? Tech Coloproctol. 2013;17(4):377–81.

23. Gouvas N, Gogos-Pappas G, Tsimogiannis K, Agalianos C, Tsimoyiannis E, Dervenis C, et al. Impact of splenic flexure mobilization on short-term outcomes after laparoscopic left colectomy for colorectal cancer. Surg Laparosc Endosc Percutan Tech. 2014;24(5):470–4.

24. Kye BH, Kim HJ, Kim HS, Kim JG, Cho HM. How much colonic redundancy could be obtained by splenic flexure mobilization in laparoscopic anterior or low anterior resection? Int J Med Sci. 2014;11(9):857–62.

25. Oliveira MA, Pereira TR, Gilbert A, Tulandi T, de Oliveira HC, De Wilde RL. Bowel complications in endometriosis surgery. Best Pract Res Clin Obstet Gynaecol. 2016;35:51–62.

26. Johnson CD, Lamont PM, Orr N, Lennox M. Is a drain necessary after colonic anastomosis? J R Soc Med. 1989;82(11):661–4.

27. Merad F, Hay JM, Fingerhut A, Yahchouchi E, Laborde Y, Pelissier E, et al. Is prophylactic pelvic drainage useful after elective rectal or anal anastomosis? A multicenter controlled randomized trial. French Associations for Surgical Research. Surgery. 1999;125(5):529–35.

28. Merad F, Yahchouchi E, Hay JM, Fingerhut A, Laborde Y, Langlois-Zantain O. Prophylactic abdominal drainage after elective colonic resection and suprapromontory anastomosis: a multicenter study controlled by randomization. French Associations for Surgical Research. Arch Surg. 1998;133(3):309–14.

29. Ricciardi R, Roberts PL, Marcello PW, Hall JF, Read TE, Schoetz DJ. Anastomotic leak testing after colorectal resection: what are the data? Arch Surg. 2009;144(5):407–11. discussion 11–2

30. Matthiessen P, Hallbook O, Rutegard J, Simert G, Sjodahl R. Defunctioning stoma reduces symptomatic anastomotic leakage after low anterior resection of the rectum for cancer: a randomized multicenter trial. Ann Surg. 2007;246(2):207–14.

31. Shiomi A, Ito M, Maeda K, Kinugasa Y, Ota M, Yamaue H, et al. Effects of a diverting stoma on symptomatic anastomotic leakage after low anterior resection for rectal cancer: a propensity score matching analysis of 1,014 consecutive patients. J Am Coll Surg. 2015;220(2):186–94.

32. Gu WL, Wu SW. Meta-analysis of defunctioning stoma in low anterior resection with total mesorectal excision for rectal cancer: evidence based on thirteen studies. World J Surg Oncol. 2015;13:9.

33. Ferrero S, Anserini P, Remorgida V, Ragni N. Body mass index in endometriosis. Eur J Obstet Gynecol Reprod Biol. 2005;121(1):94–8.

34. Siassi M, Hohenberger W, Losel F, Weiss M. Quality of life and patient's expectations after closure of a temporary stoma. Int J Color Dis. 2008;23(12):1207–12.

35. Pakkastie TE, Luukkonen PE, Jarvinen HJ. Anastomotic leakage after anterior resection of the rectum. Eur J Surg. 1994;160(5):293–7. discussion 9–300

36. Grabham JA, Moran BJ, Lane RH. Defunctioning colostomy for low anterior resection: a selective approach. Br J Surg. 1995;82(10):1331–2.

37. Morino M, Parini U, Giraudo G, Salval M, Brachet Contul R, Garrone C. Laparoscopic total mesorectal excision: a consecutive series of 100 patients. Ann Surg. 2003;237(3):335–42.

38. Nesbakken A, Nygaard K, Lunde OC, Blucher J, Gjertsen O, Dullerud R. Anastomotic leak following mesorectal excision for rectal cancer: true incidence and diagnostic challenges. Color Dis. 2005;7(6):576–81.

39. Eckmann C, Kujath P, Schiedeck TH, Shekarriz H, Bruch HP. Anastomotic leakage following low anterior resection: results of a standardized diagnostic and therapeutic approach. Int J Color Dis. 2004;19(2):128–33.

40. Leroy J, Jamali F, Forbes L, Smith M, Rubino F, Mutter D, et al. Laparoscopic total mesorectal excision (TME) for rectal cancer surgery: long-term outcomes. Surg Endosc. 2004;18(2):281–9.

41. Sartori CA, Dal Pozzo A, Franzato B, Balduino M, Sartori A, Baiocchi GL. Laparoscopic total mesorectal excision for rectal cancer: experience of a single center with a series of 174 patients. Surg Endosc. 2011;25(2):508–14.

42. Belghiti J, Ballester M, Zilberman S, Thomin A, Zacharopoulou C, Bazot M, et al. Role of protective defunctioning stoma in colorectal resection for endometriosis. J Minim Invasive Gynecol. 2014;21(3):472–9.

43. Bonin E, Bridoux V, Chati R, Kermiche S, Coget J, Tuech JJ, et al. Diverting stoma-related complications following colorectal endometriosis surgery: a 163-patient cohort. Eur J Obstet Gynecol Reprod Biol. 2019;232:46–53.

44. Ferreira H, Smith AV, Vilaca J. Ghost ileostomy in anterior resection for bowel endometriosis: technical description. J Minim Invasive Gynecol. 2019;2019:S1553-4650(19)31180-X.

45. Miccini M, Amore Bonapasta S, Gregori M, Barillari P, Tocchi A. Ghost ileostomy: real and potential advantages. Am J Surg. 2010;200(4):e55–7.

46. Wiggins T, Markar SR, Arya S, Hanna GB. Anastomotic reinforcement with omentoplasty following gastrointestinal anastomosis: a systematic review and meta-analysis. Surg Oncol. 2015;24(3):181–6.

47. Hanacek J, Havluj L, Drahonovsky J, Urbankova I, Krepelka P, Feyereisl J. Interposition of the mesorectal flap as prevention of rectovaginal fistula in patients with endometriosis. Int Urogynecol J. 2019;30(12):2195–8.

48. Vesale E, Boudy AS, Zilberman S, Bendifallah S, Ileko A, Darai E. Rectovaginal fistula prevention after enbloc colorectal resection and hysterectomy for deep endometriosis. Gynecol Obstet Fertil Senol. 2019;47(4):378–80.

49. Boudy AS, Vesale E, Arfi A, Owen C, Jayot A, Zilberman S, et al. Prevesical peritoneum interposition to prevent risk of rectovaginal fistula after en bloc colorectal resection with hysterectomy for endometriosis: results of a pilot study. J Gynecol Obstet Hum Reprod. 2020;49(2):101649.

50. Darai E, Ackerman G, Bazot M, Rouzier R, Dubernard G. Laparoscopic segmental colorectal resection for endometriosis: limits and complications. Surg Endosc. 2007;21(9):1572–7.

51. Lim PC, Kang E, Park do H. Robot-assisted total intracorporeal low anterior resection with primary anastomosis and radical dissection for treatment of stage IV endometriosis with bowel involvement: morbidity and its outcome. J Robot Surg. 2011;5(4):273–8.

52. Ercoli A, D'Asta M, Fagotti A, Fanfani F, Romano F, Baldazzi G, et al. Robotic treatment of colorectal endometriosis: technique, feasibility and short-term results. Hum Reprod. 2012;27(3):722–6.

53. Neme RM, Schraibman V, Okazaki S, Maccapani G, Chen WJ, Domit CD, et al. Deep infiltrating colorectal endometriosis treated with robotic-assisted rectosigmoidectomy. JSLS. 2013;17(2):227–34.

54. Morelli L, Perutelli A, Palmeri M, Guadagni S, Mariniello MD, Di Franco G, et al. Robot-assisted surgery for the radical treatment of deep infiltrating endometriosis with colorectal involvement: short- and mid-term surgical and functional outcomes. Int J Color Dis. 2016;31(3):643–52.

55. Ercoli A, Bassi E, Ferrari S, Surico D, Fagotti A, Fanfani F, et al. Robotic-assisted conservative excision of retrocervical-rectal deep infiltrating endometriosis: a case series. J Minim Invasive Gynecol. 2017;24(5):863–8.

56. Graham A, Chen S, Skancke M, Moawad G, Obias V. A review of deep infiltrative colorectal endometriosis treated robotically at a single institution. Int J Med Robot. 2019;15(4):e2001.

Long-Term Follow-Up of Patients Undergoing Surgical Treatment of Bowel Endometriosis

Basma Darwish, Benjamin Merlot, Isabella Chanavaz-Lacheray, Myriam Noailles, Damien Forestier, and Horace Roman

15.1 Introduction

Surgical treatment involved in the management of Deep infiltrating Endometriosis of the Bowel may be classified into those involving a radical approach described by a segmental resection of the involved bowel followed by intestinal anastomosis, or a conservative approach where the bowel nodule is either removed by disc excision or shaving [1–4].

Surgery is often considered the best management option in women with symptomatic bowel endometriosis. However, only a few RCTs have been conducted on the effect of surgery for symptomatic disease, and long-term outcomes are poorly defined.

Outcomes of surgery are related to postoperative complications [5, 6], functional outcomes and recurrence of DIER [7–9].

B. Darwish
Department of Gynecology, Bahrain Defense Force Hospital, Riffa, Bahrain

B. Merlot · I. Chanavaz-Lacheray · M. Noailles
D. Forestier
Endometriosis Center, Clinique Tivoli-Ducos, Bordeaux, France

H. Roman (✉)
Endometriosis Center, Clinique Tivoli-Ducos, Bordeaux, France

Aarhus Medical University, Aarhus, Denmark

15.1.1 Postoperative Functional Outcomes

15.1.1.1 Conservative Versus Radical Surgical Treatment

Adopting a conservative approach to the surgical management of deep endometriosis infiltrating the rectum, by employing shaving or disc excision, appears to yield improved digestive functional outcomes. However, data available in literature includes comparative studies that were not randomized, and thus introduces a possible bias regarding the presumed superiority of conservative techniques due to the inclusion of patients with more severe deep endometriosis who underwent colorectal resection.

In our 2-arm randomized trial, ENDORE [1], which enrolled 60 patients with deep endometriosis infiltrating the rectum up to 15 cm from the anus, measuring more than 20 mm in length, involving at least the muscular layer in depth and up to 50% of rectal circumference, the study aimed at comparing functional outcomes following conservative versus radical treatment of large deep infiltrating endometriosis of the rectum in terms of constipation (1 stool/>5 consecutive days), frequent bowel movements (≥3 stools/day), defecation pain, anal incontinence, dysuria or bladder atony requiring self-catheterization 24 months (2 years) postoperatively [1]. It also evaluated the Visual Analog Scale (VAS), Knowles–Eccersley–Scott-Symptom Questionnaire (KESS), the

© Springer Nature Switzerland AG 2020
S. Ferrero, M. Ceccaroni (eds.), *Clinical Management of Bowel Endometriosis*,
https://doi.org/10.1007/978-3-030-50446-5_15

Gastrointestinal Quality of Life Index (GIQLI), the Wexner scale, the Urinary Symptom Profile (USP) and the Short Form 36 Health Survey (SF36) as secondary endpoints. Recently, a 5-year assessment in only 55 women managed in Rouen, using the same endpoints was reported by the same team [10].

Although previous case series and comparative observational studies suggested better overall functional outcomes following conservative surgery, our trial did not show a statistically significant superiority of conservative surgery for midterm functional digestive and urinary outcomes in this specific population of women with large involvement of the rectum [1, 11].The differences between the frequencies of functional symptoms composing the primary endpoint, as well as the values of GIQLI, KESS, and SF36 scores in the two arms suggest that the functional outcomes of the two surgical approaches are very close. (Table 15.1) The improvement becomes significant 6 months after the surgery, then it appears stable during at least 5 years after the surgery (Table 15.2).

However, exhaustive assessment of overall digestive function using standardized questionnaires showed that complete removal of large deep endometriosis infiltrating the rectum does not guarantee relief from digestive complaints 1 year after the surgery, whatever the surgical technique used [12, 13]. In the ENDORE trial, the presumption that on average half of all patients managed by segmental resection would report significant abnormal postoperative bowel function, was confirmed. Conversely, the hypothesis that conservative surgery would result in much better functional outcomes when compared to radical surgery was not proven. The presumption was based on a small number of retrospective case series which reported data on postoperative functional outcomes. However, these retrospective studies may have compared patients with more severe disease managed by colorectal resection and patients with smaller digestive nodules managed by shaving. This unbalanced distribution may have pointed to better postoperative outcomes in patients managed conservatively. Removal of deep rectal nodules

by shaving or disc excision does preserve the mesorectum, rectal vascularization and nerves, as the procedure exclusively concerns the anterior rectal wall and does not modify the overall length of the rectum. However, this did not have a major positive impact on postoperative rectal function, when compared to colorectal resection. Several explanations might be considered. Deep endometriosis infiltrating the rectum may also involve uterosacral ligaments, vagina, parametrium, inferior hypogastric plexus and splanchnic nerves. Complete resection of large endometriosis lesions may induce postoperative dysfunction of vegetative nerves [14–18]. Despite the employment of nerve-sparing techniques [19], it is obvious that inferior hypogastric plexus and splanchnic nerves may be altered by either the disease or iatrogenically by the surgeon, resulting in various concerns with bowel and bladder function or vaginal dryness [17]. Furthermore, recent studies have shown that patients with colorectal endometriosis may preoperatively present with rectal or bladder dysfunction [20], i.e., anal and urethral sphincter hypertonia, and these troubles may be irreversible and not restored by removal of nodules. Moreover, the present data suggest that in patients presenting with deep colorectal endometriosis, microscopically complete excision of rectal endometriosis may be unachievable because of bowel occult microscopic endometriosis implants located far from macroscopic nodules [21, 22]. Bowel occult microscopic endometriosis was found in 14.6% of specimen resection margins. No impact on either pelvic or digestive symptoms was observed after 1-year follow-up postoperatively [23].

15.1.1.2 Functional Outcomes Following Rectal Surgery for Endometriosis

Surgical management of rectal endometriosis whatever the technique employed is followed by improvement in standardized gastrointestinal, urinary and quality of life scores, as early as 6 months after surgery. No further significant improvement was then observed from 6 to 24 months postoperatively [10].

Table 15.1 Clinical assessment 5 years after surgery

Parameter	Conservative surgery ($n = 27$)	Radical surgery ($n = 28$)	P
Rectal nodule recurrence	1 (3.7%)	0	1
Assessment of digestive and urinary function			
Patients presenting primary outcome	12 (44.4%)	17 (60.7%)	0.29
Digestive symptoms:			
< =than 1 stool/5 days	4 (14.8%)	3 (11.1%)	1
Defecation pain	6 (22.2%)	8 (29.6%)	0.76
> = 3 stools/day	5 (18.5%)	8 (29.6%)	0.53
Involuntary gas or stool loss	2 (7.4%)	5 (18.5%)	0.42
GIQLI score	119 (99–130)	116 (97–126)	0.67
KESS score	10 (6–15)	7.5 (4–15)	0.65
Wexner score	0 (0–1)	0 (0–2)	0.98
How long are you able to defer defecation?			0.86
<5 min	6 (23.1%)	5 (19.2%)	
5–10 min	6 (23.1%)	6 (23.1%)	
10–15 min	1 (3.9%)	3 (11.5%)	
>15 min	13 (50%)	13 (50%)	
USP of dysuria	0 (0–1)	0 (0–0)	0.39
Bladder self-catheterization	0	0	1
Short Form 36 Health Survey score:			
Physical functioning	95 (85–100)	95 (85–100)	0.99
Physical role functioning	100 (50–100)	100 (50–100)	0.82
Bodily pain	84 (58–100)	85 (45–90)	0.44
General health perceptions	63 (46–83)	63 (38–75)	0.18
Vitality	63 (30–75)	55 (30–60)	0.18
Social functioning	75 (50–100)	88 (75–100)	0.48
Emotional role functioning	100 (67–100)	100 (67–100)	0.90
Mental health	74 (56–80)	68 (56–76)	0.63
Physical Score	85 (61–95)	82 (63–91)	0.32
Mental Score	72 (61–90)	76 (58–83)	0.66
Do you consider your bowel movements as being normal?			1
No	12 (44.4%)	13 (46.4%)	
Yes	15 (55.6%)	15 (53.6%)	
Assessment of postoperative pelvic pain			
Patients with menstruation during preceding 6 months	9 (33%)	15 (45%)	0.77
Among whom, patients with dysmenorrhoea	4/9 (44%)	8/15 (53%)	1.00
VAS of dysmenorrhoea	3 (2–4)	4 (3–6)	0.86
Months until first recurrence of dysmenorrhoea	12 (5–18)	10 (4–18)	1.00
Patients having sexual intercourse after surgery during preceding 6 months	24 (89%)	32 (97%)	0.32
Among whom, patients with dyspareunia	8/24 (33%)	9/32 (28%)	0.77
VAS of dyspareunia	4 (3–6)	4 (3–7)	1.00
Patients with intermenstrual pelvic pain during preceding 6 months	6 (22%)	10 (3%)	0.57
VAS of intermenstrual pelvic pain	4 (3–5)	4 (3–6)	0.83

Published in Hum Reprod 2019;34(12):2362–2371. doi:https://doi.org/10.1093/humrep/dez217. Under Open Access License

Data are *n*(%) or median (Q1–Q3); *GIQLI* Gastrointestinal Quality of Life Index, *KESS* Knowles-Eccersley-Scott-Symptom, *USP* Urinary Symptom Profile Score, *VAS* Visual Analogue Scale

Table 15.2 Evolution of gastrointestinal and QOL scores during the 5 year-follow up

	Baseline			1-year assessment			2-year assessment			3-year assessment			4-year assessment			5-year assessment			Trends		
	CS ($n = 27$)	RS ($n = 28$)	P	CS ($n = 27$)	RS ($n = 28$)	P	CS ($n = 27$)	RS ($n = 28$)	P	CS ($n = 27$)	RS ($n = 28$)	P	CS ($n = 27$)	RS ($n = 28$)	P	CS ($n = 27$)	RS ($n = 28$)	P	$P*$	$P**$	$P***$
GICQLI Score	89 (82–105)	94 (87–108)	0.40	116 (105–127)	119 (102–127)	0.59	111 (97–135)	121 (99–128)	0.72	113 (98–125)	118 (96–126)	0.71	109 (93–131)	112 (96–122)	0.90	119 (99–130)	116 (97–126)	0.67	<0.001	<0.001	0.36
KESS Score	14 (9–18)	10 (7–18)	0.26	9 (5–15)	9 (6–18)	0.47	10 (5–15)	9 (5–17)	0.97	10 (6–14)	9 (6–18)	0.88	90.5 (6–17)	9 (6–16)	0.96	10 (6–15)	7.5 (4–15)	0.65	0.006	0.64	0.18
WEXNER Score	0 (0–3)	0 (0–4)	.46	0 (0–1)	0 (0–0.5)	.59	0 (0–1)	0 (0–2)	.55	0 (0–1)	0 (0–1)	.83	0 (0–1)	0 (0–1)	.38	0 (0–1)	0 (0–2)	0.98	0.26	0.022	0.39
USP of dysuria	0 (0–2.5)	0 (0–1.5)	0.25	0 (0–1)	0 (0–0)	0.26	0 (0–1)	0 (0–0)	0.12	0 (0–1)	0 (0–0)	0.19	0 (0–1)	0 (0–0)	0.05	0 (0–1)	0 (0–0)	0.34	0.39	0.09	0.73
Short Form 36 Health Survey Score	52 (44–67)	49 (41–62)	0.60	84 (63–91)	74 (64–87)	0.34	87 (70–92)	80 (63–84)	0.24	73 (56–88)	71 (60–84)	0.75	75 (57–88)	72 (57–83)	0.41	72 (61–90)	79 (61–86)	0.60	<0.001	<0.001	0.97
Physical functioning	80 (55–90)	85 (63–95)	0.55	95 (85–100)	90 (83–100)	0.53	95 (90–100)	95 (83–100)	0.89	95 (90–100)	100 (83–100)	0.90	95 (85–100)	95 (80–100)	0.53	95 (85–100)	95 (85–100)	0.99	0.01	0.034	0.94
Physical role functioning	38 (0–75)	50 (13–75)	0.72	100 (50–100)	100 (63–100)	0.79	100 (75–100)	100 (88–100)	0.62	100 (50–100)	100 (50–100)	0.67	100 (50–100)	75 (50–100)	0.53	100 (50–100)	100 (50–100)	0.82	0.001	0.003	0.96
Bodily pain	41 (32–51)	51 (32–62)	0.31	79 (62–100)	74 (51–92)	0.36	84 (62–100)	74 (61–92)	0.23	73 (45–100)	76 (56–90)	0.96	83 (68–100)	78 (45–90)	0.44	84 (58–100)	85 (45–90)	0.44	<0.001	0.001	0.86
General health perceptions	65 (47–80)	60 (42–70)	0.28	77 (62–87)	72 (52–85)	0.22	75 (57–90)	67 (50–82)	0.33	65 (46–79)	63 (40–73)	0.64	63 (46–83)	58 (46–75)	0.26	63 (46–83)	63 (38–75)	0.18	0.007	0.14	0.85
Vitality	38 (30–60)	35 (20–45)	0.09	63 (45–75)	55 (35–70)	0.29	60 (40–75)	50 (43–63)	0.38	45 (30–70)	55 (30–68)	0.76	48 (30–80)	50 (25–65)	0.41	63 (30–75)	55 (30–60)	0.18	0.004	<0.001	0.47
Social functioning	56 (50–75)	56 (50–63)	0.33	100 (75–100)	88 (63–100)	0.12	100 (75–100)	75 (63–100)	0.21	88 (63–100)	75 (50–94)	0.33	88 (75–100)	75 (50–100)	0.08	75 (50–100)	88 (75–100)	0.48	0.015	<0.001	0.17
Emotional role functioning	67 (0–100)	33 (0–67)	0.61	100 (67–100)	100 (83–100)	0.93	100 (67–100)	100 (67–100)	0.67	100 (33–100)	100 (50–100)	0.83	100 (33–100)	100 (67–100)	0.76	100 (67–100)	100 (67–100)	0.90	0.14	<0.001	0.82
Mental health	46 (36–60)	48 (34–60)	0.77	80 (60–88)	64 (52–76)	0.10	76 (60–88)	64 (56–76)	0.18	68 (48–80)	64 (48–78)	0.99	68 (44–84)	68 (56–76)	0.48	74 (56–80)	68 (56–76)	0.63	<0.001	<0.001	0.48

Physical Score	60 (49–65)	58 (41–71)	0.88	86 (57–94)	80 (62–94)	0.73	90 (75–96)	85 (73–91)	0.34	84 (53–93)	81 (58–88)	0.58	79 (62–94)	71 (61–89)	0.33	85 (61–95)	82 (63–91)	0.32	<0.001	0.006	0.99
Mental Score	48 (34–68)	48 (30–58)	0.29	85 (60–91)	73 (59–86)	0.22	81 (68–90)	75 (58–80)	0.29	68 (42–86)	68 (50–81)	0.86	73 (51–91)	72 (54–79)	0.42	72 (61–90)	76 (58–83)	0.66	0.003	<0.001	0.55
How long are you able to defer defecation?			0.07			0.57			0.87			0.14			0.77			0.86	0.51	0.79	0.25
<5 min	6 (22.2%)	1 (3.6%)		2 (7.7%)	4 (14.3%)		5 (19%)	6 (18 %)		2 (7.7%)	7 (25.9%)		4 (15.4%)	5 (20%)		6 (23.1%)	5 (19.2 %)				
5–10 min	6 (22.2%)	8 (28.6%)		8 (30.8%)	8 (28.6%)		4 (15 %)	8 (24 %)		8 (30.8%)	6 (22.2%)		5 (19.2%)	4 (16%)		6 (23.1 %)	6 (23.1 %)				
10–15 min	4 (14.8%)	1 (3.6%)		0 (0%)	2 (7.1%)		3 (11 %)	4 (12 %)		1 (3.9%)	4 (14.8%)		1 (3.9%)	3 (12%)		1 (3.9 %)	3 (11.5 %)				
>15 min	11 (41%)	18 (64%)		16 (61.5%)	14 (50%)		15 (56%)	15 (45%)		15 (58%)	10 (37%)		16 (61.5%)	13 (52%)		13 (50%)	13 (50%)				
"Do you consider your bowel movements as being normal?"			–	–					0.78			0.78			0.26			1.0	<0.001	<0.001	0.39
No	27 (100%)	28 (100%)		–	–	–	10 (37%)	12 (42.9%)		12 (44%)	14 (50%)		12 (40%)	18 (64%)		12 (44.4%)	13 (46.4%)				
Yes	0	0		–	–	–	17 (63%)	16 (57.1%)		15 (56%)	14 (50%)		15 (60%)	10 (49%)		15 (55.6%)	15 (53.6%)				

The results are expressed as Median value (Q1–Q3) and *N* (%); *CS* conservative surgery, *RS* radical surgery. *P value of the trend of score related to conservative surgery, including baseline values;**P value of the trend of scores related to radical surgery, including baseline values; ***P value of the comparison of trends related to respectively conservative and radical surgery, including baseline values
value—including baseline (excluding baseline)

The ENDORE study showed an immediate and significant postoperative improvement in the scores used to assess main and secondary endpoints, which remained stable for up to 24 months (except for the constipation score). Both the overall and the gastrointestinal quality of life scores (SF36 and GIQLI) improved significantly within 6 months after surgery. Anal continence (Wexner score) also improved, and pelvic pain related to endometriosis (Biberoglou & Behrman score) was significantly reduced. Other authors reported similar trends in patients managed by colorectal resection for deep endometriosis by the open route [24].

The trial also demonstrated that severe baseline constipation increases the likelihood of postoperative abnormal bowel movements. Conversely, constipation may be impaired from 6 to 24 months. This observation may be related to preoperative injuries of splanchnic nerves and inferior hypogastric plexus, which are not relieved by endometriotic nodules removal. Patients should receive this information prior to surgery for rectal endometriosis. Moreover, it may be useful in the decision of the shared therapeutic choice.

In previous retrospective studies, we observed that surgery for rectal endometriosis may not significantly improve baseline constipation, regardless of the surgical technique used, i.e., rectal shaving [25, 26], disc excision [27], or colorectal resection [28]. This information should be discussed preoperatively, particularly with patients for whom constipation is one of the symptoms indicating surgery. The mechanism of this symptom may be multifactorial. Constipation by slow stool progression through the left colon and rectum may be a result of the dysfunction of splanchnic nerves and inferior hypogastric plexus, by either deep endometriosis or excessively radical surgery [7, 14, 15, 17, 18]. Despite the use of nerve-sparing techniques [19], the function of the inferior hypogastric plexus and splanchnic nerves may not be systematically preserved, resulting in bowel and bladder function discomfort [17]. This is most likely when patients with colorectal endometriosis present preoperatively with rectal or bladder dysfunction [20], i.e., anal and urethral sphincter hypertonia, which may bear witness to irreversible nerve dysfunction.

15.1.2 Postoperative Complications

Surgery of the DIER may be challenging, and Clavien–Dindo 3 postoperative complications may involve up to 27% of patients [1] However, it may be emphasized that postoperative complications do not negatively impact on neither 1 year-outcomes [29] nor postoperative pregnancy rate [11, 30]. Thus, the fear of postoperative complications should not balance the expected benefit in terms of pelvic pain, bowel movements, quality of life, and ability to conceive [29]. Studies have revealed a higher risk of rectovaginal fistula and leakage in women managed by colorectal resection when compared to those receiving shaving [27]. Bowel stenosis might be more frequent following colorectal resection, as it is more likely to occur after circular colorectal anastomosis [1, 31] than after semicircular disc excision or shaving, and sometimes linked to the inflammatory status of the pelvis.

15.1.3 Recurrence

In a systematic review and meta-analysis focusing on the likelihood of recurrence comparing three-surgical approaches for DE with colorectal involvement i.e., rectal shaving, discoid resection, and segmental colorectal resection, when comparing the recurrence rate independently to the recurrence diagnosis based on clinical examination, imaging or histology, no significant differences are shown between the three groups. Considering histologically proven recurrences, a recent meta-analysis found that the risk of recurrence is significantly higher after rectal shaving compared to both segmental resection (RR 4.76, 95% CI: 2.16–10.49, I2 = 0%) and disc excision (RR 3.81, 95% CI 1.27–11.43, I2 = 0%) [32].

In the ENDORE randomized trial, overall 5 year-recurrence rate of 1.8% demonstrates that surgical removal of the DIER is a valid procedure with excellent long-term remission. Furthermore, recurrence rates were comparable between the conservative and radical surgery arms (3.7% vs. 0%) (P = 1). In the literature, the main argument supporting the radical approach in DIER is the presumed excess of recurrence after conservative procedures [8]. Meta-analysis as well as the only randomized trial demonstrates that this argument is not valid, at least during the first 5 years after the procedure. Furthermore, 25 bowel resections have to be performed in order to prevent a single bowel resection for recurrence following rectal shaving [28].

Risk factors of recurrence after endometriosis surgery are still unclear. Indeed, Guo et al. [33] and Bozdag et al. [34], based on two reviews highlighted those are often conflicting. In details, it appears that young age at the time of surgery, left-sided lesions, high rAFS score, the size of the cysts, important preoperative pain, the absence of pregnancy or a preoperative medical treatment and the radicality of the surgery appears to be main risk factors for recurrence. In this specific setting, specific risk of colorectal recurrence is a major issue and data are lacking [32].

It should be emphasized that the interpretation of recurrence data may be misled by the inappropriate choice of surgical technique: a poor indication of rectal shaving increases the risk of recurrence, hence the wide range of reported recurrence. No data is available on the treatment of bowel endometriosis, but experience shows that revision surgeries are complex because of loss of dissection planes resulting in greater risk of complication. Therefore, the best surgical technique should be chosen initially in order to decrease the risk of recurrence, taking into consideration the patient's age and thus time of exposure to recurrence. Moreover, in case of recurrence, medical management versus revision surgery should be considered as an option. In conclusion, the long-term follow-up of patients included in the randomized trial ENDORE will further be able to add an idea of the recurrence rate between conservative and radical techniques.

15.1.4 Fertility

Surgical management for rectal endometriosis is followed by high pregnancy rates, with a majority of natural conceptions [11] Surgical management enables natural conception in women with deep endometriosis of the rectum, for whom the likelihood of preoperative conception is not found to exceed 13% [35, 36] Several studies have focused on postoperative fertility outcomes in women managed for colorectal endometriosis. In a recent review of series of patients presenting with bowel involvement, exclusively managed by colorectal resection (n = 1320), the postoperative rates of natural conception and overall conception were 28.6% (95% CI: 25–32.3) and 46.9% (95% CI: 42.9–50.9), respectively [37]. In a prospective trial [38] conducted in patients having undergone colorectal resection for deep endometriosis, the postoperative rates of natural conception, overall conception and ART induced conception were 24% (13/54), 50% (27/54), and 26% (14/54). In our database, 65% of patients operated for associated colorectal endometriosis and ovarian endometriomas conceived after surgery and 60% of these pregnancies were natural [36]. We previously estimated that ~74.5% of pregnancies occurred during the first 3 years after surgery [36].

In ENDORE randomized trial which enrolled patients with deep endometriosis infiltrating the rectum, 81% of them were able to get pregnant, 59% of which were natural conceptions. The probabilities of achieving pregnancy at 12, 24, 36, and 48 months postoperatively were 33.4% (95% CI: 20.6–51.3%), 60.6% (44.8–76.8%), 77% (61.5–89.6%), and 86.8% (72.8–95.8%) respectively [1]. Furthermore, in women with preoperative proven infertility, pregnancy rate was 75% with a majority of natural conceptions. Skilled surgical management for symptomatic large deep endometriosis nodules infiltrating the rectum in young women is followed by a high pregnancy rate at least 4 years after surgery.

15.2 Conclusion

Long-term postoperative functional outcomes, pain improvement and recurrence rates are comparable between radical and conservative techniques employed to treat the DIER. The benefits of surgery in symptomatic patients with DIER, become significant 6 months after surgery [10], and remain stable for 5 years after the surgery. Conservative and radical rectal surgery is an efficient and lasting treatment of patients suffering from pain and digestive troubles due to DIER.

The overall low recurrence rate demonstrates that surgical removal of the DIER is a valid procedure with excellent long-term remission with comparable recurrence rates between the conservative and radical surgical approaches.

Complete removal of large deep endometriosis infiltrating the rectum does not guarantee normal postoperative bowel movements [13, 14, 39, 40], even though [29], the quality of life reveals significant and lasting improvement. Patients should receive this information prior to surgery for rectal endometriosis, particularly when they are embarrassed by severe preoperative constipation.

Surgery of the DIER may be challenging, and Clavien–Dindo 3 postoperative complications may involve up to 27% of patients [1]. However, it may be emphasized that postoperative complications do negatively impact on neither 1 year-outcomes [29] nor postoperative pregnancy rate [11, 30]. Postoperative complications in skilled hands do not carry long-term negative impacts. Thus, the fear of postoperative complications should not out way the expected benefit in terms of pelvic pain, bowel movements, quality of life, and ability to conceive.

High conception rates, with a majority of spontaneous conceptions [11], prove that surgical management of DIER accomplishes both clinical improvement and conception, thus it can safely be recommended to young women experiencing pelvic or digestive complaints along with pregnancy wish. Symptomatic patients may benefit from laparoscopic surgery for DIER with favorable long-term outcomes.

References

1. Roman H, Bubenheim M, Huet E, Bridoux V, Zacharopoulou C, Daraï E, Collinet P, Tuech JJ. Conservative surgery versus colorectal resection in deep endometriosis infiltrating the rectum: a randomized trial. Hum Reprod. 2018;33:47–57.
2. Abrao MS, Petraglia F, Falcone T, Keckstein J, Osuga Y, Chapron C. Deep endometriosis infiltrating the recto-sigmoid: critical factors to consider before management. Hum Reprod Update. 2015;21:329–39.
3. Donnez J, Squifflet J. Complications, pregnancy and recurrence in a prospective series of 500 patients operated on by the shaving technique for deep rectovaginal endometriotic nodules. Hum Reprod. 2010;25:1949–58.
4. Fanfani F, Fagotti A, Gagliardi ML, et al. Discoid or segmental rectosigmoid resection for deep infiltrating endometriosis: a case-control study. Fertil Steril. 2010;94:444–9.
5. Donnez O, Roman H. Choosing the right surgical technique for deep endometriosis: shaving, disc excision, or bowel resection? Fertil Steril. 2017;108:931–42.
6. Abo C, Moatassim S, Marty N, Saint Ghislain M, Huet E, Bridoux V, Tuech JJ, Roman H. Postoperative complications after bowel endometriosis surgery by shaving, disc excision, or segmental resection: a three-arm comparative analysis of 364 consecutive cases. Fertil Steril. 2018;109:172–8.
7. Roman H, Vassilieff M, Tuech JJ, et al. Postoperative digestive function after radical versus conservative surgical philosophy for deep endometriosis infiltrating the rectum. Fertil Steril. 2013;99:1695–704.
8. Meuleman C, Tomassetti C, D'Hoore A, et al. Surgical treatment of deeply infiltrating endometriosis with colorectal involvement. Hum Reprod Update. 2011;17:311–26.
9. Afors K, Centini G, Fernandes R, Murtada R, Zupi E, Akladios C, Wattiez A. Segmental and discoid resection are preferential to bowel shaving for medium-term symptomatic relief in patients with bowel endometriosis. J Minim Invasive Gynecol. 2016;23(7):1123–9.
10. Roman H, Bubenheim M, Huet E, Bridoux V, Zacharopoulou C, Collinet P, Daraï E, Tuech JJ. Baseline severe constipation negatively impacts functional outcomes of surgery for deep endometriosis infiltrating the rectum: results of the ENDORE randomized trial. J Gynecol Obstet Hum Reprod. 2019; https://doi.org/10.1016/j.jogoh.2019.03.013.
11. Roman H, Chanavaz-Lacheray I, Ballester M, Bendifallah S, Touleimat S, Tuech JJ, Farella M, Merlot B. High postoperative fertility rate following surgical management of colorectal endometriosis. Hum Reprod. 2018;33:1669–76.
12. Kupelian AS, Cutner A. Segmental bowel resection for deep infiltratingendometriosis. BJOG. 2016;123:1368.
13. Riiskjaer M, Greisen S, Glavind-Kristensen M, Kesmodel US, Forman A, Seyer-Hansen M. Pelvic organ function before and after laparoscopic bowel resection for rectosigmoid endometriosis: a prospective, observational study. BJOG. 2016;123:13607.
14. Possover M. Pathophysiologic explanation for bladder retention in patients after laparoscopic surgery for deeply infiltrating rectovaginal and/or parametric endometriosis. Fertil Steril. 2011;101:754–8.
15. Bonneau C, Zilberman S, Ballester M, et al. Incidence of pre- and postoperative urinary dysfunction associated with deep infiltrating endometriosis: relevance of urodynamic tests and therapeutic implications. Minerva Ginecol. 2013;65:385–405.
16. Roman H, Bridoux V, Tuech JJ, et al. Bowel dysfunction before and after surgery for endometriosis. Am J Obstet Gynecol. 2013;209:524–30.

17. Darwish B, Roman H. Nerve sparing and surgery for deep infiltrating endometriosis: pessimism of the intellect or optimism of the will. Semin Reprod Med. 2017;35:72–80.
18. de Resende JA Jr, Cavalini LT, Crispi CP, de Freitas Fonseca M. Risk of urinary retention after nerve-sparing surgery for deep infiltrating endometriosis: a systematic review and meta-analysis. Neurourol Urodyn. 2017;36:57–61.
19. Ceccaroni M, Clarizia R, Bruni F, et al. Nerve-sparing laparoscopic eradication of deep endometriosis with segmental rectal and parametrial resection: the Negrar method. A single-center, prospective, clinical trial. Surg Endosc. 2012;26:2029–45.
20. Mabrouk M, Ferrini G, Montanari G, et al. Does colorectal endometriosis alter intestinal functions? A prospective manometric and questionnaire-based study. Fertil Steril. 2012;97:652–6.
21. Badescu A, Roman H, Barsan I, Soldea V, Nastasia S, Aziz M, Puscasiu L, Stolnicu S. Patterns of bowel invisible microscopic endometriosis reveal the goal of surgery: removal of visual lesions only. J Minim Invasive Gynecol. 2018;25(3):522–527.e9. https://doi.org/10.1016/j.jmig.2017.10.026.
22. Badescu A, Roman H, Aziz M, Puscasiu L, Molnar C, Huet E, Sabourin JC, Stolnicu S. Mapping of bowel occult microscopic endometriosis implants surrounding deep endometriosis nodules infiltrating the bowel. Fertil Steril. 2016;105(2):430-4.e6. https://doi.org/10.1016/j.fertnstert.2015.11.006.
23. Roman H, Hennetier C, Darwish B, Badescu A, Csanyi M, Aziz M, Tuech JJ, Abo C. Bowel occult microscopic endometriosis in resection margins in deep colorectal endometriosis specimens has no impact on short-term postoperative outcomes. Fertil Steril. 2016;105(2):423-9.e7.   https://doi.org/10.1016/j.fertnstert.2015.09.030.
24. Dousset B, Leconte M, Borghese B, et al. Complete surgery for low rectal endometriosis. Long-term results of a 100-case prospective study. Ann Surg. 2010;251:887–95.
25. Marty N, Touleimat S, Moatassim-Drissa S, Millochau JC, Vallee A, Stochino Loi E, Desnyder E, Roman H. Rectal shaving using plasma energy in deep infiltrating endometriosis of the rectum: four years of experience. J Minim Invasive Gynecol. 2017;24(7):1121–7.
26. Roman H, Moatassim-Drissa S, Marty N, Milles M, Vallée A, Desnyder E, Stochino Loi E, Abo C. Rectal shaving for deep endometriosis infiltrating the rectum: a 5-year continuous retrospective series. Fertil Steril. 2016;106(6):1438–1445.e2.
27. Roman H, Darwish B, Bridoux V, Chati R, Kermiche S, Coget J, Huet E, Tuech JJ. Functional outcomes after disc excision in deep endometriosis of the rectum using transanal staplers: a series of 111 consecutive patients. Fertil Steril. 2017;107:977–86.
28. Roman H, Milles M, Vassilieff M, et al. Long-term functional outcomes following colorectal resection versus shaving for rectal endometriosis. Am J Obstet Gynecol. 2016;215:762.e1–9.
29. Riiskjær M, Forman A, Kesmodel US, Andersen LM, Ljungmann K, Seyer-Hansen M. Pelvic pain and quality of life before and after laparoscopic bowel resection for rectosigmoid endometriosis: a prospective. Observ Study Dis Colon Rectum. 2018;61:221–9.
30. Ferrier C, Roman H, Alzahrani Y, d'Argent EM, Bendifallah S, Marty N, Perez M, Rubod C, Collinet P, Daraï E, Ballester M. Fertility outcomes in women experiencing severe complications after surgery for colorectal endometriosis. Hum Reprod. 2018;33:411–5.
31. Maytham GD, Dowson HM, Levy B, Kent A, Rockall TA. Laparoscopic excision of rectovaginal endometriosis: report of a prospective study and review of the literature. Color Dis. 2010;12(11):1105–12. https://doi.org/10.1111/j.1463-1318.2009.01993.x. Review.
32. Bendifallah S, Vesale E, Darai E, Thomassin-Naggara I, Bazot M, Tuech JJ, Abo C, Roman H. Recurrence after surgery for colorectal endometriosis: systematic review and meta-analysis. J Minim Invasive Gynecol. 2019;27(2):441–451.e2.
33. Guo S-W. Recurrence of endometriosis and its control. Hum Reprod Update. 2009;15(4):441–61.
34. Bozdag G. Recurrence of endometriosis: risk factors, mechanisms and biomarkers. Womens Health Lond Engl. 2015;11(5):693–9.
35. Vercellini P, Pietropaolo G, De Giorgi O, Daguati R, Pasin R, Crosignani PG. Reproductive performance in infertile women with rectovaginal endometriosis: is surgery worthwhile? Am J Obstet Gynecol. 2006;195:1303–10.
36. Roman H. Colorectal endometriosis and pregnancy wish: why doing primary surgery. Front Biosci (Schol Ed). 2015;7:83–93.
37. Cohen J, Thomin A, Mathieu d'Argent E, Laas E, Canlorbe G, Zilberman S, Belghiti J, Thomassin-Naggara I, Bazot M, Ballester M, et al. Fertility before and after surgery for deep infiltrating endometriosis with and without bowel involvement: a literature review. Minerva Ginecol. 2014;66:575–87.
38. Meuleman C, Tomassetti C, Wolthuis A, Van Cleynenbreugel B, Laenen A, Penninckx F, Vergote I, D'Hoore A, D'Hooghe T. Clinical outcome after radical excision of moderate-severe endometriosis with or without bowel resection and reanastomosis. A prospective cohort study. Ann Surg. 2014;259:522–31.
39. Erdem S, Imboden S, Papadia A, Lanz S, Mueller MD, Gloor B, Worni M. Functional outcomes after rectal resection for deep infiltrating pelvic endometriosis: long-term results. Dis Colon Rectum. 2018;61:733–42.
40. Soto E, Catenacci M, Bedient C, Jelovsek JE, Falcone T. Assessment of long-term bowel symptoms after segmental resection of deeply infiltrating endometriosis: a matched cohort study. J Minim Invasive Gynecol. 2016;23:753–9.

Hormonal Treatment of Bowel Endometriosis

Simone Ferrero, Fabio Barra, Alessandro Loddo, and Erkut Attar

16.1 Introduction

When bowel endometriosis causes a severe stenosis of the intestinal lumen associated with sub-occlusive or occlusive symptoms (such as nausea and vomiting during the menstrual cycle, small-caliber stools), colorectal surgery is the only reasonable treatment. However, most of the patients affected by bowel endometriosis do not suffer subocclusive or occlusive symptoms, but they may complain severe pain and intestinal symptoms (such as abdominal bloating, intestinal cramping, diarrhea, constipation, cyclical rectal bleeding, and passage of mucus in stools). Hormonal therapies have been shown to be safe, well tolerated, and effective in the long-term treatment of pain symptoms caused by deep pelvic endometriosis [1–3]. Over the last ten years, several studies investigated the efficacy of these therapies in the treatment of symptoms caused by bowel endometriosis. Targeted and local hormonal therapies can also be developed for the treatment of bowel endometriosis as the molecular mechanisms underlying deep pelvic endometriosis becomes more evident. The aim of this chapter is to review the role of hormonal therapies in the treatment of bowel endometriosis. In addition, to discuss the futuristic and preventive treatments under the influence of recent developments in the pathogenesis of endometriosis.

16.2 Background for the Use of Hormonal Therapies in the Treatment of Bowel Endometriosis

Histological studies demonstrate that intestinal endometriotic lesions contain not only ectopic endometrial-like mucosa but also extensive fibrosis and smooth muscle fibers [3–5]. Based on this, it has been believed that these nodules may be unresponsive to hormonal changes. However, hormonal therapies may act on two of three components of deep endometriosis: the ectopic endometrial tissue and the smooth muscle fibers [3]. Although progestins may have some anti-inflammatory activity on the fibrosis associated with deep endometriosis, it seems unlikely that hormonal therapies have a major influence on the fibrosis associated with deep endometriosis.

S. Ferrero (✉) · F. Barra
Academic Unit of Obstetrics and Gynecology,
IRCCS Ospedale Policlinico San Martino,
Genova, Italy

Department of Neurosciences, Rehabilitation, Ophthalmology, Genetics, Maternal and Child Health (DiNOGMI), University of Genova, Genova, Italy

A. Loddo
Department of Obstetrics and Gynecology,
University of Cagliari, Cagliari, Italy

E. Attar
Department of Obstetrics and Gynecology, Yeditepe University Medical School, Istanbul, Turkey

© Springer Nature Switzerland AG 2020
S. Ferrero, M. Ceccaroni (eds.), *Clinical Management of Bowel Endometriosis*,
https://doi.org/10.1007/978-3-030-50446-5_16

Responsiveness of deep endometriotic lesions to gonadal steroids is a prerequisite for medical therapy. Progesterone receptors (PRs) are present in ectopic glands infiltrating the muscular layer of the bowel wall; while, estrogen receptors (ERs) are not present in bowel endometriosis [6]. In contrast, both ERs and PRs have been demonstrated in other deep infiltrating endometriotic nodules [6]. Notably, independently of the cycle's phase, PRs are significantly more abundant than ERs [6]. Interestingly, GnRH-a suppresses the expression of ERs and PRs in the smooth muscle component of rectovaginal endometriosis [7]. A recent study measured the expression of ERα and PR in deep endometriotic lesions of untreated women and during various types of hormonal therapies [8]. Epithelial staining for PR was lower in treated patients, whichever treatment considered (combined oral contraceptive, progestins, or GnRH-a). Hormonal treatment for at least 3 months did not significantly alter neither the pattern nor the intensity of ERα immunoreactive epithelial staining. In the stromal compartment of the ectopic endometrium, stromal staining intensity for PR or ERα was not modified by treatment. Hormonal therapies improve irritative-type symptoms caused by bowel endometriosis; this phenomenon may be explained by the resolution of cyclic inflammation due to intra- and peri-lesional micro-hemorrhages [9].

ary symptoms and low Endometriosis Health Profile (EHP)-30 scores. Moreover, the Short Form (SF)-36 scores remained constant and comparable to the background population. The authors observed progression of length of endometriotic nodules in nine patients, and progression of width in six patients; these changes occurred without worsening of symptoms or quality of life. In a recent retrospective study based on medical record review, 238 women with ultrasonographic diagnosis of rectosigmoid endometriosis who did not wish to conceive were offered a 6-month hormonal treatment (progestins, combined contraceptives and GnRH-a) [11]. Over the course of follow-up, 143 (60.1%) women continued the medical treatment while 95 (39.9%) had worsening of pain symptoms or intestinal lesion growth, with surgical resection performed in 54 cases. Women satisfied with hormonal therapy were older and had smaller rectosigmoid nodules compared to those who failed to respond to medical treatment. Similar significant reduction in pain scores for dysmenorrhea, chronic pelvic pain, cyclic dyschezia, and dysuria was observed in both groups; however, greater reduction in pain scores for dyspareunia was noted in the patients who underwent surgery. The authors concluded that, given this background, surgery should be reserved for patients with symptoms unresponsive to hormonal therapy.

16.3 Use of Hormonal Therapies in the Treatment of Bowel Endometriosis

A prospective cohort study investigated the role of hormonal therapies (oral contraceptives, progestin, or the levonorgestrel-releasing intrauterine device) in treating symptoms caused by rectosigmoid endometriosis [10]. Only patients who did not previously undergo surgery for bowel endometriosis were included in the study. The patients were follow-up for a mean of 4 years; 80 patients completed the follow-up. Only 6% of participants needed surgery during the study period. Otherwise, patients had station-

16.4 Progestins

Progestins are of the first-line therapies for the treatment of pain symptoms caused by deep endometriosis [2]. They are usually well tolerated and efficacious in improving pain symptoms [12]. Several progestins have been used to treat the symptoms caused by bowel endometriosis. The levonorgestrel-releasing IUD (LNG-IUD) is as effective as GnRH-a in the treatment of endometriosis-associated pain. Insertion of an LNG-IUD alleviates pain and reduces the size of lesions in patients with endometriosis of the rectovaginal septum [13].

16.4.1 Norethisterone Acetate

A prospective study investigated the efficacy of norethisterone acetate (NETA) in treating pain and intestinal symptoms of patients with colorectal endometriosis [14]. Subjects of the study ($n = 40$) had the diagnosis of colorectal endometriosis based on multidetector computerized tomography enteroclysis and had an estimated bowel stenosis <60%. Patients with subocclusive symptoms were excluded from the study. Study patients received NETA 2.5 mg/day continuously, starting on the first day of the menstrual cycle for 12 months. In case of breakthrough bleeding after two months of treatment, the dose of NETA was increased by 2.5 mg/day. Eighty percentage of the patients completed the 12-month treatment. The treatment significantly ameliorated chronic pelvic pain, deep dyspareunia, and dyschezia. The treatment caused the disappearance of symptoms related to the menstrual cycle such as dysmenorrhea, constipation during the menstrual cycle, diarrhea during the menstrual cycle and cyclical rectal bleeding. The severity of diarrhea, intestinal cramping, and passage of mucus significantly improved during treatment. In contrast, the administration of NETA did not change the intensity of constipation, abdominal bloating, and feeling of incomplete evacuation after bowel movements. Furthermore, the treatment significantly decreases the use of anti-inflammatory drugs while the use of laxative did not significantly change during the treatment. A prospective study including 18 patients showed that 6-month treatment with NETA significantly decrease the volume of rectovaginal endometriotic nodules infiltrating the rectum. In addition, a further decrease in the volume of these nodules is observed after 12 months of treatment [15].

16.4.2 Dienogest

A prospective cohort study including 30 women evaluated the effectiveness of 12-month treatment with dienogest (DNG, 2 mg/day) in treating pain caused by intestinal and posterior fornix deep infiltrating endometriosis. The therapy sig-nificantly decreased the intensity of dysmenorrhea, pelvic pain, dyspareunia, and intestinal pain. The treatment significantly improved quality of life assessed by the brief version of the World Health Organization QoL measure (WHOQOL-BREF). The changes in the volume of the endometriotic nodules were monitored by transvaginal ultrasonography; the volume of the nodules was calculated by measuring three measurements (depth × length × extension × 0.52). No significant change in the volume of the bowel endometriotic nodules was observed after 12-month treatment with DNG (before, 2.18 ± 2.99 cm^3; after, 2.21 ± 4.06 cm^3; $p = 0.23$). In addition, there was no significant correlation between the improvement in pain symptoms and the decrease in the volume of endometriotic nodules [16].

A recent report described the case of a patient with previous surgery for ovarian endometriosis at 40 years that was using oral contraceptive pill. At 44 years, the patient had positive fecal occult blood test. Colonoscopy revealed a submucosal tumor-like elevation occupying almost 50% of the rectal lumen. Biopsy specimens revealed the diagnosis of rectal endometriosis. The patient was treated with DNG; although the mass did not regress in size, her abdominal pain quickly improved. After 6 years of treatment, the patient was free of abdominal pain or obstruction to defecation [17]. Recently, a retrospective study based on a prospectively collected database investigated the efficacy of 36-month therapy with DNG for treating pain intestinal symptoms of patients with rectosigmoid endometriosis [18]. Eighty-three patients were included in the study. At 1-year follow-up, DNG significantly ameliorated dysmenorrhea, chronic pelvic pain, dyspareunia, dyschezia, and intestinal symptoms. The improvement of the intestinal symptoms was demonstrated by the Gastrointestinal Quality of Life Index (GIQLI). A statistical increase of the GIQLI score was observed from baseline to 12 months of treatment. A further improvement of the GIQLI score was observed at 24 months while it remained stable during the third year of treatment. A progressive increase in quality of life (assessed by the Endometriosis Health

Profile-30) was observed in the first two years of therapy. Improvements of patients' symptoms and quality of life were maintained until the end of the study. Discontinuation because of adverse effects was more frequent in the first year of therapy (47.3%) in comparison to the second year (14.3%) and third year of therapy (12.5%). At 36-month follow-up, 34 women were still using DNG. The regimen was well tolerated, and the frequency and amount of irregular bleeding decreased as treatment progressed. The volume of the endometriotic nodules was assessed by transvaginal ultrasonography. After 6 months of treatment, the volume of the nodules significantly decreased when compared with baseline values. After the end of the first year of treatment, there was a further significant reduction in the volume of the nodules. Between 24 and 36 months of treatment, the volume of endometriotic nodules remained stable. At the end of the study, there was a decrease in the volume of the nodules of at least 10% in 52.9% of patients, the nodules remained stable in 35.3% and in 11.8% of the patients there was an increase in the volume compared to baseline values.

DNG may also be used following GnRH-a suppression of endometriotic lesions. Kitawaki et al. showed that a treatment with a GnRH-a followed by long-term DNG therapy maintains the relief of endometriosis-associated pelvic pain for at least 12 months. This regimen reduces the amount of irregular uterine bleeding that often occurs during the early phase of dienogest therapy [19].

16.4.3 Desogestrel

A large patient preference prospective study compared the efficacy of a 12-month treatment with desogestrel-only contraceptive pill (DSG; 75 µg/day) and the sequential vaginal ring (15 µg ethinylestradiol and 120 µg etonogestrel through days 1–21) in treating symptoms caused by rectovaginal endometriosis infiltrating the rectum. The diagnosis of rectal endometriosis was based on magnetic resonance imaging. Only women with estimated colorectal stenosis <60% were included in the study. At 12-month follow-up the rate of satisfied patients was higher in patients treated with DSG (61.7%) than in those treated with the vaginal ring (36.1%). When only changes in intestinal symptoms were considered, the satisfaction rate was higher in patients treated with DNG (50.0%) than in those treated with the vaginal ring (31.3%). One hundred and forty-three women were included in the study. The continuous treatment with DSG had the advantage of causing the disappearance of symptoms associated with menstruation (such as dysmenorrhea, constipation during menstruation, diarrhea during menstruation and cyclical rectal bleeding). Among patients treated with DSG, at 12-month follow-up, there was a significant amelioration in the intensity of all pain and intestinal symptoms (except abdominal bloating) compared with baseline. Among patients treated with the vaginal ring, the severity of all pain and intestinal symptoms (except diarrhea during menstruation and passage of mucus) significantly decreased compared with baseline. Notably, at 12-month follow-up the intensity of chronic pelvic pain, dyschezia, deep dyspareunia, diarrhea, intestinal cramping, feeling of incomplete evacuation, and passage of mucus was lower in patients treated with DSG than in those treated with the vaginal ring; there was no significant difference in the intensity of constipation and abdominal bloating between the two study groups. The 12-month treatment caused a similar decrease in the volume of the nodule in patients treated with DSG (28.0%) and in those treated with the vaginal ring (27%). Interestingly, an increase in the size of endometriotic nodule was observed in 11.1% of patients treated with DSG and in 8.5% of those treated with the vaginal ring. The major limitation of this study was that the vaginal ring was administered sequentially while DSG requires a continuous administration [20]. Because of this study design, it is not possible to establish if the differences in the outcome were caused by the sequential administration of one therapy or by the use of different drugs.

A prospective study including 26 patients showed that 6-month treatment with DSG significantly decrease the volume of rectovaginal endometriotic nodules infiltrating the rectum. A further decrease was observed after 12-month of treatment [15].

16.5 Combined Estroprogestin Combinations

Combined estroprogestin combinations are one of the most commonly used and efficacious therapies for endometriosis related pain. They can be administered either sequentially or continuously; the continuous administration is particularly suitable for patients suffering menstrual related symptoms (such as dysmenorrhea and menstrual migraine).

A prospective study evaluated the efficacy of a 12-month treatment with continuous low-dose combined oral contraceptive (15 µg ethinylestradiol and 60 µg gestodene) in treating symptoms caused by colorectal endometriosis. Twenty-six women were included in the study. The diagnosis of colorectal endometriosis was based on rectal endoscopic ultrasonography. The treatment causes a substantial decrease in the volume of the intestinal nodules (mean reduction in the largest diameter, 26%; mean reduction in the volume, 62%). The treatment improved dysmenorrhea, dyspareunia, painful defecation and non-menstrual pelvic pain. At the end of the 12-month treatment, 69% of the patients were either very satisfied or satisfied, while only 16% were either dissatisfied or very dissatisfied [21].

A prospective study including 30 patients showed that 6-month treatment with a sequential oral contraceptive pill significantly decreases the volume of rectovaginal endometriotic nodules infiltrating the rectum; a further decrease in the volume of these nodules was observed after 12 months of treatment [15].

16.6 Gonadotrophin-Releasing Hormone Agonists

Case reports described the use of GnRH-a in the treatment of selected cases of bowel endometriosis. A patient had the diagnosis of rectal endometriosis based on computed tomography, magnetic resonance imaging and colonoscopy. Intestinal symptoms (rectal bleeding and constipation) persisted despite treatment with danazol (800 mg/day) for eight months. Since the patient desired to avoid surgery, she was treated with leuprolide acetate (1.0 mg subcutaneously daily) and she quickly became asymptomatic. In addition, a decrease in the size of the rectal nodule from a 3–4 cm lesion to a 2–3 cm lesion was observed. After 15-month hormonal treatment, the patient was still symptom free, but she underwent surgery because the long-term treatment with GnRH-a was not supported by the medical literature [22]. Another case report described a patient with histologically proved sigmoid endometriosis (1.8 cm) presenting as a polypoid lesion complaining abdominal and pelvic pain, rectal bleeding and anemia. The patient was treated with leuprolide acetate 3.75 mg, i.e., every 4 weeks for 3 months. Symptoms promptly improved after the first injection. An oral contraceptive was subsequently prescribed but was immediately interrupted because of the occurrence of severe migraine. After 6 months, colonoscopy demonstrated a flat pale lesion and biopsy confirmed the absence of endometriosis. No recurrence was documented by colonoscopy at 2-year follow-up. Three years later, the patient underwent hysterectomy because of uterine myomas. Surgery did not reveal endometriosis in the pelvic organs and on the intestinal serosa. A colonoscopy showed a small asymptomatic endometriotic polyp in the sigma which disappeared after treatment with leuprolide acetate depot 3.75 mg for 3 months; it is difficult to assess whether it was a recurrence or a new endometriotic lesion [23].

An open-label prospective study investigated the efficacy of GnRH-a in treating pain and intestinal symptoms of 18 patients with colorectal endometriosis. Bowel endometriosis was diagnosed by multidetector computerized tomography enema. Patients with a stenosis of the bowel lumen >60% and with pain and endometriotic lesions located on the cecum and ileum were excluded from the study. Patients were treated with intramuscular injections of depot triptorelin

(11.25 mg every 3 months) and oral tibolone (2.5 mg daily) for 12 months. The mean estimated size of the intestinal nodules was 2.2 cm. At 12-month follow-up, 72.2% of the patients were very satisfied or satisfied, 11.1% were uncertain, and 16.7% were dissatisfied. As expected, the treatment significantly improved pain symptoms (dysmenorrhea, non-menstrual pelvic pain, deep dyspareunia and dyschezia). 61.1% of the patients had an improvement in intestinal symptoms. Patients suffering diarrhea were significantly more likely to have improvement in symptoms than those complaining constipation. At 6- and 12-month follow-up, there was a significant improvement in intestinal cramping, abdominal bloating and passage of mucus. Furthermore, the treatment significantly decreased the number of anti-inflammatory drugs used by the patients. After the completion of the 12-month treatment, 38.9% of the patients wished to continue the combined treatment with triptorelin and tibolone [24].

A prospective study including ten patients with rectovaginal endometriotic nodules infiltrating the rectum showed that a 12-month treatment with triptorelin (11.25 mg every 3 months) and tibolone (2.5 mg/day) significantly decreases the volume of rectovaginal nodules infiltrating the rectum [15].

16.7 Aromatase Inhibitors

The aromatase enzyme mediates the conversion of androstenedione to estrone and of testosterone to estradiol. It has been demonstrated that aromatase is expressed in endometriotic implants, thus providing the ectopic tissue with excessive proliferative stimulus [25, 26]. These biological findings prompted performance of several studies in women with endometriosis using aromatase inhibitors (AI) to treat pain symptoms [27]. When AI are administered to women of reproductive age, the decrease in estrogen levels promotes the secretion of gonadotropins causing stimulatory effects on the ovary. Therefore, AI must by combined with additional drugs (such as progestins or combined estroprogestin combinations) that effectively downregulate the ovaries.

A prospective study assessed the efficacy of 6-month treatment with letrozole (2.5 mg/day) and NETA (2.5 mg/day) in improving pain and intestinal symptoms of six patients with colorectal endometriosis. All patients completed the 6-month treatment. At 3-month follow-up, the intensity of non-menstrual pelvic pain, dyspareunia and dyschezia was significantly decreased compared with baseline; a further improvement was observed at 6-month follow-up. The double-drug treatment improved symptoms mimicking diarrhea-predominant irritable bowel syndrome, intestinal cramping, abdominal bloating, and passage of mucus in the stools. At the completion of treatment, one woman (17%) was very satisfied, three women (50%) were satisfied, one woman (17%) was uncertain, and one woman (17%) was dissatisfied [28].

An ultrasonographic prospective study demonstrated the letrozole (2.5 mg/day) combined with NETA (2.5 mg/day) significantly decrease the volume of rectovaginal nodules infiltrating the rectum. At 6-month follow-up the volume of these nodules was significantly decreased compared with baseline; furthermore, at 12-month follow-up, the volume of the nodules was lower than at 6-month follow-up [15].

In a randomized controlled trial, anastozole alone was used in one arm of the study and anastrozole plus a GnRH-a was used in the other arm. Although, combination regimen suppressed the follicle development in ovaries, it caused significant bone loss. However, pain recurred later in the group who used the combination treatment [29].

Adding an oral contraceptive or progestin to the treatment also prevents bone loss in long-term use of AIs. Vitamin D and calcium combination can also be added to this treatment regimen to prevent bone loss.

16.8 Progression of Bowel Endometriosis During Hormonal Treatment

No study has systematically investigated the progression of bowel endometriosis in patients receiving long-term hormonal treatment. A case report demonstrated that bowel endometriosis may progress during the use of an oral contraceptive pill [30]. A 25-year-old woman suffering dysmenorrhea and deep dyspareunia, who had no intestinal symptom, was diagnosed with a 2.5 cm rectovaginal nodule. Multidetector computerized tomography enteroclysis revealed the presence of a small sigmoid endometriotic nodule of the serosal surface that did not infiltrate the muscularis propria. The patient was treated with continuous oral contraceptive pill (DSG 150 µg and ethinylestradiol 20 µg). After four years, the patient complained pain and persistent gastrointestinal symptoms of increasing severity (constipation and dyschezia). Magnetic resonance enema revealed the presence of a large sigmoid nodule in the same site where multidetector computerized tomography enteroclysis previously revealed the small serosal sigmoid nodule. The patient was treated by laparoscopic segmental bowel resection. Another case report confirmed that hormonal treatment may not prevent the progression of colorectal endometriosis [31]. A 26-year-old woman underwent surgery because of ovarian endometriomas. During surgery, an intestinal endometriotic nodule was diagnosed. Bowel surgery was not performed because the patient had few intestinal complains and the nodule was not diagnosed preoperatively. Postoperative computed tomographic colonography revealed a short rigid area 40 cm above the anus, where the wall appeared thickened by up to 14 mm and the bowel lumen was reduced down to 17 mm. Endorectal ultrasound found a normal rectum and sigmoid colon. The patient was treated with continuous cyproterone acetate (50 mg/day) and add back therapy with estradiol (0.5 mg/day, percutaneously). The treatment was modified 2 years after the surgery because of mood disorders, and a combined contraceptive pill (150 µg levonorgestrel + 30 µg ethinylestradiol per day) was administered continuously. Four years later, the patient presented constipation alternating with diarrhea, bloating, dyschezia, and pelvic pain. MRI revealed endometriosis infiltrating the sigmoid colon measuring 6–8 cm, with a thickened wall including T1 spots, indicating active endometriosis of the bowel. CTC revealed abnormal sigmoid colon from 42 to 50 cm above the anus, with a digestive tract diameter reduced from 10 mm down to the virtual lumen, along with an overall rigid appearance. Thus, the patients underwent laparoscopic rectosigmoid resection.

16.9   Comparison Between Hormonal Therapy and Surgery

A parallel cohort study compared the degree of patient satisfaction in women with symptomatic colorectal endometriosis who choose medical or surgical treatment [9]. Patients were allowed to choose the preferred treatment. Participants choosing the hormonal therapy used a low-dose monophasic oral contraceptive pill or a progestin (NETA 2.5 mg once a day or DNG 2 mg once a day). Fifty patients (57%) used the medical treatment and 37 (43%) underwent surgery. Among patients choosing the hormonal treatment, 12 used a low-dose OCP and 38 a progestin (29 NETA and 9 DNG). The median follow-up was 40 months for women choosing the medical treatment and 45 months for those undergoing surgery. Thirty-seven patients (74%) treated by hormonal therapy experienced adverse effects; in three patients these adverse effects were severe enough to cause withdrawal from the study. Surgery was performed by laparoscopy in nine patients and by laparotomy in 28 patients; all patients underwent segmental colorectal resection. There was no major intraoperative complication. There were six major postoperative complications requiring immediate or delayed re-intervention (intestinal anastomosis dehiscence, $n = 2$; hemoperitoneum, $n = 2$; rectovaginal fistula, $n = 1$; colostomy occlusion, $n = 1$). Furthermore, one patient developed severe dysfunctional constipation. At 12-month follow-up, 78% of women who choose the medical treatment were satisfied or very satisfied with treatment compared with 76% of patients who choose surgery. At final follow-up, 72% of patients treated with hormonal therapy and 65% of those treated by surgery were satisfied or very satisfied. All intestinal symptoms improved in both study groups with the exception of diarrhea in operated patients. Pain symptoms (dysmenorrhea, dyspareunia, non-menstrual pelvic pain, and dyschezia) improved in both study groups but the magnitude of the improvement was more pronounced in women treated by hormonal therapy. The quality of life and the psychological status improved in both study groups. The sexual function was assessed using the Female Sexual Function Index (FSFI); the total FSFI score improved only in women who chose medical treatment.

A French randomized controlled trial (MESURE trial, NCT01973816) including women with deep endometriosis involving the rectum and not intending to get pregnant is comparing medical and surgical treatment of rectovaginal endometriosis. In this trial, patients receiving the hormonal therapy are treated with triptorelin (11.25 mg every 3 months) and add back therapy (estradiol 0.5% percutaneous gel) for 6 months, followed by cyproterone acetate (50 mg daily) and add back therapy (estradiol 0.5% percutaneous gel) for 18 months. Patients treated by surgery (rectal shaving, rectal disc excision or colorectal resection based on the choice of the surgeon) receive daily cyproterone acetate (50 mg daily) and add back therapy (estradiol 0.5% percutaneous gel) for 18 months in order to prevent recurrence of endometriosis [32].

16.10 Futuristic and Preventive Hormonal Treatments

Bidirectional relationship between the microbiome and endometriosis has begun to be characterized by recent studies. Laboratory and clinical studies demonstrate that there are indeed differences in the microbiome composition of hosts with and without endometriosis. Gut microbiota shifts (lower lactobacilli concentrations and higher gram-negative bacteria levels) in endometriosis. Clinical interest in the human intestinal microbiota has increased considerably. The gut microbiome in patients with endometriosis may have a large number of β-glucuronidase producing bacteria which may lead to increased levels of estrogen metabolites. In postmenopausal women,

the absence of estrogen alters intestinal microbial composition and structure, leading to decreased microbial diversity. Similarly, GnRH-a has been shown to impact the local microbiota of the uterus demonstrating the ability of hormonal regulation to modulate microbiota composition [33]. We previously showed that a histone-deacetylase inhibitor, sodium butyrate inhibits aromatase activity in a promoter dependent manner in endometriotic cells in culture [34]. Epigenetic influences have also been shown to affect the course of endometriosis [35]. Aromatase, Steroid Factor-1, COX-2, and Homeobox A10 also have epigenetic modifications in endometriosis. DNA methyltransferases, estrogen and progesterone receptors, micro-RNAs, and histone deacetylators have shown differential expression in endometriosis compared with normal endometrium [36]. Future targeted uses of these works may include histone-deacetylase inhibitors for prevention and treatment of endometriosis.

In normal endometrium, progesterone acts on stromal cells to induce the expression of the enzyme 17beta-hydroxysteroid dehydrogenase type 2 (17beta-HSD-2), which metabolizes the biologically active estrogen E2 to estrone E1. Recent data support the role of progesterone resistance in deep pelvic endometriosis [37]. The molecular basis of progesterone resistance in endometriosis may be related to an overall reduction in the levels of PRs and the lack of the PRB [38]. PR deficiency also leads to defective retinoid synthesis in endometriotic cells. It has been shown that fenretinide, a synthetic retinoid analogue that reverses the pathological loss of retinoid availability targeting the retinoic acid signaling pathway may also be a promising treatment for women with endometriosis [39]. Thus, single use or combination of these natural compounds may also have a protective effect in endometriosis.

16.11 Conclusion

The studies presented in this chapter demonstrate that hormonal therapies can improve not only pain, but also intestinal symptoms caused by bowel endometriosis. This finding is not surprising because intestinal nodules are histologically similar to other deep endometriotic nodules. Furthermore, patients with bowel endometriosis usually have endometriotic lesions located in other sites of the abdominal cavity. Therefore, it is likely that the improvement of pain symptoms is caused by the activity of hormonal therapies on all endometriotic lesions. Basic and clinical research paved the way to the development of new promising targeted hormonal therapies in prevention and treatment of endometriosis.

Obviously, hormonal therapy cannot be prescribed to all women affected by bowel endometriosis. Patients with subocclusive symptoms (such as nausea and vomiting during the menstrual cycle, reduced bowel movements or pass gas) should be informed of the potential risk of bowel occlusion and, in general, they should undergo surgery. Patients with suspicion of intestinal malignancy should obviously undergo colonoscopy with biopsy and, in case of diagnostic doubts, surgery. Finally, hormonal therapies are contraceptive or, at least, they interfere with conception; therefore, these therapies cannot be prescribed to patients wishing to conceive.

In the other patients, hormonal therapies must be considered the first-line treatment for symptoms caused by intestinal endometriosis. In fact, surgery is associated with potential serious complications such as temporary ileostomy, postoperative uterine retention, rectovaginal fistula, iatrogenic ureteral injuries, and de novo constipation. In addition, hormonal therapy is efficacious in improving symptoms in about two-thirds of women with bowel endometriosis [9]. Patients must be thoroughly informed on potential benefits, risks, and drawbacks of medical therapies. Patients receiving long-term hormonal therapy must be monitored during treatment because intestinal nodules may progress despite the use of these therapies [20, 30, 31]. The growth of intestinal nodules may increase the stenosis of the bowel lumen and, theoretically, it can expose the patients to the risk of subocclusion or occlusion. Furthermore, retrocervical endometriotic nodules infiltrating the rectum can extend toward the ureters thus causing ureteral stenosis, hydronephrosis and potential loss of renal function [40]. Patients receiving hormonal therapies must be

informed that this treatment induces only temporary relief of symptoms which usually recur few months after discontinuation of therapies; thus, these therapies are not expected to be definitively curative [41]. Based on this, patients choosing the hormonal therapy should continue the treatment for many years, ideally until a pregnancy is desired or the physiologic menopause ensues [3]. Finally, patients choosing between hormonal and surgical treatment should consider that postoperative hormonal therapy is usually recommended to decrease the risk of recurrence of pain after surgical excision of deep endometriosis. Although no study has specifically investigated the role of endocrine therapies to prevent the recurrence of pain after surgical treatment of bowel endometriosis.

References

1. Vercellini P, Crosignani PG, Somigliana E, Berlanda N, Barbara G, Fedele L. Medical treatment for rectovaginal endometriosis: what is the evidence? Hum Reprod. 2009;24(10):2504–14.
2. Ferrero S, Alessandri F, Racca A, Leone Roberti Maggiore U. Treatment of pain associated with deep endometriosis: alternatives and evidence. Fertil Steril. 2015;104(4):771–92.
3. Vercellini P, Buggio L, Somigliana E. Role of medical therapy in the management of deep rectovaginal endometriosis. Fertil Steril. 2017;108(6):913–30.
4. Donnez J, Nisolle M, Gillerot S, Smets M, Bassil S, Casanas-Roux F. Rectovaginal septum adenomyotic nodules: a series of 500 cases. Br J Obstet Gynaecol. 1997;104(9):1014–8.
5. Remorgida V, Ragni N, Ferrero S, Anserini P, Torelli P, Fulcheri E. How complete is full thickness disc resection of bowel endometriotic lesions? A prospective surgical and histological study. Hum Reprod. 2005;20(8):2317–20.
6. Noel JC, Chapron C, Bucella D, Buxant F, Peny MO, Fayt I, et al. Estrogen and progesterone receptors in smooth muscle component of deep infiltrating endometriosis. Fertil Steril. 2010;93(6):1774–7.
7. Kitano T, Matsumoto T, Takeuchi H, Kikuchi I, Itoga T, Sasahara N, et al. Expression of estrogen and progesterone receptors in smooth muscle metaplasia of rectovaginal endometriosis. Int J Gynecol Pathol. 2007;26(2):124–9.
8. Brichant G, Nervo P, Albert A, Munaut C, Foidart JM, Nisolle M. Heterogeneity of estrogen receptor alpha and progesterone receptor distribution in lesions of deep infiltrating endometriosis of untreated women or during exposure to various hormonal treatments. Gynecol Endocrinol. 2018;34(8):651–5.

9. Vercellini P, Frattaruolo MP, Rosati R, Dridi D, Roberto A, Mosconi P, et al. Medical treatment or surgery for colorectal endometriosis? Results of a shared decision-making approach. Hum Reprod. 2018;33(2):202–11.

10. Egekvist AG, Marinovskij E, Forman A, Kesmodel US, Graumann O, Seyer-Hansen M. Conservative treatment of rectosigmoid endometriosis: a prospective study. Acta Obstet Gynecol Scand. 2019;98(9):1139–47.

11. Andres MP, Mendes RFP, Hernandes C, Araujo SEA, Podgaec S. Hormone treatment as first line therapy is safe and relieves pelvic pain in women with bowel endometriosis. Einstein (Sao Paulo). 2019;17(2):eAO4583.

12. Barra F, Scala C, Ferrero S. Current understanding on pharmacokinetics, clinical efficacy and safety of progestins for treating pain associated to endometriosis. Expert Opin Drug Metab Toxicol. 2018;14(4):399–415.

13. Fedele L, Bianchi S, Zanconato G, Portuese A, Raffaelli R. Use of a levonorgestrel-releasing intrauterine device in the treatment of rectovaginal endometriosis. Fertil Steril. 2001;75(3):485–8.

14. Ferrero S, Camerini G, Ragni N, Venturini PL, Biscaldi E, Remorgida V. Norethisterone acetate in the treatment of colorectal endometriosis: a pilot study. Hum Reprod. 2010;25(1):94–100.

15. Ferrero S, Leone Roberti Maggiore U, Scala C, Di Luca M, Venturini PL, Remorgida V. Changes in the size of rectovaginal endometriotic nodules infiltrating the rectum during hormonal therapies. Arch Gynecol Obstet. 2013;287(3):447–53.

16. Leonardo-Pinto JP, Benetti-Pinto CL, Cursino K, Yela DA. Dienogest and deep infiltrating endometriosis: the remission of symptoms is not related to endometriosis nodule remission. Eur J Obstet Gynecol Reprod Biol. 2017;211:108–11.

17. Kazama S, Hiramatsu T, Kuroda K, Hongo K, Watanabe Y, Tanaka T, et al. A case of unique endoscopic findings of intestinal endometriosis exposed to the mucosa: aggregation of papillary protruded bulges from the submucosal elevation of the rectum. Clin J Gastroenterol. 2019;12(2):166–70.

18. Barra F, Scala C, Maggiore ULR, Ferrero S. Long-term administration of dienogest for the treatment of pain and intestinal symptoms in patients with rectosigmoid endometriosis. J Clin Med. 2020;9(1):154.

19. Kitawaki J, Kusuki I, Yamanaka K, Suganuma I. Maintenance therapy with dienogest following gonadotropin-releasing hormone agonist treatment for endometriosis-associated pelvic pain. Eur J Obstet Gynecol Reprod Biol. 2011;157(2):212–6.

20. Leone Roberti Maggiore U, Remorgida V, Scala C, Tafi E, Venturini PL, Ferrero S. Desogestrel-only contraceptive pill versus sequential contraceptive vaginal ring in the treatment of rectovaginal endometriosis infiltrating the rectum: a prospective open-label comparative study. Acta Obstet Gynecol Scand. 2014;93(3):239–47.

21. Ferrari S, Persico P, Dip F, Vigano P, Tandoi I, Garavaglia E, et al. Continuous low-dose oral contraceptive in the treatment of colorectal endometriosis evaluated by rectal endoscopic ultrasonography. Acta Obstet Gynecol Scand. 2012;91(6):699–703.

22. Markham SM, Welling DR, Larsen KS, Snell MJ. Endometriosis of the rectum treated with a long term GnRH agonist and surgery. N Y State J Med. 1991;91(2):69–71.

23. Porpora MG, Pallante D, Ferro A, Crobu M, Cerenzia P, Panici PL. Intestinal endometriosis without evident pelvic foci treated with gonadotropin-releasing hormone agonist. Eur J Obstet Gynecol Reprod Biol. 2006;125(2):265–6.

24. Ferrero S, Camerini G, Ragni N, Menada MV, Venturini PL, Remorgida V. Triptorelin improves intestinal symptoms among patients with colorectal endometriosis. Int J Gynaecol Obstet. 2010;108(3):250–1.

25. Attar E, Bulun SE. Aromatase inhibitors: the next generation of therapeutics for endometriosis? Fertil Steril. 2006;85(5):1307–18.

26. Bulun SE. Endometriosis. N Engl J Med. 2009;360(3):268–79.

27. Ferrero S, Venturini PL, Ragni N, Camerini G, Remorgida V. Pharmacological treatment of endometriosis: experience with aromatase inhibitors. Drugs. 2009;69(8):943–52.

28. Ferrero S, Camerini G, Ragni N, Venturini PL, Biscaldi E, Seracchioli R, et al. Letrozole and norethisterone acetate in colorectal endometriosis. Eur J Obstet Gynecol Reprod Biol. 2010;150(2):199–202.

29. Soysal S, Soysal ME, Ozer S, Gul N, Gezgin T. The effects of post-surgical administration of goserelin plus anastrozole compared to goserelin alone in patients with severe endometriosis: a prospective randomized trial. Hum Reprod. 2004;19(1):160–7.

30. Ferrero S, Camerini G, Venturini P, Biscaldi E, Remorgida V. Progression of bowel endometriosis during treatment with the oral contraceptive pill. Gynecol Surg. 2011;8(3):311–3.

31. Millochau JC, Abo C, Darwish B, Huet E, Dietrich G, Roman H. Continuous amenorrhea may be insufficient to stop the progression of colorectal endometriosis. J Minim Invasive Gynecol. 2016;23(5):839–42.

32. Roman H. Medical versus surgical treatments of rectal endometriosis (MESURE). https://www.clinicaltrials.gov/ct2/show/NCT01973816?term=endometriosis+AND+France&draw=4&rank=24.

33. Khan KN, Fujishita A, Masumoto H, Muto H, Kitajima M, Masuzaki H, et al. Molecular detection of intrauterine microbial colonization in women with endometriosis. Eur J Obstet Gynecol Reprod Biol. 2016;199:69–75.

34. Attar E, Yilmaz MB, Innes J, Utsunomiya H, Demura M, Bulun SE. Sodium Butyrate is a tissue specific inhibitor of aromatase expression in endometriosis. 53rd annual scientific meeting of the Society for Gynecologic Investigation, Toronto, Canada; 2006.

35. Demura M, Bulun SE. CpG dinucleotide methylation of the CYP19 I.3/II promoter modulates cAMP-

stimulated aromatase activity. Mol Cell Endocrinol. 2008;283(1–2):127–32.

36. Grimstad FW, Decherney A. A review of the epigenetic contributions to endometriosis. Clin Obstet Gynecol. 2017;60(3):467–76.

37. Kamergorodsky G, Invitti AL, D'Amora P, Parreira RM, Kopelman A, Bonetti TCS, et al. Progesterone's role in deep infiltrating endometriosis: progesterone receptor and estrogen metabolism enzymes expression and physiological changes in primary endometrial stromal cell culture. Mol Cell Endocrinol. 2020;505:110743.

38. Bulun SE, Cheng YH, Yin P, Imir G, Utsunomiya H, Attar E, et al. Progesterone resistance in endometriosis: link to failure to metabolize estradiol. Mol Cell Endocrinol. 2006;248(1–2):94–103.

39. Pavone ME, Malpani SS, Dyson M, Kim JJ, Bulun SE. Fenretinide: a potential treatment for endometriosis. Reprod Sci. 2016;23(9):1139–47.

40. Barra F, Scala C, Biscaldi E, Vellone VG, Ceccaroni M, Terrone C, et al. Ureteral endometriosis: a systematic review of epidemiology, pathogenesis, diagnosis, treatment, risk of malignant transformation and fertility. Hum Reprod Update. 2018;24(6):710–30.

41. Ferrero S, Remorgida V, Venturini PL. Current pharmacotherapy for endometriosis. Expert Opin Pharmacother. 2010;11(7):1123–34.

Fertility and Infertility in Patients with Bowel Endometriosis

17

Simone Ferrero, Antoine Watrelot, and Gedis Grudzinskas

17.1 Introduction

Colorectal endometriosis is often associated with other lesions involving the uterosacral ligaments, torus uterinus, parametrium, vagina and ovaries, and pelvic adhesions, which often affect ovaries and tubes and thus may impair fertility. However, the impact of colorectal endometriosis alone on fertility is unclear [1].

Three techniques may be used to treat bowel endometriosis: bowel shaving, disc resection, and colorectal segmental resection and anastomosis. The term "bowel shaving" is used to describe the resection of rectosigmoid deep endometriosis leaving the mucosa intact. Disc excision refers to the entire resection of the intestinal wall, including the mucosa, and is followed by the closure of the intestinal defect by sutures or using staplers. Finally, segmental resection refers to the excision of the affected colonic segment, followed by colorectal anastomosis. The choice of surgical technique is dependent on the characteristics of bowel endometriotic nodules, such as the largest diameter of the nodule, presence of multiple nodules in the same bowel segment, depth of infiltration of endometriosis in the intestinal wall and degree of stenosis of the intestinal lumen. Also, when the sigmoid colon is involved, typically only disc resection and segmental resection may be performed but not shaving. The experience and preferences of the surgeon have relevant roles in choosing the type of surgery as some surgeons prefer to perform segmental resection [2]. Nevertheless, shaving and disc excision are reported to be associated with a lower rate of complications compared with segmental bowel resection [3–6]. A general tendency nowadays is to try to be less invasive and to prefer whenever it is possible to perform shaving instead of bowel resection. It is also considered that in asymptomatic patients (approximately 4.5%) expectant management should be the preferred option [7].

S. Ferrero
Academic Unit of Obstetrics and Gynecology, IRCCS Ospedale Policlinico San Martino, Genova, Italy

Department of Neurosciences, Rehabilitation, Ophthalmology, Genetics, Maternal and Child Health (DiNOGMI), University of Genova, Genova, Italy
e-mail: simone.ferrero@unige.it

A. Watrelot
Hôpital Privé Natecia, Lyon, France
e-mail: watrelot@watrelot.org

G. Grudzinskas (✉)
London, UK
e-mail: gedis@grudzinskas.co.uk

17.2 Spontaneous Fertility in Women with Bowel Endometriosis

Very limited data is available on the spontaneous fertility of patients with colorectal endometriosis. A prospective Italian study investigated the

© Springer Nature Switzerland AG 2020
S. Ferrero, M. Ceccaroni (eds.), *Clinical Management of Bowel Endometriosis*,
https://doi.org/10.1007/978-3-030-50446-5_17

pregnancy rate and the time to conception in 105 infertile women with rectovaginal endometriosis who underwent surgery or expectant management [8]. The 24-month cumulative pregnancy rate was similar in the two study groups: 44.9% in patients who underwent surgery and 46.8% in those who underwent expectant management. The authors concluded that, although surgery for rectovaginal endometriosis in infertile women did not increase fecundability, it increased the pain-free interval. However, the authors did not discriminate between the patients with and those without bowel involvement. Furthermore, all surgical procedures were performed by laparotomy. A single-center Italian prospective cohort study investigated the pregnancy rate in patients with colorectal endometriosis diagnosed with the use of magnetic resonance enema [9]. The median age of the patients was 33 years (range, 24–41 years). During follow-up, 17 patients left the study because of the change of partner, health problems, or change of plans. Twenty-five patients (27.8%) conceived spontaneously; the median time required to conceive being ten months (range, 2–32 months). Seventeen patients (18.8%) conceived following intrauterine insemination or in vitro fertilization (IVF), the median time to conceive was 21 months (range, 9–46 months). The total pregnancy rate in the study population was 46.7% (42/90; 95% CI, 36.1–57.5%) after a median follow-up of 28.2 months (range, 2–70 months). After the first pregnancy, there were four conceptions among the ten patients who tried to conceive again. Therefore, the authors concluded that patients with colorectal endometriosis should be informed on the possibility to conceive either spontaneously or by assisted reproductive technology (ART) without undergoing surgical excision of endometriosis. Another Italian retrospective study investigated the spontaneous pregnancy rate of women with rectovaginal endometriosis with/without ovarian endometrioma and treated by expectant management ($n = 284$) or by surgery ($n = 221$) [7]. 13.7% of the patients treated by expectant management and 15.8% of those treated by surgery had rectosigmoid endometriosis. At 1-year fol-low-up, the crude and cumulative spontaneous pregnancy rates were lower in patients undergoing expectant management (17.3% and 23.8%, respectively) than in those who underwent surgery (35.7% and 39.5%). However, the authors did not report data on the reproductive outcomes of the subgroups of patients with rectosigmoid endometriosis.

17.3 Fertility Outcomes After Surgical Treatment Endometriosis Leaving In Situ Colorectal Endometriosis

Patients with bowel endometriosis may have only mild intestinal symptoms and sometimes are pain-free. These patients, considering the potential complications of colorectal surgery, may request excision of pelvic deep endometriotic lesions only without removing bowel nodules. In other patients, bowel endometriosis may be an expected finding at the time of surgery and, thus, with a lack of preoperative informed consent, intestinal lesions are not excised. These patients may refuse second surgery aimed to treat bowel endometriosis. Only two studies evaluated the spontaneous pregnancy rate in women treated with surgical excision of deep infiltrating endometriosis but leaving colorectal endometriosis in situ. A prospective Italian trial reported a 21% pregnancy rate at a mean follow-up of 26.9 months in 40 patients with bowel endometriosis who underwent deep endometriosis removal without bowel lesion resection [10]. Notably, this pregnancy rate was significantly lower than that of patients who underwent colorectal segmental resection (35%). A Spanish retrospective study reported a 70.0% pregnancy rate in ten women with bowel endometriosis who underwent surgical excision of deep endometriosis without bowel lesion resection [11]. The different results of these two studies do not allow estimation of the pregnancy rate of patients treated for deep endometriosis leaving colorectal endometriosis in situ.

Patients with bowel endometriosis, when treated by a general gynecologist, may undergo diagnostic laparoscopy or laparoscopic treatment of ovarian endometrioma. No data are available on the spontaneous fertility of these patients. A prospective multicenter study investigated the pregnancy rate after IVF in 75 infertile patients with colorectal endometriosis. Three-quarters of the patients had undergone prior surgery for endometriosis (including diagnostic laparoscopy and cystectomy for endometriomas), but no patient had surgical excision of deep endometriosis [12]. The cumulative pregnancy rate per patient after one, two and three ICSI–IVF cycles were 29.3%, 52.9%, and 68.6%, respectively. AMH serum level lower than 2 ng/ml, patient age over 35 years, and the presence of adenomyosis were associated with a decrease in pregnancy rates.

17.4 Risk of Bowel Occlusion in Patients Wishing to Conceive

Previously, pregnancy was considered to have a beneficial effect on endometriosis [13]. However, over the last 15 years, several reports described complications caused by bowel endometriosis in patients wishing to conceive either spontaneously or by in vitro fertilization (IVF). Hormonal therapies are widely used to treat pain and intestinal symptoms caused by bowel endometriosis [14–17]. Bowel occlusion may occur in women who discontinue long-term hormonal treatments because of the desire to conceive [18]. Infertile women with bowel endometriosis may postpone surgery and quickly undergo ART because of the potential risk of surgical complications and the presumed absence of benefit of primary surgery on pregnancy rate post-ART. Also, ART instead of surgery may shorten the interval to conception. However, patients with bowel endometriosis undergoing ART may suffer from severe complications. In a study evaluating the complications after 1500 oocyte retrievals (311 in patients with endometriosis), Govaerts et al. observed that two

patients had a worsening of intestinal symptoms caused by bowel endometriosis and one patient required intestinal resection [19]. Anaf et al. reported four cases of severe bowel symptoms caused by sigmoid endometriosis during ovarian stimulation [20]. Before treatment, the sigmoid nodules were diagnosed by laparoscopy in three patients. These patients did not complain of intestinal symptoms, and their lesions did not cause stenosis of the intestinal lumen visible at colonoscopy, leading to a decision not to treat sigmoid endometriosis before ART. Two patients had three cycles of ovarian stimulation, one patient had one cycle, and one patient had seven cycles before the occurrence of severe intestinal symptoms. Roman et al. reported a series of 12 patients with bowel endometriosis desiring to conceive in whom postponing surgery was considered to be responsible for bowel occlusion ($n = 2$) or sub-occlusion ($n = 10$) [21]. The diagnosis of bowel endometriosis was based on magnetic resonance imaging. The major intestinal symptoms were bloating, defecation pain, constipation, liquid stools, and a feeling of incomplete stool evacuation. 58.3% of the patients had infertility treatments before bowel occlusion or sub-occlusion (16.7% underwent intrauterine insemination and 41.7% underwent IVF). The median length of the digestive tract stenosis was 50 mm (range, 20–100 mm). In eight patients (66.7%), virtual colonoscopy revealed a virtual intestinal lumen. The median length of the resected colorectal specimen was 120 mm (range, 60–200 mm).

Furthermore, patients with bowel endometriosis undergoing ART must be informed that bowel occlusion or perforation may also occur during pregnancy and in the postpartum period [22, 23].

17.5 Fertility Outcomes After Surgical Treatment of Bowel Endometriosis

Over the past 15 years, several studies reported fertility outcomes after surgical treatment of bowel endometriosis. A single-center prospective study including 46 patients investigated the pregnancy rate after segmental bowel resection for rectosigmoid endometriosis performed either by laparoscopy or laparotomy [24]. The pregnancy rate was significantly higher in women who underwent bowel resection by laparoscopy (57.6%) than in those who underwent laparotomy (23.1%). Women who conceived were significantly younger than those who did not conceive; only 26.7% of women aged > or =35 years conceived after bowel resection. Uterine adenomyosis was more frequently present in women who did not conceive than in those who conceived. Subsequently, an Italian nonrandomized study investigated the influence of bowel endometriosis on spontaneous fertility and whether its removal improves the chance of conception [10]. The study included three groups of infertile patients: patients who underwent surgery for endometriosis with colorectal segmental resection ($n = 60$), women with evidence of bowel endometriosis who underwent endometriosis removal without bowel resection ($n = 40$), and women who underwent surgery for moderate or severe endometriosis with at least one endometrioma and deep infiltrating endometriosis but without bowel involvement ($n = 55$). After a mean follow-up of 27 months, the pregnancy rate was 35% after surgery with segmental colorectal resection, 21% after surgery without colorectal resection, and 70% in patients without bowel endometriosis. Therefore, this study suggested that the presence of bowel endometriosis negatively influences the reproductive outcome in infertile women. Also, this study suggested that, when surgery is performed, the complete removal of endometriosis, including bowel endometriosis, seems to offer better results in terms of postoperative fertility. Subsequently, the same authors investigated fertility and clinical outcome after laparoscopic excision of deep endometriosis and bowel resection in 62 infertile women [25]. The study was based on a prospectively collected database. The median length of follow-up was 19.6 months (range, 6–48 months). Twelve patients did not try to conceive during the follow-up period. The total cumula-

tive pregnancy rate was 34%. All women who conceived were younger than 35 years. Fifty-two percentage of patients younger than 35 years conceived spontaneously after surgery. Five of 14 patients who underwent ART conceived. Among women trying to conceive spontaneously younger than 30 years, the cumulative pregnancy rate was 58%, and for women aged 30–34 years, the rate was 45%. A prospective French study evaluated fertility, pregnancy outcomes, and their determinant factors after laparoscopic segmental colorectal resection for endometriosis [26]. The study included 83 women who underwent colorectal resection for endometriosis (77 patients treated by laparoscopy and six by laparotomy); 55 women wished to conceive after surgery. The mean age of the study population was 31.7 years (range 21–45). The mean follow-up after surgery was 34 months (6–68 months). Twenty-four (43.6%) of the 55 patients conceived during the follow-up and four women conceived twice. Twenty-nine pregnancies were obtained, including 20 spontaneous pregnancies (69%) and nine pregnancies by ART (31%). The median time to conceive after colorectal resection was 11 months (range: 2–68). The time to conceive was shorter for spontaneous pregnancies than for those obtained by ART (6 months vs. 20 months). A significant correlation was found between pregnancy rate and patient age. Reduction in pregnancy rate was correlated to the presence of adenomyosis, high ASRM total score, and conversion to laparotomy. The higher pregnancy rate observed after laparoscopy compared with open surgery might be explained by the lower incidence of postoperative pelvic adhesions. A French randomized controlled study investigated the outcomes of colorectal resection for endometriosis performed by laparoscopy or by open surgery [27]. This study showed that the pregnancy rate was higher in patients treated by laparoscopy. A sub-analysis of the previous randomized controlled study investigated whether the surgical route of colorectal resection for endometriosis is a determinant factor for fertility [28]. The study included 52 patients (29 had no history of infertility, and 23 were infertile). After surgery, 13 of the 29 patients (44.8%) without infertility and 15 of the 23 patients (65.2%) with infertility wished to conceive. The mean follow-up was 29 months (range, 6–52 months). Among the 28 patients wishing to conceive, 11 (39.3%) became pregnant. All patients who conceived spontaneously were aged <35 years. The median time to conceive after colorectal resection was 14 months (range, 1–24 months); the median time to conceive spontaneously was 7.5 months (range, 1–18 months) and by ART 21 months (range, 14–24 months). The overall cumulative pregnancy rate at 52 months was 45.1%. For patients with or without infertility, the cumulative pregnancy rate was 37.6% and 55.6%, respectively, and the cumulative spontaneous pregnancy rate was 13.3% and 36.5%, respectively. Notably, all the spontaneous pregnancies were observed in the laparoscopy group. A prospective study including 203 women investigated the clinical outcome of women requiring laparoscopic excision of moderate-severe endometriosis in women with and without bowel resection and re-anastomosis [29]. One hundred forty-eight women (73%) wanted to conceive after surgery; the proportion of women with pregnancy wish was similar in patients who underwent bowel resection (71%; $n = 54/76$) and in those who did not undergo bowel surgery (74%; $n = 94/127$). At 24-months follow-up, the pregnancy rate was similar in patients who underwent bowel resection (50%) and in those who did not undergo bowel surgery (51%). Among 48 women with at least one patent tube, 38% became pregnant spontaneously. Unfortunately, in this study, it was not possible to distinguish between women with proven infertility and those wishing to conceive without proven infertility. A review assessed the impact of various locations of deep endometriosis on spontaneous fertility and the benefit of surgery and ART on fertility outcomes [30]. Among women with deep endometriosis with bowel involvement without surgical management ($n = 115$), the pregnancy rate after ART was 29% (95% CI, 20.7–37.4%). For women with bowel involvement treated by surgery

($n = 1320$), the spontaneous pregnancy rate was 28.6% (95% CI, 25–32.3%), the overall pregnancy rate being 46.9% (95% CI, 42.9–50.9%). Thus, the authors concluded that, for patients with bowel endometriosis, the low spontaneous and relatively high overall pregnancy rate suggests the potential benefit of combining surgery and ART. An Italian retrospective study investigated the feasibility and safety of laparoscopic segmental bowel resection for deep infiltrating endometriosis [31]. Among 72 patients who tried to conceive spontaneously, 61% achieved pregnancy with a mean interval of 8.4 ± 4.1 months. Among the 28 patients who failed to conceive, six achieved viable pregnancies by IVF. More recently, a systematic review with meta-analysis evaluated the impact of colorectal endometriosis on fertility and the contribution of assisted reproduction techniques and colorectal surgery on fertility outcomes in women with and without preexisting infertility [1]. The overall pregnancy rate after colorectal resection was 51.1% (95% CI, 48–54%). Data on spontaneous conception after surgical treatment of endometriosis with colorectal endometriosis were available in 26 studies published from 1990 to 2015, including 1968 patients. Among the 855 women with proven infertility or wishing to conceive without proven infertility, 31.4% (95% CI, 28–34%) became pregnant spontaneously. The spontaneous pregnancy rate in women with and without proven infertility was 31.4% and 31.1%, respectively. These results support the potential benefit of colorectal surgery on spontaneous pregnancy rate when compared to the pregnancy rate in women treated by expectant management. In this review, the differential benefit of ART on the overall pregnancy rate was 19.8%. When considering pregnancy rate after ART in women with and without proven infertility, the values were 21.4% and 15.5%, suggesting a greater benefit for patients with proven infertility. When comparing IUI and IVF-ICSI, the contribution of IUI appears minimal, which supports routine first-line management by IVF-ICSI. However, the authors of this review highlighted the absence of randomized controlled trials conducted to verify the effect of bowel surgery on the likelihood of postoperative conceptions achieved naturally or by ART. Another systematic review investigated the influence of surgery for bowel endometriosis on fertility [32]. No randomized controlled study was identified. The review included four retrospective studies and three prospective observational uncontrolled studies. The authors highlighted the poor quality of the available data. However, the results of this review indicated the possibility that surgery for bowel endometriosis may improve the spontaneous pregnancy rate, and the positive effects on ART outcomes could not be excluded. A French retrospective matched cohort study compared the impact of first-line ART and first-line colorectal surgery followed by ART on fertility outcomes in women with colorectal endometriosis-associated infertility [33]. The study included 110 women (55 women in each group). The median age of the study population was 32 years (range, 24–39), and the median duration of infertility was 3 years (range, 1–9). 58.2% of the patients had undergone prior surgery for endometriosis, including diagnostic laparoscopy and cystectomy for endometriomas, but none for deep infiltrating endometriosis or colorectal surgery. Hence, none of the patients had rectal shaving, full-thickness nodule resection, or segmental resection. The pregnancy rate was 60% in women who underwent colorectal surgery before IVF and 36% in those undergoing immediate ART. The live birth rate was 49% (33/67) in the former group and 20% (14/69) in the latter. The cumulative live birth rates were significantly higher for women who underwent first-line surgery followed by ART compared with first-line ART in the subset of women with good prognosis (age <=35 years and AMH >=2 ng/mL and no adenomyosis) and women with AMH serum level <2 ng/ml. Therefore, the authors concluded that first-line surgery might be a good option for women with colorectal endometriosis-associated infertility. Furthermore, surgical treatment of bowel endometriosis exposes women to the risk of severe complications (such as rectovaginal fistula, anastomotic leakage with the risk of peri-

tonitis, pelvic abscess, uretero-hydronephrosis, urinary fistula, and bowel obstruction and diverting stoma). Patients with postoperative complications may need to be managed in the intensive care unit. A French retrospective cohort study investigated the fertility outcomes in women wishing to conceive after experiencing a severe complication from surgical removal of colorectal endometriosis [34]. Fifty-three women were included in the study, and fertility outcome was available for 48 women. A protective diverting stoma was created in more than one-third of cases. The median follow-up was 5 years (range: 1–12). Twenty women achieved pregnancy; the overall pregnancy rate was 41.2%, 80% conceived spontaneously, and 20% following ART. Four women conceived at least twice, resulting in 26 pregnancies in total. Of the 17 women who underwent an ART procedure, four (23.5%) became pregnant. The median time between surgery and the first pregnancy was 3 years (range: 1–6), the live birth rate was 29.2% (14/48). The 5-year cumulative pregnancy rate was 46%. A lower cumulative pregnancy rate was observed in women who experienced anastomotic leakage (with or without rectovaginal fistula) or deep pelvic abscess (with or without anastomotic leakage). The authors concluded that the occurrence of a severe postoperative complication has little impact on fertility outcomes, in contrast to bacterial contamination of the pelvis. More recently, Hudelist et al. reported the fertility outcome of patients with rectosigmoid endometriosis treated by full-thickness disc excision or segmental bowel resection [35]. Sixty-one women were infertile before surgery and 12 women were not infertile preoperatively and tried to conceive during follow-up. 63.9% of the infertile patients (39/61) conceived during follow-up. The postsurgical conception interval was seven months in patients treated by segmental resection (range, 2–51 months) and 5 months (range 1–48 months) in those treated by disc resection. There was a 58.3% (7/12) pregnancy rate in patients who were not infertile preoperatively (four spontaneous pregnancies and three by ART).

17.6 Conclusion

Despite the numerous published studies on bowel endometriosis, as there is a lack of data on the fecundability of patients with untreated colorectal endometriosis, risk factors for infertility thereby remain poorly identified [1, 9]. Consequently, interpretation of fertility outcomes after colorectal surgery for deep endometriosis is difficult. Firstly, colorectal surgery can be performed by various techniques (shaving, disc excision, and colorectal resection). The majority of published studies report the pregnancy rate after colorectal resection, but the fertility outcomes after discoid resection or rectal shaving are mostly unknown. There is evidence that laparoscopic colorectal surgery is less likely to negatively impact fertility compared with open surgery [24, 26, 27]. Secondly, it is challenging to clarify if the postoperative conceptions are due to the removal of bowel endometriosis or to the excision of genital-pelvic deep endometriosis [2]. Furthermore, several authors do not distinguish between patients with true infertility from those wishing to conceive without proven infertility (unknown fertility status) and for whom ART is rapidly proposed [1]. Finally, the overall quality of the studies investigating the impact of bowel surgery on fertility outcomes is poor [2].

When counseling patients with bowel endometriosis, several factors must be considered including, first of all, the severity of pain and for fertility: ovarian reserve (and particularly previous surgery for ovarian endometrioma), tubal patency, and sperm characteristics. The assessment of ovarian reserve is particularly relevant also for women without an immediate desire to conceive because they may be advised to performed oocyte or ovarian tissue cryopreservation.

Patients with bowel endometriosis undergoing IVF must be informed of the potential risk of complications (such as bowel occlusion) during ovarian stimulation, oocyte collection, and pregnancy [2, 20, 21, 23, 28]. This risk may be higher in patients undergoing several ovarian stimulations. However, the real incidence of endometriosis-related bowel occlusion may be underreported due to publication bias. Patients experiencing bowel occlusion are often treated in a nearby general surgery department and not referred to specialist endometriosis centers. Before conception, patients with bowel endometriosis should be assessed in a referral center to evaluate the presence of bowel stenosis and hydroureteronephrosis. Finally, delaying surgery may lead to an increase in the area of the intestinal wall infiltrated by the endometriotic nodule. Despite a shortfall in epidemiological studies focusing on the progression of deep endometriosis, it is evident that patients undergoing colorectal resection at the age of 30 years would not have required the same surgical procedure if they had been treated several years earlier [36]. This progression of bowel endometriosis may be particularly relevant for those surgeons who systematically attempt to conserve the bowel by shaving or disc excision, which seems to be the general tendency. Furthermore, the lateral progression of deep infiltrating endometriosis may lead to involvement and stenosis of the ureters [37]. Finally, untreated bowel and deep endometriosis are associated with the persistence of pain and intestinal complaints. However, ART has some advantages in patients with bowel endometriosis because it shortens the delay in conception, which may be particularly relevant in patients with poor ovarian reserve. Also, primary ART avoids the negative impact of prior postoperative complications (such as anastomotic leakage or deep pelvic abscess) on fertility (Table 17.1).

Based on the available data, bowel surgery should be performed to relieve pain and intestinal symptoms caused by endometriosis and preferably through laparoscopy. In contrast, the usefulness of bowel surgery to improve the likelihood of conception still needs to be established in women who could otherwise avoid intestinal surgery [2].

Table 17.1 Advantages and disadvantages of primary surgery and primary IVF in patients with bowel endometriosis and pregnancy wish

Primary surgery	Primary IVF
Advantages	
Improvement in pain and intestinal symptoms	Shorter time to conceive
Decreased risk of endometriosis-related complications (such as bowel occlusion, ureteral stenosis)	
Potential reduction in medical expenses because no IVF is performed in patients who conceive spontaneously	
Delay in the attempts to conceive	
Disadvantages	
Risk of postoperative complications (anastomotic leakage, deep pelvic abscess) which negatively impact on spontaneous conception, risk of diverting stoma	Potential endometriosis-related complications (such as bowel occlusion, ureteral stenosis) during ovarian stimulation, oocyte collection, and pregnancy
Damage to ovarian reserve in patients with endometriomas associated with deep endometriosis (and potential risk of ovarian failure)	Possible progression of deep endometriosis
Higher psychological impact of advanced colorectal surgery in nulliparous women	Persistence of pain and intestinal symptoms

References

1. Darai E, Cohen J, Ballester M. Colorectal endometriosis and fertility. Eur J Obstet Gynecol Reprod Biol. 2017;209:86–94.
2. Vercellini P, Vigano P, Frattaruolo MP, Borghi A, Somigliana E. Bowel surgery as a fertility-enhancing procedure in patients with colorectal endometriosis: methodological, pathogenic and ethical issues. Hum Reprod. 2018;33(7):1205–11.
3. Roman H, Milles M, Vassilieff M, Resch B, Tuech JJ, Huet E, et al. Long-term functional outcomes following colorectal resection versus shaving for rectal endometriosis. Am J Obstet Gynecol. 2016;215(6):762e1–9.
4. Roman H, Bubenheim M, Huet E, Bridoux V, Zacharopoulou C, Darai E, et al. Conservative surgery versus colorectal resection in deep endometriosis infiltrating the rectum: a randomized trial. Hum Reprod. 2018;33(1):47–57.
5. Donnez O, Roman H. Choosing the right surgical technique for deep endometriosis: shaving, disc excision, or bowel resection? Fertil Steril. 2017;108(6):931–42.
6. Nezhat C, Li A, Falik R, Copeland D, Razavi G, Shakib A, et al. Bowel endometriosis: diagnosis and management. Am J Obstet Gynecol. 2018;218(6):549–62.
7. Leone Roberti Maggiore U, Scala C, Tafi E, Racca A, Biscaldi E, Vellone VG, et al. Spontaneous fertility after expectant or surgical management of rectovaginal endometriosis in women with or without ovarian endometrioma: a retrospective analysis. Fertil Steril. 2017;107(4):969–76.e5.
8. Vercellini P, Pietropaolo G, De Giorgi O, Daguati R, Pasin R, Crosignani PG. Reproductive performance in infertile women with rectovaginal endometriosis: is surgery worthwhile? Am J Obstet Gynecol. 2006;195(5):1303–10.
9. Ferrero S, Leone Roberti Maggiore U, Scala C, Tafi E, Venturini P, Racca A. Fertility in patients with untreated colorectal endometriosis. Fertil Steril. 2016;103(3):e-269–e70.
10. Stepniewska A, Pomini P, Bruni F, Mereu L, Ruffo G, Ceccaroni M, et al. Laparoscopic treatment of bowel endometriosis in infertile women. Hum Reprod. 2009;24(7):1619–25.
11. Acien P, Nunez C, Quereda F, Velasco I, Valiente M, Vidal V. Is a bowel resection necessary for deep endometriosis with rectovaginal or colorectal involvement? Int J Womens Health. 2013;5:449–55.
12. Ballester M, d'Argent EM, Morcel K, Belaisch-Allart J, Nisolle M, Darai E. Cumulative pregnancy rate after ICSI-IVF in patients with colorectal endometriosis: results of a multicentre study. Hum Reprod. 2012;27(4):1043–9.
13. Martin DC, Ling FW. Endometriosis and pain. Clin Obstet Gynecol. 1999;42(3):664–86.
14. Ferrero S, Camerini G, Ragni N, Venturini PL, Biscaldi E, Seracchioli R, et al. Letrozole and norethisterone acetate in colorectal endometriosis. Eur J Obstet Gynecol Reprod Biol. 2010;150(2):199–202.
15. Ferrero S, Camerini G, Ragni N, Venturini PL, Biscaldi E, Remorgida V. Norethisterone acetate in the treatment of colorectal endometriosis: a pilot study. Hum Reprod. 2010;25(1):94–100.
16. Ferrero S, Camerini G, Venturini P, Biscaldi E, Remorgida V. Progression of bowel endometriosis during treatment with the oral contraceptive pill. Gynecol Surg. 2011;8(3):311–3.
17. Ferrero S, Camerini G, Ragni N, Menada MV, Venturini PL, Remorgida V. Triptorelin improves intes-

tinal symptoms among patients with colorectal endometriosis. Int J Gynaecol Obstet. 2010;108(3):250–1.

18. Roman H, Friederich L, Khalil H, Marouteau-Pasquier N, Hochain P, Marpeau L. Treating severe endometriosis by pregnancy: a risky business. Gynecol Obstet Fertil. 2007;35(1):38–40.

19. Govaerts I, Devreker F, Delbaere A, Revelard P, Englert Y. Short-term medical complications of 1500 oocyte retrievals for in vitro fertilization and embryo transfer. Eur J Obstet Gynecol Reprod Biol. 1998;77(2):239–43.

20. Anaf V, El Nakadi I, Simon P, Englert Y, Peny MO, Fayt I, et al. Sigmoid endometriosis and ovarian stimulation. Hum Reprod. 2000;15(4):790–4.

21. Roman H, Puscasiu L, Lempicki M, Huet E, Chati R, Bridoux V, et al. Colorectal endometriosis responsible for bowel occlusion or subocclusion in women with pregnancy intention: is the policy of primary in vitro fertilization always safe? J Minim Invasive Gynecol. 2015;22(6):1059–67.

22. Setubal A, Sidiropoulou Z, Torgal M, Casal E, Lourenco C, Koninckx P. Bowel complications of deep endometriosis during pregnancy or in vitro fertilization. Fertil Steril. 2014;101(2):442–6.

23. Leone Roberti Maggiore U, Ferrero S, Mangili G, Bergamini A, Inversetti A, Giorgione V, et al. A systematic review on endometriosis during pregnancy: diagnosis, misdiagnosis, complications and outcomes. Hum Reprod Update. 2016;22(1):70–103.

24. Ferrero S, Anserini P, Abbamonte LH, Ragni N, Camerini G, Remorgida V. Fertility after bowel resection for endometriosis. Fertil Steril. 2009;92(1):41–6.

25. Stepniewska A, Pomini P, Scioscia M, Mereu L, Ruffo G, Minelli L. Fertility and clinical outcome after bowel resection in infertile women with endometriosis. Reprod Biomed Online. 2010;20(5):602–9.

26. Darai E, Carbonnel M, Dubernard G, Lavoue V, Coutant C, Bazot M, et al. Determinant factors of fertility outcomes after laparoscopic colorectal resection for endometriosis. Eur J Obstet Gynecol Reprod Biol. 2010;149(2):210–4.

27. Darai E, Dubernard G, Coutant C, Frey C, Rouzier R, Ballester M. Randomized trial of laparoscopically assisted versus open colorectal resection for endometriosis: morbidity, symptoms, quality of life, and fertility. Ann Surg. 2010;251(6):1018–23.

28. Darai E, Lesieur B, Dubernard G, Rouzier R, Bazot M, Ballester M. Fertility after colorectal resection for endometriosis: results of a prospective study comparing laparoscopy with open surgery. Fertil Steril. 2011;95(6):1903–8.

29. Meuleman C, Tomassetti C, Wolthuis A, Van Cleynenbreugel B, Laenen A, Penninckx F, et al. Clinical outcome after radical excision of moderate-severe endometriosis with or without bowel resection and reanastomosis: a prospective cohort study. Ann Surg. 2014;259(3):522–31.

30. Cohen J, Thomin A, Mathieu D'Argent E, Laas E, Canlorbe G, Zilberman S, et al. Fertility before and after surgery for deep infiltrating endometriosis with and without bowel involvement: a literature review. Minerva Ginecol. 2014;66(6):575–87.

31. Malzoni M, Di Giovanni A, Exacoustos C, Lannino G, Capece R, Perone C, et al. Feasibility and safety of laparoscopic-assisted bowel segmental resection for deep infiltrating endometriosis: a retrospective cohort study with description of technique. J Minim Invasive Gynecol. 2016;23(4):512–25.

32. Iversen ML, Seyer-Hansen M, Forman A. Does surgery for deep infiltrating bowel endometriosis improve fertility? A systematic review. Acta Obstet Gynecol Scand. 2017;96(6):688–93.

33. Bendifallah S, Roman H, Mathieu d'Argent E, Touleimat S, Cohen J, Darai E, et al. Colorectal endometriosis-associated infertility: should surgery precede ART? Fertil Steril. 2017;108(3):525–31.e4.

34. Ferrier C, Roman H, Alzahrani Y, d'Argent EM, Bendifallah S, Marty N, et al. Fertility outcomes in women experiencing severe complications after surgery for colorectal endometriosis. Hum Reprod. 2018;33(3):411–5.

35. Hudelist G, Aas-Eng MK, Birsan T, Berger F, Sevelda U, Kirchner L, et al. Pain and fertility outcomes of nerve-sparing, full-thickness disk or segmental bowel resection for deep infiltrating endometriosis – a prospective cohort study. Acta Obstet Gynecol Scand. 2018;97(12):1438–46.

36. Roman H. Colorectal endometriosis and pregnancy wish: why doing primary surgery. Front Biosci (Schol Ed). 2015;7:83–93.

37. Barra F, Scala C, Biscaldi E, Vellone VG, Ceccaroni M, Terrone C, et al. Ureteral endometriosis: a systematic review of epidemiology, pathogenesis, diagnosis, treatment, risk of malignant transformation and fertility. Hum Reprod Update. 2018;24(6): 710–30.

MIX
Papier aus verantwortungsvollen Quellen
Paper from responsible sources
FSC® C105338

If you have any concerns about our products,
you can contact us on
ProductSafety@springernature.com

In case Publisher is established outside the EU,
the EU authorized representative is:
Springer Nature Customer Service Center GmbH
Europaplatz 3, 69115 Heidelberg, Germany

Printed by Libri Plureos GmbH
in Hamburg, Germany